THE HYPERCARNIVORE DIET

EAT MEAT, GET HEALTHY. PLANTS OPTIONAL.
First Edition

DON MATESZ

THE HYPERCARNIVORE DIET

Eat Meat, Get Healthy. Plants Optional.

Don Matesz, M.A., M.S., L.Ac.

INTEGRITY PRESS
2018

THE HYPERCARNIVORE DIET

First Edition

ISBN-13: 978-1985619883

ISBN-10: 1985619881

CONTENTS

NOTICE

Diet has a powerful effect on health and fitness. If you are seriously ill or on medications, consult a health care provider knowledgable about nutrition and its health effects and about your medications before you make any changes to your diet or exercise program. You remain always responsible for your choices, actions, and their consequences. This book serves as educational information only and does not substitute for the guidance of a health care professional familiar with your unique situation. Nothing herein is to be construed as a diagnosis or treatment plan for any individual's unique physical condition.

ACKNOWLEDGEMENTS

Thanks to my wife Tracy for encouragement, support and help editing this book.

Thanks to Ted Naiman, M.D. and Shawn Baker, M.D. for sharing information on social media that helped me do research for this book.

Thanks to Ray Audette for writing *Neanderthin* and sharing knowledge resources with me.

Many others too numerous to mention have played a role in my education leading up to completion of this project. I am grateful to all.

Any errors that appear in this book despite my best effort to exclude them are my responsibility alone.

Don Matesz, Aug 19, 2018.

PREFACE

> Before there is truth there must be a true human.
>
> Chuang Tzu

I have had deep doubts about writing this book. I have made my dietary experiments public, and endured a lot of ridicule for having changed my mind and my practices back and forth between plant- and animal-based diets a few times. I don't have any reason to think anyone will want to read this or have any confidence in what I have to say. Nevertheless, I feel compelled by Nature to write, so I do.

People have vilified me for changing positions, yet it is very clear that our culture as a whole holds contradictory and confusing attitudes towards and approaches to foods and diets. My journey has just re-presented the most basic conflict between plant-based and animal-based approaches to eating, but we also have cooked vs. raw and a plethora of supposedly ideal diets represented by hundreds of books published every year.

What passes for science today has offered no real help in clearing this confusion. You can find 'scientific' papers ostensibly providing evidence supporting both plant-based and animal-based, high- and low- carbohydrate diets. You can find vociferous 'authorities' with high-ranking conventional credentials on either side.

However, one critically thinking scientist, John Ioannidis has studied research and mathematically proven that most published research findings are false.[1] He notes that published research findings are

---

[1] Ioannidis JPA (2005) Why Most Published Research Findings Are False. PLoS Med 2(8): e124. https://doi.org/10.1371/journal.pmed.0020124

often declared conclusive based on "statistical significance" teased out of the data by what exercise scientist Dr. Ralph Carpinelli has called "numerological abracadabra,"[2] but these findings are rarely if ever confirmed by other independent teams.

Science is supposed to involve competing laboratories exactly repeating experiments of one another in order to confirm or refute claimed findings. However, this rarely happens. Physicist Richard Feynman recounted an interaction with a student that illustrates why scientists avoid replication experiments, in spite of replication being one of the supposed cornerstones of science:

> "Other kinds of errors are more characteristic of poor science. When I was at Cornell, I often talked to the people in the psychology department. One of the students told me she wanted to do an experiment that went something like this—I don't remember it in detail, but it had been found by others that under certain circumstances, X, rats did something, A. She was curious as to whether, if she changed the circumstances to Y, they would still do, A. So her proposal was to do the experiment under circumstances Y and see if they still did A.

> "I explained to her that it was necessary first to repeat in her laboratory the experiment of the other person—to do it under condition X to see if she could also get result A—and then change to Y and see if A changed. Then she would know that the real difference was the thing she thought she had under control.

> "She was very delighted with this new idea, and went to her professor. And his reply was, no, you cannot do that, because the experiment has already been done and you would be

---

[2] Carpinelli RN. Critical review of a meta-analysis for the effect of single and multiple sets of resistance training on strength gains. Med Sport 2012;16(3): 122-130.

wasting time. This was in about 1935 or so, and it seems to have been the general policy then to not try to repeat psychological experiments, but only to change the conditions and see what happens."[3]

Thus, since a premium is placed on publishing "original research" and "new" data, results of previous research reports are accepted without question or confirmation. The result is that the scientific literature is filled with reports of findings taken to be true, but never confirmed to be true.

Ioannidis notes that the vast majority of published studies suffer from bias consisting of "various design, data, analysis, and presentation factors that tend to produce research findings when they should not be produced." He shows that "the majority of modern biomedical research is operating in areas with very low pre- and post- study probability for true findings," so common research findings "may often be simply accurate measures of the prevailing bias." In his words:

> "For example, let us suppose that no nutrients or dietary patterns are actually important determinants for the risk of developing a specific tumor. Let us also suppose that the scientific literature has examined 60 nutrients and claims all of them to be related to the risk of developing this tumor with relative risks in the range of 1.2 to 1.4 for the comparison of the upper to lower intake tertiles. Then the claimed effect sizes are simply measuring nothing else but the net bias that has been involved in the generation of this scientific literature. Claimed effect sizes are in fact the most accurate estimates of the net bias. It even follows that between 'null fields,' the fields that claim stronger effects (often with accompanying claims of medical or public

---

[3] Feynman RP. Cargo Cult Science. Some remarks o science, pseudoscience, and learning how to not fool yourself. Caltech's 1974 commencement address. <http://calteches.library.caltech.edu/51/2/CargoCult.htm>

health importance) are simply those that sustained the worst biases."

Ioannidis and Schoenfeld[4] have shown that in 80% of epidemiological studies linking 40 different foods to cancer risk (increased or decreased), the statistical support was weak or nonnominally significant. In 75% of studies that claimed an increased risk related to a food, and 76% of studies that claimed a decreased risk related to a food, the statistical support for the claims was weak or nonnominally significant. Also, there was no standardized, consistent selection for evaluating exposure to the foods, making it difficult to combine data from multiple studies to generate conclusions. Although it is statistically most likely that no relationship would be found and such relationships are spurious, the data from these studies did not fall into the expected Bell curve with a large peak of null results. Ioannidis and Schoenfeld remarked:

> "The credibility of studies in this and other fields is subject to publication and other selective outcome and analysis reporting biases, whenever the pressure to publish fosters a climate in which 'negative' results are undervalued and not reported. Ingredients viewed as 'unhealthy' may be demonized, leading to subsequent biases in the design, execution and reporting of studies. Some studies that narrowly meet criteria for statistical significance may represent spurious results, especially when there is large flexibility in analyses, selection of contrasts, and reporting. When results are overinterpreted, the emerging literature can skew perspectives and potentially obfuscate other truly significant findings. This issue may be especially problematic in areas such as cancer epidemiology, where randomized trials may be exceedingly difficult and expensive to conduct; therefore, more reliance is placed on

---

[4] Schoenfeld JD, Ioannidis JPA. Is everything we eat associated with cancer? A systematic cookbook review. Am J Clin Nutr 2013 January 1;97(1):127-134. <https://academic.oup.com/ajcn/article/97/1/127/4576988>

observational studies, but with a considerable risk of trusting false-positive or inflated results."[2]

Simply put, most research reports claiming to have found evidence that some food or nutrient promotes or causes a common disease have not found such evidence, but are simply reports of what the authors and reviewers of the report believe, regardless of the actual lack of evidence for their beliefs. This applies to findings in exercise science as well. Research reports claiming to have found strong evidence that some complicated or time-consuming exercise method produces much better results ("large effect sizes") compared to simpler and briefer methods are probably reports of what the authors and reviewers of the report want to believe (i.e. their bias). And, the more certainty they claim for their findings, the less likely the findings are true.

Ioannidis has also noted:

> "Nutritional intake is notoriously difficult to capture with the questionnaire methods used by most studies. A recent analysis showed that in the National Health and Nutrition Examination Survey, an otherwise superb study, for two thirds of the participants the energy intake measures inferred from the questionnaire are incompatible with life. More sophisticated measurements based on biochemical, web, camera, mobile, or sensor tools may not necessarily reduce bias. Caution about the reliability of measurements should extend to inferences that depend on them."[5]

Ioannidis goes on to remark that many findings are entirely implausible. We can find in many peer-reviewed epidemiological studies the suggestion that we can cut our risk of cancer in half with just a couple of servings a day of a single nutrient or food. However, Ioannidis notes that dozens of randomized trials have shown single

---

[5] Ioannidis JPA. Implausible results in human nutrition research. Definitive solutions won't come from another million observational papers or small randomized trials. BMJ 2013;347:f6698 doi: 10.1136/bmj.f6698

nutrients or foods are unlikely to either reduce or elevate *relative* risk by more than 10 percent, and most show the *relative* risk reduction or increase to be less than 5 percent if not zero.[3] He also adds that the respective absolute risk differences "would be trivial."

Almost all studies report *relative* risk reduction or increase, and this always dramatically inflates the actual risk. For example, the Cochrane Review reported that in 11 epidemiological studies of 53, 300 people comparing low saturated fat consumption (less than 10% of calories from saturated fat) to "usual" saturated fat consumption (more than 10% of calories), the relative risk reduction was 17%, but in every 10, 000 individuals, there were only 138 fewer "combined cardiovascular events" in 52 months of follow-up,[6] which is an absolute event reduction of only 1.4%. The relative risk reduction for cardiovascular death was 5%, but the absolute event reduction was only 10 fewer per 10,000, which is only 0.1% absolute event reduction. The relative coronary heart disease event reduction was reported as 13%, but the absolute reduction was only 80 fewer per 10, 000, which is an absolute event reduction of only 0.8%. These are essentially null results, i.e. there was no absolute benefit to restricting saturated fat consumption to less than 10% of calories.

Hence, Ioannidis wrote that most nutritional research shows that:

> "Observational studies and even randomized trials of single nutrients seem hopeless, with rare exceptions. Even nominal confounding or other biases create noise that exceeds any genuine effect. Big datasets just confer spurious precision status to noise."[3]

Ioannidis went on to explain that to identify nutrition interventions that produce a mere 5-10% *relative* risk reduction in overall mortality in the general population (not just high risk patients), we

---

[6] Hooper L, Martin N, Abdelhamid A, Davey Smith G. Reduction in saturated at intake for cardiovascular disease. Cochrane Databased of Systematic Reviews 2015. <http://cochranelibrary-wiley.com/doi/10.1002/14651858.CD011737/epdf>

would need randomized trials including about 75, 000 subjects, with long-term follow-up, linkage to death registries, careful efforts to ensure adherence, and freedom from conflicts of interest and allegiance bias in sponsors and conductors of the study. It is unlikely that any such study will ever be conducted and given that it would only identify a 5-10% *relative* risk reduction, which would be a trivial *absolute* risk reduction, it is difficult to justify the enormous expense of time and resources it would involve.

In short, current science is not a reliable guide to the optimal dietary choices, and future science is very unlikely to be any greater help.

In his books *Against Method* and *Science in a Free Society*, philosopher Paul Feyerabend has shown that, contrary to the *fairytale* we are told about science, history shows that scientists do not have a magic method for discovering the truth about Nature, and that science does not necessarily produce results superior to or more desirable than non-scientific methods of inquiry.[7]

> "According to the fairytale the success of science is the result of a subtle but carefully balanced combination of inventiveness and control. Scientists have *ideas*. And they have special *methods* for improving ideas. The theories of science have passed the test of method. They give a better account of the world than ideas which have not passed the test."[8]

> "But the fairytale is false. There is no special method that guarantees success or makes it probable. Scientists don't solve problems because they possess a magic wand – methodology – but because they have studied a problem for a long time, because they know the situation fairly well,

---

[7] For a concise introduction to Feyerabend's arguments, read his essay: "'Science.' The Myth and its Role in Society. Inquiry;18:167-81. You can download it from my website: **http://www.fullrangestrength.com/support-files/ feyerabendmyth.pdf**

[8] Ibid.

because they are not too unintelligent, and because the excesses of one scientific school are almost always balanced by the excesses of some other school. (Besides, scientists only rarely solve their problems, they make lots of mistakes, and many of their solutions are quite useless.) Basically there is hardly any difference between the process preceding that which leads to the announcement of a new scientific law and the process preceding passage of a new law in society: one informs either all citizens, or those immediately concerned, one collects 'facts' and prejudices, one discusses the matter, and one finally votes."[9]

That's why we often hear scientists talking about the "consensus" in their discipline. Most will agree to the "consensus" because not doing so puts them at odds with their colleagues, who determine whether they get funding or employment, or not.

For example, if a majority of highly indoctrinated, biased scientists ridden with conflicts of interest (e.g. stock holdings in corporations that produce cholesterol-reducing drugs) agrees with the statement "High blood cholesterol promotes cardiovascular disease," then everyone is supposed to genuflect to their supreme wisdom and refrain from questioning their authority.

Unfortunately, career scientists have a perverse motivation to fail to solve problems. Solving a practical problem – e.g. curing cancer – will eliminate the need for research, and thus put the researcher out of his job. Failure to solve the problem produces job security: "More research is needed."

My cognitive and dietary reversals – which so disturbed some of my audience – only reflected my attempts to reconcile the conflicting and contradictory science of nutrition. Some 'authorities' including T. Colin Campbell and Michael Greger claim the science proves that humans need no animal foods, and any intake of cholesterol-containing animal products is detrimental to health, increasing one's

---

[9] Ibid.

risk for cardiovascular disease, cancer, arthritis and a myriad of other conditions; a position which resonates with the official dietary guidelines from the USDA and other national advisory bodies (which unbeknownst to many, receive financial support from industries that pedal plant products). A few renegades claim the science proves otherwise, that cholesterol intake has little or no bearing on one's risk for any common disease.

Yet our culture has put science on a pedestal. Everyone is required to worship science as the only human enterprise capable of providing the 'final solution' to all human problems. Philosophy, logic and common sense have fallen by the wayside. As Feyerabend notes:

> "Even human relations are dealt with in a scientific manner, as is shown by education programs, proposals for prison reform, army training, and so on. Almost all scientific subjects are compulsory in our schools. While the parents of a six-year-old child can decide to have him instructed in the rudiments of Protestantism, or in the rudiments of the Jewish faith, or to omit religious instruction altogether, they do not have a similar freedom in the case of the sciences. Physics, astronomy, history *must* be learned. They cannot be replaced by magic, astrology, or by a study of legends."[10]

Highly intelligent people who receive high degrees of indoctrination in conventional educational institutions are particularly susceptible to putting faith in science, simply because they receive the most indoctrination and reinforcement. One simply cannot graduate without accepting and 'mastering' the claims of science. Disputing 'science' will result in loss of face, ridicule, and failure to graduate to the next level of indoctrination. In contrast, as Feyerabend points out, accepting the *scientific faith* will make one a member of the 'club of intelligents,' and possibly even a *bigshot* with special privileges:

---

[10] Ibid.

"This is where the fairytale assumes its decisive function. It conceals, by a recitation of 'objective' criteria, the freedom of decision which creative scientists and the general public have, even inside the most rigid and advanced parts of science, and thus protects the bigshots (Nobel prize winners, heads of laboratories, educators, etc.) from the masses (laymen, experts in non-scientific fields, experts in other fields): only those citizens count who were subjected to the pressures of scientific institutions (they have undergone a long process of education), who succumbed to these pressures (they have passed their examinations), and who are now firmly convinced of the truth of the fairytale. This is how scientists have deceived themselves and everyone else about their business, but without any real disadvantage; they have more money, more authority, more sex appeal than they deserve, and even the most stupid procedures and the most laughable results in their domain are surrounded with an aura of excellence. It is time to cut them down to size, to give them a more modest position in society."[11]

I first had the benefit of Feyerabend's perspective more than 30 years ago, when I was earning my undergraduate and Master's degrees in philosophy (I had a minor concentration in philosophy of science). Yet after graduation with honors, this perspective had little impact on my relationship to science. As a testament to the power of the science-based education/indoctrination I received, like any other student attending public schools, from the age of 5 years on, I continued to have some *faith* in science, particularly the 'science of nutrition' until early 2017, when in late February, I had an experience that released me from any remaining *faith* I had in science as an independently reliable source of diet and nutrition guidance.

Over the course of some 36 years I had studied human nutrition and experimented with diets ranging from 100 percent plant-based to

---

[11] Ibid.

(very briefly) 100 percent animal-based. My main personal goal was to find a way of eating that would cure me of eczema and psoriasis lesions that started in childhood and got worse as I became an adult. No one else in my family had this supposedly genetic condition.

My first wife Rachel Albert and I experimented with plant-based diets, mostly macrobiotic vegetarian and vegan at times, for many years. Over our years together, we had gone back and forth between including and excluding animal products multiple times, but always continued to eat large amounts of vegetables and/or fruits because we believed that they were good for us. It seemed that all the 'authorities' agreed on this, whether they espoused a plant-based diet, or a meat-based diet.

The dominant ideology maintained that if one had any diet-related illness, it could not be caused by fruits or vegetables, and probably was caused by eating animal foods. After all, according to this ideology, we are just 'slightly modified' chimpanzees, so must be, like chimps, adapted to a plant-based diet (a claim I will in this book demonstrate to be false).

If I was eating animal products when my skin conditions worsened or some other undesired condition appeared, I always suspected but was not sure that the animal products caused the problem. I suspected because in the 'scientific' nutrition paradigm widely accepted around me, and heavily promoted by the mass media, animal products are the most likely toxic foods, the cause of heart disease, cancer and other ailments, because of their (supposedly) toxic contents of protein, cholesterol, and saturated fats.

In contrast, some conditions I experienced during my many experiments never occurred except when I was restricting animal products and eating large amounts of fibrous plant foods. For example, I always got gas, bloating, flatulence and loose acidic stools on plant-based diets. I also lost libido, muscle mass and tolerance for hard exercise, and my skin and hair were very dry and flakey all over, not just where I had psoriatic lesions. This was a direct and immediate experience, not a hypothetical "well, maybe this blood lipid level will cause you to have a heart attack 40 years from now."

After years of eating plant based diets and suffering with the digestive discomfort and weakness, Rachel and I got to a point where we thought we had had enough. Over the years I had read several books that convinced me that a paleolithic diet rich in animal products *and* abundant in fruits and vegetables was the best alternative to a strictly plant-based diet. Rachel and I embarked on what we thought was a practically paleolithic diet path and eventually published *The Garden of Eating: A Produce-Dominated Diet & Cookbook*.

Cutting out grains and beans definitely helped my digestion and eating animal protein enabled me to regain lost muscle mass and exercise tolerance. However, this pseudo-paleo diet approach did not improve my most stubborn psoriatic lesions, and sometimes it seemed they were even worse. Also, after some time I developed some more alarming issues: skin tags, lipomas, and intermittent urinary difficulties consistent with prostatitis (I was in my 40s).

During this time my father was diagnosed with prostate cancer, and Rachel started noticing fibrocystic changes in her breasts. I became concerned with these issues. Because of my previous indoctrination, particularly my familiarity with the clinical work of John McDougall, M.D. and the research work of T. Colin Campbell, Ph.D., author of *The China Study*, part of me still believed that prostatitis, fibrocystic breast changes, and prostate cancer are caused by eating animal protein and fat. My belief was strong enough to cause me to try to convince Rachel that we needed to once again remove animal products from our diet.

She wasn't interested in that and friction between us on this issue exacerbated tensions that already existed between us. Eventually we got a divorce.

After the divorce I tried eating a plant-based diet again for a short period, but the return of the digestive discomfort dissuaded me from continuing for more than a few months. I returned to *The Garden of Eating Diet*: a meat-based practically paleo diet with large amounts of fruits, vegetables and nuts.

Sometime around 2009-2010, I came across some websites and online forums – mainly, ZeroingInOnHealth.com, by Charles Washington – where people were reporting their positive experiences with a completely carnivorous diet. These reports convinced me to try eliminating plants from my diet 6 out of every 7 days (I reserved Saturdays for eating some plants for pleasure and socializing). On the other days I ate meat and animal fats, but got most of my fat from cheese.

However, I abandoned this after a month because I had constipation and cramps and strongly believed that I needed fruits and vegetables in my diet for digestive health. I didn't eat enough fat and consumed very little salt, since I still believed the story (lie) that our paleolithic ancestors ate a low sodium diet. I still believed that our paleolithic ancestors ate lots of fruits and vegetables, and that one of the 'mistakes' of my parents' generation was its relatively limited inclusion of vegetables and fruits in their diet. I had great difficulty entertaining the hypothesis that my daily indulgence in carbohydrate-rich fruits and roots might be causing some of the issues I was experiencing on my practically paleo diet. After all, advocates of the paleolithic diet argued that as primates allegedly closely related to the frugivorous, folivorous chimps, we are naturally adapted to a diet rich in fruits and vegetables. Although my chronic skin conditions persisted whether I ate animal products or not – and therefore persisted as long as I ate a plant based diet – I just was unable to take the carnivorous diet seriously. I believed that science including evolutionary considerations had proven that we should eat as much fruits and vegetables as practical.

However, my devotion to vegetables was not Natural. When I was a child, like most children, I was not a spontaneous vegetable lover. However, like most people, I was cajoled, bribed and coerced into eating vegetables. "Finish your vegetables or you don't get dessert." Adults told me how important it was for me to eat vegetables. They even produced Popeye cartoons which convinced my immature mind that eating spinach will turn anyone into a superhero. How could vegetables and fruits be harmful?

Early in 2010, I met my current wife Tracy, and she adopted my pseudo-paleo diet habits, which included a fair amount of heavy cream and butter along with daily consumption of carbohydrate-rich fruits and starchy vegetables (dates, bananas, sweet potatoes, white potatoes, etc.). As the year progressed Tracy progressively gained body fat, and started having premenstrual breast tenderness and lumps, and overall her breasts became unnaturally large and uneven in size.

Then, one day in 2010, Rachel called to tell me that she had received a diagnosis of breast cancer. I was floored. She wanted me to help her decide how to eat to increase her chances of reversing this condition, to provide acupuncture and herbal medicine, and to help her deal with oncologists and other health care providers and understand and evaluate her treatment options, both conventional and 'alternative.'

At the time, I knew of some, very little, preliminary research supporting use of a low carbohydrate, high protein or ketogenic diet to treat cancer or support cancer treatment. Initially I thought that a high protein ketogenic diet might be the best path for her.[12] However, at the time research support for that approach was very limited.

On the other hand, a part of me still believed that the preponderance of research linked breast and prostate cancer risk with diets rich in meat and animal fat. That was in fact the dominant view at the time.

Moreover, I had studied the natural history of cancer, and learned

---

12 Ho VW, Leung K, Hsu A, Luk B, et al., "A Low Carbohydrate, High Protein Diet Slows Tumor Growth and Prevents Cancer Initiation," Cancer Research 2011 July;71(13): DOI: 10.1158/0008-5472.CAN-10-3973 <http://cancerres.aacrjournals.org/content/71/13/4484.full-text.pdf>

14

that by the time any malignant tumor becomes detectable by current techniques, it has been actively growing for about 10 years since the first cells went rogue, and has already metastasized. Doing the math I figured that Rachel's cancer had started as a single rogue cell when we were married and after we had been eating a meat-rich paleoid diet for several years.

Leading paleo diet promoters recommended eating a large amount of fruits and vegetables because a large number of epidemiological studies purported to find that this produce had anti-cancer effects, but no paleo diet promoters I was aware of believed that meat had anti-cancer effects. In *The Garden of Eating*, I had written:

> "When 150 scientists reviewed 4500 research studies of the influence of dietary variables on 18 different cancers, vegetables were found to provide a convincing protective effect for 5 cancers, a probable preventive effect for 4 others, and a possible preventive effect for another 7. For fruits the analysis revealed 4 convincing, probable, and possible preventive relationships. For cereal grains there were no convincing or probable preventive relationships, and only 1 possible preventive effect (that for cancer of the esophagus).[13]

> "The World Cancer Research Fund and American Institute for Cancer Research recommend 400 grams (nearly 1 pound) of fruits and vegetables daily, providing at least 10 percent of daily calories, to prevent cancer.[14] If you follow our plan you will consume more than 1200 grams of fruits and vegetables daily, providing more than 30 percent of your daily energy intake, and gain a substantial cancer-preventive effect."

---

13 World Cancer Research Fund & American Institute for Cancer Research, 1997.

14 Munoz de Chavez M, Chavez A. Diet that prevents cancer: recommendations from the American Institute for Cancer Research. Int J Cancer Suppl (United States)1998;11:85-9.

Thus, I had accepted the opinion of these authorities, that fruits and vegetables had only strong anti-cancer properties, and no cancer-promoting properties, so the plants in our palaeoid diet could not have been responsible for promoting Rachel's breast cancer. Since her cancer most likely began as a single rogue cell when we were eating a produce-rich paleo diet, and supposedly cancer-promoting animal meat and fat were major components of that diet, I was led by my premises to the conclusion that the meat portion of the palaeoid diet must have been the culprit.

I had studied writings of John McDougall, M.D., and T. Colin Campbell, Ph.D., wherein they claimed that cancer could be reversed by a plant-based diet devoid of animal protein, and I found that idea hard to shake. McDougall boasts that he published the first ever study accepted in a scientific journal regarding the treatment of breast cancer with diet.[15] He argues that excess calories, animal fats, vegetable fats, and cholesterol all promote cancer, while fiber and various phytonutrients inhibit it. One of McDougall's patients, Ruth Heidrich, claims to have reversed aggressive, metastatic breast cancer with a lumpectomy and a 100% plant-based diet.[16]

Campbell agrees on all those points and also claims to have proven in animal studies that restricting animal protein intake will reverse cancer[17] (he doesn't draw attention to the fact that his research team also proved that this only happens if the diet is deficient in one or more essential amino acids[18]).

---

[15] McDougall J. Preliminary study of diet as an adjunct therapy for breast cancer. Breast 1984;10:18.

[16] Heidrich R. A Race for Life: From Cancer to the Ironman. Heidrich & Assoc, 1990.

[17] Campbell TC. The China Study. Benbella Books, 2006.

[18] Schulsinger DA, Root MM, Campbell TC. Effect of dietary protein quality on development of aflatoxin B1-induced hepatic preneoplastic lesions. J Natl Cancer Inst. 1989 Aug 16;81(16):1241-5. PubMed PMID: 2569044.

In addition, one of my friends, Gordon Saxe, M.D., Ph.D., had by that time conducted multiple intervention studies suggesting that a whole foods plant based diet can stall or even reverse prostate cancer.[19, 20, 21, 22]

So, I had my father with prostate cancer, myself with intermittent prostatitis symptoms, Rachel with breast cancer, and Tracy with weight gain and pre-menstrual breast cysts and tenderness similar to what Rachel had developed during our years together eating the pseudo-paleo diet. I was afraid I was going to develop prostate cancer, and Tracy was going to develop breast cancer. I lacked evidence and hence conviction that an animal-based diet could prevent and treat cancer, but believed I had evidence – including some from studies conducted by a friend of mine – that animal fat and protein promote cancer, whereas a whole foods plant-based diet can reverse or support reversal of breast and prostate cancer.

As a consequence of this line of reasoning, I chose to publish my "Farewell to Paleo" post on June 14, 2011 on my Primal Wisdom

[19] Saxe GA, Major JM, Nguyen JY, Freeman KM, Downs TM, Salem CE. Potential attenuation of disease progression in recurrent prostate cancer with plant-based diet and stress reduction. Integr Cancer Ther. 2006 Sep;5(3):206-13. PubMed PMID:16880425.

[20] Berkow SE, Barnard ND, Saxe GA, Ankerberg-Nobis T. Diet and survival after prostate cancer diagnosis. Nutr Rev. 2007 Sep;65(9):391-403. Review. PubMed PMID:17958206.

[21] Saxe GA, Hébert JR, Carmody JF, Kabat-Zinn J, Rosenzweig PH, Jarzobski D, Reed GW, Blute RD. Can diet in conjunction with stress reduction affect the rate of increase in prostate specific antigen after biochemical recurrence of prostate cancer? J Urol. 2001 Dec;166(6):2202-7. PubMed PMID: 11696736.

[22] Saxe GA, Major JM, Westerberg L, Khandrika S, Downs TM. BIOLOGICAL MEDIATORS OF EFFECT OF DIET AND STRESS REDUCTION ON PROSTATE CANCER. *Integrative cancer therapies*. 2008;7(3):130-138. doi: 10.1177/1534735408322849.

blog.[23] I returned to a whole foods strictly plant based diet, in spite of my repeated previous experience that such a diet would give me much digestive distress and cause me to lose a lot of muscle and exercise tolerance. I chose to trust in authorities and to eat to lower my cholesterol, rather than to trust my body signals and direct experience.

Sure enough, I promptly lost about 15-20 pounds, mostly muscle mass, and the gas, bloating, loose stools, and anal itching returned. In 2007, on *The Garden of Eating Diet*, my total cholesterol, LDL, HDL and triglycerides were 231, 138, 85 and 47 mg/dL respectively. At the time, I was unaware of the importance of having a low remnant cholesterol, but it was only 8 mg/dL, a value indicating very low cardiovascular disease risk (I discuss remnant cholesterol in Chapter 4). On the whole foods strictly plant based diet my total and LDL cholesterol dropped, but so did my HDL, and my triglycerides went up; in 2012 they were 180, 105, 53, and 105 respectively, and the remnant cholesterol increased by 2.6 times to 21. The reversal of the triglyceride/HDL ratio and the increase in remnant cholesterol indicated the whole foods plant based diet was not improving my health, but I was doggedly pursuing a total cholesterol under 150 because all the doctors advocating the whole foods plant based diet claim that such a cholesterol level makes one "heart attack proof."

On November 25, 2016, after 5 years on a strictly plant-based diet I had my last vegan blood test. I received the results in December. My total cholesterol had finally dropped to 154 mg/dL. According to promoters of plant-based diets, I should have been as healthy as possible, no longer burdened with supposedly toxic high cholesterol, now virtually heart attack and cancer proof.

In fact my health and fitness were suffering. Every day I was plagued with the digestive discomfort – bloating, cramping and loose stools – that I had always had with any diet high in plant foods. Although physician advocates of plant-based diets had explained that this gas is just the price one pays for eating a healthy, fiber-rich

---

[23] By July 2018 the post had 165,000 views.

plant-based diet that promotes abundant growth of supposedly beneficial gut flora, I was tired of it. In addition, I had started experiencing acid reflux after my starchy bean and grain meals.

My skin was drier than ever and flaking all over (especially elbows). New psoriasis lesions were emerging, and old ones were re-emerging or getting worse. In five years my eyesight had gone from better than 20/20 to worse. My waist had increased by several inches in circumference even though I was lighter than when on the meat-rich *Garden of Eating Diet*. In other words, I had gained fat and lost muscle, in spite of doing intense bodyweight strength training several times weekly. My progress in the training was painfully slow.

In August of 2015 I injured my knee doing bodyweight strength training; in February of 2017 it was still not healed. I had also strained my back a couple of times during the 5 vegan years, and it just did not fully heal either. I was limping around like an invalid for 18 months. People were remarking that I seemed to have aged beyond my years. Later I learned that during these 5 years of eating a "nutrient-dense" whole foods plant-based vegan diet, I also developed caries in two teeth, despite regularly taking vitamin D supplements and getting plenty of sun exposure.

Moreover, the lab report showing my cholesterol was only 154 mg/dL also found that I was suffering from deficiencies. My blood phosphorus and globulin protein levels were significantly below the normal range. The cereals and legumes upon which I had based my diet for several years are poor sources of phosphorus because in these foods it is bound by by phytates. The low globulin level suggested I was not getting enough protein, in spite of the fact that I was eating legumes and soy products providing much more than recommended levels of protein. Both Tracy and I took a zinc taste challenge test, and we both tested probably deficient. Zinc deficiency is a well-established issue for plant-based dieters.

In addition, my LDL, HDL, and triglycerides were 78, 60, and 78 mg/dL respectively, so my remnant cholesterol was 16, twice the level found when I was eating the high fat, high protein and also too high carbohydrate *Garden of Eating Diet* in 2007.

And for a couple of months, I had been craving meat.

During 2016, I also became aware of other strong evidence, discussed in Chapter 2, that humans do in fact have an evolved innate drive to eat meat, specific biological adaptations to meat-eating, and requirements for nutrients either exclusively supplied by animal products or so poorly supplied by plants or endogenous synthesis that we must eat meat to obtain adequate amounts (e.g. taurine, choline, arachidonic acid, and docosahexaenoic acid).

After I received those lab test results, from December 2016 and into February of 2017, I initially tried to correct the developed deficiencies and reverse my declining health and fitness by tweaking my plant-based diet, eating more high protein plant foods and taking some supplements.

However, one afternoon in February 2017, Tracy and I were sitting in our Chinese medicine and acupuncture office eating a whole foods plant based lunch. I was contemplating all I knew about human nutrition and all I had experienced up to that point, when suddenly my perspective shifted away from lab values, supposedly scientific research, and the opinions of authorities like McDougall and Campbell, and towards my direct, immediate experience.

I paid attention to how the food I was eating tasted to me, I thought about how it made my gut feel, and I remembered a Truth recorded by Ray Audette in his book *Neanderthin*:

A creature can't require what in Nature it can't acquire.

And then, while finishing that vegan meal consisting largely of legumes and cereals, the following question arose in my mind:

"Why did I eat that?"

As soon as the question was asked, the following inner conversation occurred in only moments:

"Because I think it is the healthiest way to eat."

"And why do I think that?"

"Because I was told to eat my vegetables, science, experts, etc. blah blah..."

"And what would you eat if there were no 'experts' to tell you what you should eat, but you, like your ancient ancestors, had to decide what was healthy without this foreign ideological input. How would you know what was healthy and what was not?"

And at that moment, I finally realized that I didn't need expert guidance or 'science' to choose the right foods. No healthy non-human animal needs a dietitian, physician, blood test, science or ideology to know what to eat. Every creature simply follows Nature, and most importantly, no creature follows a "balanced" diet.

I realized that Nature, the Creator, has given each of us senses of sight, smell, taste, hunger, and satisfaction, and these have no other purpose than to enable us to decide what Natural, unprocessed foods are good for us and what is not.

A True Human would eat in harmony with his True Nature, following his biology, not any ideology.

He would eat whatever he could acquire from Nature using his strength and wit.

He would eat what is by its Nature pleasing to his senses of sight, smell, and taste.

He would eat Natural foods that he can easily digest, with no discomfort, not 'foods' that only exist or are edible or digestible only because they have been highly processed by human artifice.

If I were a True Human in abundant Nature, not encumbered by ideology nor lost in the jungle of thought, and not trying to control the food supply, or avoid some hypothetical future fate, I would eat what by Nature I prefer to eat: meat, fat and any other tasty animal product I could acquire.

I wouldn't eat grains or beans, because they are not edible or palatable in their Natural state, and because when I do eat them they give me gut distress (gas, bloating, cramping, loose stools).

I would limit my intake of vegetables to a palatable few, because they don't satisfy my taste or hunger and in large amounts they too give me bloating.

I would have a limited intake of fruits or nuts, because these also gave me trouble, and because Nature provides few that are edible and tasty in any season, and none in some seasons.

I would eat nothing that needs processing, extensive cooking and doctoring to just to become edible or more or less palatable.

I would eat only when hungry and stop eating when I felt satisfied or the food I was eating no longer tasted good to me.

This came to me:

"I am sure Nature, the Creator, gave me these senses to help me make right choices. I know from experience that experts can be lost in ideology and ignorant of Nature, they can lie and mislead. But Nature is what is. Nature is Truth. My job is to align my thoughts and actions with Reality, with Nature, not with 'authorities.'"

And so, after years of trying to figure things out by consulting experts, I *came to my senses*, had a *gut realization,* and *began* to trust my True Nature – both outer and inner – to guide me to my right diet.

I started cutting unpalatable plant foods out of my diet and based my diet on meat, fat, eggs and selected dairy products, complemented by very small amounts of vegetables, berries and fruits. I had been eating lots of nuts and seeds, but after my realization I quickly learned that most nuts and seeds either irritate my mouth or give me gas (or both), so I started avoiding them.

Within days, I was free of the bloating, flatulence, and loose stools. Within a week, my mood and sleep started to improve. Within a few weeks, I had lost some of the excess fat from around my waist, and I finally saw some improvement in the psoriasis lesions in my ears and on my scalp that had never responded to macrobiotic, vegetarian, vegan, whole foods omnivorous, or paleo diets rich in vegetables, fruits and/or nuts and seeds.

The transition to a hypercarnivorous diet did result in some initial difficulty with defecation. For about 5 months I had a bowel elimination only two or three times a week, which in itself is no cause for alarm, but sometimes would have a little trouble getting stools started. After years of eating a low-fat diet and having loose stools more or less explode out, propelled by gasses and irritating acids produced by fiber fermentation, I had sluggish bile production and flow and wasn't used to having to bear down to move the stool. However, I had seen our carnivorous cat strongly bear down to defecate, so I deduced that bearing down is required by Nature, and my ability to do it was impaired.

The one time previously I had tried a very low plant food diet, I had called this "constipation" and taken it as a sign that I needed to eat more plants. This time I refused that interpretation, because accepting it in the past led me right back into the foods that cause me chronic intestinal distress. I learned from LIFE WITHOUT BREAD by Wolfgang Lutz, M.D. that my colon had been damaged and weakened by years of a high fiber diet.   •

I also knew that bile release after fatty meals stimulates bowel movement, but eating a low fat diet for years had impaired my bile flow and gall bladder function. I refused to go back to eating foods that always gave me bloating, cramping and flatulence. I knew that I just needed to improve my bile flow and gall bladder function and let my intestines heal. I started taking digestive bitters, artichoke extract, and 300-600 mg of magnesium daily to support normal bile flow and keep things moving in the meantime.

After six months, for the first time in over 40 years, the skin lesions were finally showing some signs of improving. Not only that, my defecation became more comfortable and easy than I could ever remember. Unless I ate types or amounts of plant foods I did not tolerate, I had no more bloating, cramping or farting, no explosive elimination and I had mostly regained the natural ability to bear down to get a stool to move out, despite eating almost no plant foods on a daily basis.

I finally broke free from the nutritional spells cast on me by 'authorities.' Now I want to help you break free yourself.

INTRODUCTION

Why We Need To Change Our Ways

Modern man has produced an advanced technological society with many wondrous luxuries. We can fly hundreds of miles in an hour, explore the depths of the ocean, and transmit audio and visual messages across the world in moments. We produce more food than ever, and we live in regions previously uninhabitable due to advanced indoor climate control. We seem to be on top of the world.

If you consider only these apparent successes, it seems logical to conclude that this technology is beneficial and the ideology that produced it has been proven correct. However, a deeper investigation reveals that this apparent progress has been accompanied by physical, mental and moral degeneration of humanity and degradation of the life-support systems of the Earth.

Rates of sexually transmitted diseases reached an unprecedented high in the U.S. in 2015.[1] About 20 million new STD infections occur every year in the U.S., half of these in young adults aged 15-24, and the organisms present in these diseases have become drug resistant.[2] These diseases can cause blindness, infertility, stillbirths, and birth defects.

In the U.S., birth defects affect 3% of babies and are the leading cause of infant death, accounting for 20% of all infant deaths.[3]

---

1 CDC, NCHHSTP Newsroom, "2015 STD Surveillance Report Press Release." **<https://www.cdc.gov/nchhstp/newsroom/2016/std-surveillance-report-2015-press-release.html>**

2 Mermin J, "Have STDs Reach Crisis Level? The Status Quo Is No Longer Enough," Huffington Post 2016 Oct 20. **<http://www.huffingtonpost.com/dr-jonathan-mermin/have-stds-reached-crisis_b_12577246.html>**

3 CDC, "Birth Defects: Data & Statistics." **<http://www.cdc.gov/ncbddd/birthdefects/data.html>**

Dental defects, malocclusions, and decay are nearly universal.[4]

About 20% of the population suffers from digestive diseases.[5]

About 9% of the U.S. population has diabetes.[6]
One-third of all U.S. deaths in 2013 were caused by heart disease, stroke, or other cardiovascular diseases.[7]

In 2016, there were about 4,620 new cases of cancer diagnosed, and 1,630 deaths from cancer treatment every day in the U.S..[8] The leading cancer sites are prostate, breast, lung, colorectal, uterus, and urinary bladder.

About 3% of the U.S. population has an autoimmune disorder.[9]

---

4 NIH, Nation Institute of Dental and Craniofacial Research, "Find Data by Topic." **<http://www.nidcr.nih.gov/DataStatistics/FindDataByTopic/>**

5 NIH, National Institute of Diabetes and Digestive and Kidney Diseases, "Digestive Diseases Statistics for the United States." **<https://www.niddk.nih.gov/health-information/health-statistics/Pages/digestive-diseases-statistics-for-the-united-states.aspx>**

6 CDC, "Diabetes Home: 2014 National Diabetes Statistics Report." **<http://www.cdc.gov/diabetes/data/statistics/2014statisticsreport.html>**

7 American Heart Association, "New statistics show one of every three U.S. deaths caused by cardiovascular disease." **<http://newsroom.heart.org/news/new-statistics-show-one-of-every-three-u-s-deaths-caused-by-cardiovascular-disease>**

8 American Cancer Society, Cancer Statistics Center. <https://cancerstatisticscenter.cancer.org/?_ga=1.232068575.1792849541.1478892116#/>

9 Dooley MA, Hogan SL, "Environmental Epidemiology and Risk Factors for Autoimmune Disease," Current Opinion in Rheumatology 2003;15(2). **<http://www.medscape.com/viewarticle/449854>**

Eight percent of U.S. children engage in non-suicidal self-injury.[10] Major depression affected 7% of all U.S. adults in 2015.[11] Between 1999 and 2014, the age-adjusted suicide rate in the U.S. increased 24%, with the rate of increase greatest in girls aged 10-14 and men aged 45-64; the rate of male suicide is 3 times that for females.[12] One percent of U.S. adults suffers from schizophrenia.[13] It is estimated that about 47% of the U.S. adult population suffers from signs of an addictive disorder.[14]

Although about 90% of U.S. individuals get married before the age of 50, about 40% to 50% of married couples in the U.S. divorce.[15] In 2012, an estimated 686,000 U.S. children were victims of abuse: 78% neglected, 18% physically abused, 9% sexually abused, and 11% subjected to other types of abuse.[16]

---

10 Barrocas, Andrea L. et al. "Rates of Nonsuicidal Self-Injury in Youth: Age, Sex, and Behavioral Methods in a Community Sample." Pediatrics 130.1 (2012): 39–45. PMC. Web. 11 Nov. 2016.

11 NIH, National Institute of Mental Health, "Major Depression Among Adults." <https://www.nimh.nih.gov/health/statistics/prevalence/major-depression-among-adults.shtml>

12 CDC National Center for Health Statistics, "Increase in Suicide in the United States, 1999-2014." <http://www.cdc.gov/nchs/products/databriefs/db241.htm>

13 NIH, National Institute of Mental Health, ""Schizophrenia." <https://www.nimh.nih.gov/health/statistics/prevalence/schizophrenia.shtml>

14 Sussman, Steve, Nadra Lisha, and Mark Griffiths. "Prevalence of the Addictions: A Problem of the Majority or the Minority?" Evaluation & the health professions 34.1 (2011): 3–56. PMC. Web. 12 Nov. 2016. <https://www.ncbi.nlm.nih.gov/pmc/articles/PMC3134413/>

15 American Psychological Association, "Marriag & Divorce." <http://www.apa.org/topics/divorce/>

16 CDC, "Child Maltreatment: Facts at a Glance, 2014." <http://www.cdc.gov/violenceprevention/pdf/childmaltreatment-facts-at-a-glance.pdf>

More than one-third of U.S. adults is obese.[17] It is projected that by 2030, half of all adults (115 million adults) will be obese in the U.S..[18] Seventeen percent of U.S. children and adolescents are obese.[19] Between the 1970s and 2008, the prevalence of obesity in the U.S. doubled for children aged 2-5 years, quadrupled for children aged 6-11 years, tripled for children aged 12-19 years, and doubled for adults.[20]

U.S. children spend more than seven and a half hours daily in front of a TV, video-game, or computer screen, and only one in three children engages in physical activity every day.[21] More than 80% of adolescents do not meet guidelines for aerobic activity for youth, and more than 80% of adults do not do recommended amounts of aerobic and strength training.[22]

Humans have driven many lands to desertification by stripping lands of trees and vegetation, intensive farming, and overgrazing animals. World-wide, about 52% of agricultural land is moderately to severely degraded, affecting 1.5 billion people.[23] Every year, 12 million hectares of cropland is lost to drought and desertification.[24] Land degradation directly affects 74% of the world's impoverished

---

17 CDC, "Overweight & Obesity." **<https://www.cdc.gov/obesity/data/ adult.html>**

18 President's Council on Fitness, Sports & Nutrition, "Facts & Statistics." **<http://www.fitness.gov/resource-center/facts-and-statistics/>**

19 Ibid.

20 Ibid.

21 Ibid.

22 Ibid.

23 UN, "Desertification." **<http://www.un.org/en/events/desertificationday/ background.shtml>**

24 Ibid.

people.[25] Modern intensive mono-crop agriculture has rapidly degraded topsoil, and if current rates of soil loss continue, all of the world's top soil could be gone by 2076.[26]

Since 1900, the U.S.A. has depleted about 1,000 cubic kilometers (264 trillion gallons) of water from underground aquifers.[27] Agricultural fertilizer run-off has created dead zones devoid of animal life in many areas of the U.S. – especially along the East Coast, in the Great Lakes, and the Gulf of Mexico which has the second largest dead zone in the world.[28]

Globalization is introducing invasive plant, animal, and pathogen species into Africa and Asia, and these threaten biodiversity and the economies, livelihoods and health of people across the world, especially those in the poorest nations which have the least capacity to deal with them.[29] International "free trade" has introduced very destructive invasive species into U.S. forests[30] and these have

---

25 Ibid.

26 Arsenault C, "Only 60 Years of Farming Left If Soil Degradation Continues," Scientific American 2016. **<https://www.scientificamerican.com/article/only-60-years-of-farming-left-if-soil-degradation-continues/>**

27 Konkow LF, "Groundwater Depletion in the United States," USGS Scientific Investigations Report 2013-5079, 63p., **<http://pubs.usgs.gov/sir/2013/5079>** (Available only online.)

28 National Ocean Service, "What is a dead zone?" **<http://oceanservice.noaa.gov/facts/deadzone.html>**

29 Early, Regan et al. "Global Threats from Invasive Alien Species in the Twenty-First Century and National Response Capacities." Nature Communications 7 (2016): 12485. PMC. Web. 12 Nov. 2016. **<https://www.ncbi.nlm.nih.gov/pmc/articles/PMC4996970/>**

30 USDA, Forest Service, "Identifying & Preventing Invasive Species Threats." **<http://www.fs.fed.us/research/invasive-species/prevention/>**

"significantly impacted United States ecosystems and cost millions of dollars to prevent, detect and control."[31]

Two centuries of so-called "free trade" has also introduced at least 25 invasive fish species and 7 invasive plant species into the Great Lakes, damaging the economy and health of people who rely on those lake for food and water.[32] More than 30 foreign invasive insects – including the Africanized Honeybee, Asian Tiger Mosquito, Mediterranean Fruit Fly, and the Fire Ant – and 4 invasive vertebrates are harming U.S. ecosystems, agriculture and people.[33] Invasive species are also having a destructive effect on European ecosystems.[34]

The social and religious traditions that inspired people for millennia have lost their influence on humanity. In modernized nations, family, community and national traditions have come under attack and are on the verge of extinction.

These are just some of the more prominent signs that our modern way of life is way off balance. We are witnessing the physical, mental, and moral degeneration of humanity and the destruction of the natural resources on which we depend for our lives. It is clear that we have lost alignment with Nature.

Who can save us? Many people hope that "experts" will take care of the problems, but we must realize that following the "experts" got us into this mess. These problems are results of our own daily

---

31 USDA Forest Service, "Invasive Species." **<http://www.fs.fed.us/research/invasive-species/>**

32 EPA, "Invasive Species in the Great Lakes." **<https://www.epa.gov/greatlakes/invasive-species-great-lakes>**

33 USDA National Invasive Species Information Center > Animals. **<https://www.invasivespeciesinfo.gov/animals/main.shtml>**

34 USDA National Invasive Species Information Center > International > Europe. **<https://www.invasivespeciesinfo.gov/international/europe.shtml>**

thoughts, words and deeds. In THE GREAT LEARNING,[35] Confucius wrote:

> "The ancients who wished to illustrate illustrious virtue throughout the kingdom, first ordered well their own states. Wishing to order well their states, they first regulated their families. Wishing to regulate their families, they first cultivated their persons. Wishing to cultivate their persons, they first rectified their hearts. Wishing to rectify their hearts, they first sought to be sincere in their thoughts. Wishing to be sincere in their thoughts, they first extended to the utmost their knowledge. Such extension of knowledge lay in the investigation of things.
>
> "Things being investigated, knowledge became complete. Their knowledge being complete, their thoughts were sincere. Their thoughts being sincere, their hearts were then rectified. Their hearts being rectified, their persons were cultivated. Their persons being cultivated, their families were regulated. Their families being regulated, their states were rightly governed. Their states being rightly governed, the whole kingdom was made tranquil and happy.
>
> "From the Son of Heaven down to the mass of the people, all must consider the cultivation of the person the root of everything besides."

You are at the root of everything. Every day the average person consumes 3-5 pounds of food. Your diet determines your own physical and mental health more than any other single factor in your control, and it also primarily determines your impact on natural resources.

Through your thoughts, words and deeds, including your food choices, you control your mind and body and your impact on your

---

35 Confucius. The Great Learning. **<http://classics.mit.edu/Confucius/ learning.html>**

family, community, nation, and Nature. By changing your daily thoughts, words, deeds, and diet, you will improve yourself and develop to your full potential, and also create a more harmonious relationship with Nature.

Starting with regeneration of your blood and the cells of your body and brain, then proceeding to develop your full physical, mental, and moral potential, you will inspire changes in your family and community. By being "The One" you are waiting for, you can do everything in your power to reverse the degeneration of humanity and Nature.

You can create a healthier world by becoming a healthier human. You can become a healthier human, a True Human, by trusting your true nature.

1 THE TRUE HUMANS

> Barbarism is the natural state of mankind. Civilization is unnatural. It is a whim of circumstance. And barbarism must always ultimately triumph.
>
> ROBERT E. HOWARD

Most civilized people have no contact with or knowledge of non-civilized people. Nevertheless, from an early age, almost all people born into civilization grow up programmed to believe that the contemporary civilized life and diet is the best.

A civilized person learns to call outsiders 'primitives,' 'savages' and 'barbarians.' In addition, if anyone suggests that civilization is not all its cracked up to be, or that a 'primitive' and 'barbaric' way of life may have some advantages over civilized people, a cadre of 'doctors of philosophy' – highly indoctrinated people charged with doctoring our philosophy – will parrot the profoundly uninformed Hobbesian mantra that without civilization life could not be other than "solitary, poor, nasty, brutish and short." They relentlessly accuse the 'heretics' of being Luddites who childishly romanticize the 'noble savage.'

Consequently, few people have the inclination or opportunity to study and learn from the barbarians, and even fewer have the honesty and courage to report the truth.

Nevertheless some men have amazingly broken free from group-think, and honestly investigated and reported on the habits and condition of the barbarians in comparison to civilized people. These heretics have reported that the barbarians are better developed, more attractive, stronger, healthier, and happier than the domesticated man. The barbarians are to us what the wolf is to the domesticated dog.

As late as the 20th century, many barbarian tribes lived immune to the diseases and disabilities common in modern civilization. These people had perfect physical development: strong bones and muscles, big skulls housing big brains, broad handsome faces, and wide smiles with 32 straight teeth free of decay.[1]

I call these people True Humans. They lived in alignment with Natural Law and consequently enjoyed not only genuine health, but also legendary physical fitness. The typical tribal man had strength far beyond what most modern individuals realize, comparable to elite athletes in civilized nations. The following account gives us some idea of the degree of muscular strength had by a typical primal man:

> "In 1805, the Lewis and Clark expedition witnessed an Indian bison kill…A small herd was stampeded over a cliff into a deep, broad ravine. As the bison fell one on top of the other, dazed and injured, hunters killed those on top with spears; the others were crushed and suffocated underneath. The ravine was twelve feet wide and eight feet deep; most of the bulls weighed over a ton, yet a team of five Indian hunters pulled nearly all the bison out of the ravine onto level ground for butchering."[2]

Since a mature bison weighed about 2000 pounds, and a team of five natives could lift each animal out of the ravine, each hunter had the ability to lift and carry a load of *at least* 400 pounds on his own up out of a hole 8 feet deep and over a short distance. This story shows how Nature favored the survival and reproduction of people who

---

[1] Price W. Nutrition and Physical Degeneration. Price-Pottenger Nutrition Foundation, 1974.

[2] Eaton SB, Konner M, and Shostak M. The Paleolithic Prescription. HarperCollins,, 1989. 190.

could develop and maintain high levels of strength and corresponding muscular development.

In contrast, among any five randomly chosen civilized men, you will not likely find even one man who can deadlift 400 pounds, let alone five. The bones of our preagricultural ancestors have much larger points of tendon attachment than modern people, indicating that they had much larger, stronger muscles.

In 1988, physicians S. Boyd Eaton and Melvin Konner, and anthropologist Marjorie Shostak published "Stone Agers in the Fast Lane: Chronic Degenerative Diseases in Evolutionary Perspective" in the American Journal of Medicine.[3] In this report they presented evidence that the genetic makeup of humanity has changed little in the past 10,000 years since the end of the last Ice Age, but "during the same period, our culture has been transformed to the point that there is now a mismatch between our ancient, genetically controlled biology and certain important aspect of our daily lives." The evidence indicates that this mismatch or discordance promotes the chronic degenerative diseases that account for nearly 75% of deaths among civilized people.

In this landmark paper and their book *The Paleolithic Prescription*[4] based upon its data, they documented the superior health and physical development and fitness of uncivilized hunters or pastoralists who consumed a diet rich in animal protein and cholesterol from either wild game meat or cattle, but rather limited in carbohydrate. They reviewed evidence that these carnivorous tribes had more robust, muscular and stronger bodies than farmers and city-folk descended from them.

---

[3] Eaton SB, Konner M, Shostak M. Stone Agers in the Fast Lane: Chronic Degenerative Diseases in Evolutionary Perspective. Am J Med 1988 April; 84:739-747.

[4] Eaton SB, Konner M, Shostak M. The Paleolithic Prescription. HarperCollins, 1989.

Testing of members of the highly carnivorous hunters or pastoralists – including Finnish Lapps, Tanzanian Masai, Canadian Igloolik Eskimos, and Kalahari San – found that they all had superior or excellent anaerobic and aerobic fitness (measured by VO2 max) whereas typical civilized Canadian Caucasians did not even have good VO2 max. Moreover, unlike civilized people, the meat-eating barbarians did not suffer from obesity, diabetes, or coronary artery disease.

Modern people lack strength (not only physical, but also mental and spiritual fortitude) and consequently, also lack the corresponding muscular and bone development. Again, our ancestors were to us what a wild wolf is to a chihuahua.

These people also had excellent vision, hearing and other sensory abilities. At a distance of half a mile, they could see things invisible to eyes of civilized people. Some were able to see with the naked eye celestial bodies that no civilized person can see without a telescope.[5]

Among these people, allergies, asthma, glandular deficiencies, obesity, infertility, diabetes, heart disease, cancer, bone diseases, and neurological degenerative diseases were either non-existent or exceedingly rare.[6, 7, 8] Both acne and myopia are rare or non-existent among uncivilized tribes and probably caused by eating high-

---

[5] Price W. Nutrition and Physical Degeneration. Price-Pottenger Nutrition Foundation, 1974. 510.

[6] Trowell HC, Burkitt DP. Western Diseases, Their Emergence and Prevention. Harvard University Press, 1981.

[7] Lindeberg S. Food and Western Diseases: Health and Nutrition from an Evolutionary Perspective. Wiley-Blackwell, 2010.

8 Cordain L, Eaton SB, Brand-Miller J, et al., "The paradoxical nature of hunter-gatherer diets: meat-based, yet non-atherogenic," Eur J Clin Nutr 2002;56(1): 542-552. DOI:101.1038/sj/ejcn/1601353. **<http://www.nature.com/ejcn/journal/ v56/n1s/pdf/1601353a.pdf>**

carbohydrate (plant-based) diets.[9, 10] These people almost never had children with birth defects. They were lean and fit throughout life.

These barbarians with broad handsome faces and strong physiques were also remarkably free of emotional, mental, social, and moral disorders. Their happiness, honesty, unselfishness, and self-control were exemplary. In many tribes, one could leave a dwelling or possessions unattended and unlocked for days or months, knowing that no primitive person would touch them. None of the truly primitive groups needed prisons.

Simply, they had none of the physical, mental, or moral disabilities, disorders or diseases common to civilized people. Consequently, like wild animals, they never needed doctors, dentists, or orthodontists. The medical and dentistry professions arise only among people who have need for their services. The absence of doctors and dentists among these barbarians attests to their freedom from diseases of civilization. Who needs a dentist when all of your teeth are straight and strong and never decay? They were able to correct the minor imbalances they did experience using food, herbal medicines or shamanic rituals and practices that produced positive neurochemical changes and altered states of consciousness.

Moreover, unlike modern civilized people, primitive people (including native Europeans prior to agriculture and forced Christianization) had a fundamentally spiritual orientation. They were interested in accumulating honor and developing awareness and spirituality by serving their people, following Nature, preserving the Earth's beauty and bounty for future generations, and engaging in shamanic awareness practices.

----

9 Cordain L, Eaton SB, Brand Miller J, Lindeberg S, Jensen C. An evolutionary analysis of the aetiology and pathogenesis of juvenile-onset myopia. Acta Opthalmol Scand 2002;80:125-135.

10 Cordain L, Lindeberg S, Hurtado M, Hill K, Eaton SB, Brand-Miller J. Acne vulgaris: A disease of western civilization. Arch Dermatol 2002;138:1584-90.

Ancient Reports of Barbarian Food and Fitness

According to the *Yellow Emperor's Classic of Internal Medicine*, apparently composed in the 3rd millenium BCE, the personal physician of Huang Qi (the Yellow Emperor), Qi Bo, reported that ancient hunter-gatherers living in harmony with Nature had better health than the civilized Chinese:

> "In ancient times, people lived simply. They hunted, fished, and were with nature all day. When the weather cooled, they became active to fend off the cold. When the weather heated up in summer, they retreated to cool places. Internally, their emotions were calm and peaceful, and they were without excessive desires. Externally, they did not have the stress of today. They lived without greed and desire, close to nature. They maintained *jing shen nei suo*, or inner peace and concentration of mind and spirit. This prevented pathogens from invading. Therefore they did not need herbs to treat their internal state, nor did they need acupuncture to treat the exterior. When they did contract disease they simply guided properly the emotions and spirit and redirected the energy flow, using the method of *zhu yuo* to heal the condition.
>
> "People today are different. Internally they are enslaved by their emotions and worries. They work too hard in heavy labor. They do not follow the rhythmic changes of the four seasons and thus become susceptible to the invasion of the thieves or winds"[11].

In 55 B.C., Caesar reported that "the people of the interior [of England] do not, for the most part, cultivate grain, but live on milk and meat, and are clothed in skins."[12]

---

[11] Ni M. The Yellow Emperor's Classic of Medicine (Shambala, 1995), chapter 13.

[12] Hawkes J. The World of the Past. Random House, 1963.

In his report on Germany first published in about 110 A.D., the Roman historian Tacitus wrote that the Germans lived on wild fruit, fresh game, and curdled milk.[13] Given the cold climate and extensive forest cover of Germany of the time, wild fruit was relatively low carbohydrate and only seasonally available.

The fifth-century historian Herodotus recounts a conversation had between the Ethiopian king and the Persian king Cambyses:

> "Finally, [the Ethiopian king] came to the wine and, having learnt the process of its manufacture, drank some and found it delicious: then, for a last question, he asked what the Persian king ate and what was the greatest age that Persians could attain. Getting in reply an account of the nature and cultivation of wheat, and hearing that the Persian king ate bread, and that people in Persia did not commonly live beyond eighty, he said he was not surprised that anyone who ate dung should die so soon, adding that Persians would doubtless die younger still, if they did not keep themselves going with that drink – and here he pointed to the wine, the one thing in which he admitted the superiority of the Persians.
>
> "The Fish-Eaters, in their turn, asked the king how long the Ethiopians lived and what they ate, and were told that most of them lived to be a hundred and twenty, and some even more, and that they ate boiled meat and drank milk."[14]

Herodotus also reported that in the 5th century these meat- and milk-eating Ethiopians were "said to be the tallest and best-looking people in the world."

---

[13] Tacitus. Germania and Agricola (Ostara Publications, 2016), p. 9.

[14] Herodotus. Snakes with Wings & Gold-digging Ants (Penguin UK, 2007).

The Inuit Diet

We live in an interglacial period of an ice age which began about 2.6 million years ago. Since then, glaciation has cycled between advancing for glacial periods of 40,000 years and retreating for interglacial periods of about 10,000 years.

The cool temperatures of the ice ages have favored the growth of grasslands and herds of large animals that eat grass and convert it to animal protein and fat, but limited the growth of other plant life. Before 10,000 years ago, most areas inhabited by humans were grasslands, steppe grassland, steppe tundra, tundra, forest steppe, or even arctic conditions. During the last glacial maximum (LGM) about 30,000 to 15,000 years ago, northeast Africa was a tropical extreme desert, and Eurasia was predominantly polar and alpine desert, steppe-tundra, forest-steppe, and tundra.

Thus, Eurasian ancestors' habitats resembled the present-day arctic and subarctic biomes. These biomes simply did (do) not support growth of edible vegetation. Consequently, our ancestors lived by hunting for relatively fat-rich, very large game animals, primarily elephants.[15] Hence the contemporary hypercarnivorous indigenous populations of the Arctic may give us more insight into how our ancestors ate during the glacial periods that prevailed during most of the last 2.6 million years.

Vilhjalmur Stefansson, an explorer and Harvard-educated ethnologist, spent 11 years in the early 20th century in arctic exploration, during 9 years of which he lived almost exclusively on meat and fish, following the example of the Inuit, commonly known as Eskimos. He documented that Inuit eat almost no plant products and often live exclusively on meat and fish for 6 to 9 months each year. He also found that he and his fellow European explorers

---

15 Ben-Dor M, Gopher A, Hershkovitz I, Barkai R, "Man the Fat Hunter," PLOS One 2011;6(12): e28689. doi:10.1371/journal.pone.0028689. <http://journals.plos.org/plosone/article?id=10.1371/journal.pone.0028689>

maintained excellent health on a carnivorous diet, and that they could reverse scurvy – vitamin C deficiency – by eating fresh meat.

Coastal Inuit have subsisted for hundreds or thousands of years on a whole foods meat-based diet living in conditions perhaps similar to those of the Ice Ages in Europe. They eat some of the fattest marine animals available: whale, seal, walrus, and so on.

Observers have reported that an average adult Eskimo would consume 4 to 8 pounds of meat in a day, and the estimated average daily macronutrient intake was 280 g protein, 135 g fat, and 54 g carbohydrate (mostly from glycogen in the meat eaten).[16] This amounts to 2551 kcal, 43% protein, 48% fat, and 8% carbohydrate. Other investigators have reported protein intakes among Inuit ranging from 43% energy to 56% energy.[17]

These reports are likely erroneous. Protein intakes this high cause protein poisoning due to the gut's limited ability to absorb and the liver's limited ability to deaminate and detoxify amino acids.[18] Stefansson reported that the Inuit diet consisted of 3 parts lean and 1 part fat, which produces a protein intake closer to 25% of energy. He reported that a diet of lean meat without sufficient fat would cause nausea and diarrhea as a prelude to what explorers called "rabbit starvation."

Medical investigators found that Eskimos living on a traditional carnivorous diet had a very high immunity to diseases common among civilized people including atherosclerosis, diabetes mellitus, appendicitis, cancer, dental caries and tuberculosis. One medical

---

[16] Heinbecker P. Studies on the metabolism of Eskimos. J Bio Chem 1928 Dec 1;80:461-475. <http://www.jbc.org/content/80/2/461>

[17] Fediuk K. Vitamin C in the Inuit diet: past and present. Master's Thesis. School of Dietetics and Human Nutrition, McGill University, Montreal, Canada, July 2000.

[18] Bilsborough S and Mann N: A Review of Issues of Dietary Protein Intake in Humans. Int J Sport Nutr and Ex Metab 2006;16:129-152.

professional described Eskimos on their native whole foods meat-based diet as "peaceful, extremely happy and healthy."[19]

In the early 20th century, John Harvey Kellogg M.D., a Seventh-Day Adventist advocate of a vegetarian diet, was a leading medical authority, and he as well as many other physicians believed that humans, as primates, had an evolved dietary requirement for fruits and vegetables just like other apes. Consequently they questioned Stefansson's report.

In response to these doubters, in 1927 Stefansson and his fellow explorer Karsten Andersen agreed to serve as subjects of a study of the effects of a 100% meat and fat diet on human health over the course of one full year. They ate beef, lamb, veal, pork, and chicken, including muscle, liver, kidney, brain, bone marrow, bacon, and fat, all from conventional markets. They used table salt according to taste, which amounted to 1 to 5 grams daily including that used in cooking. They also took coffee, black tea, meat broths, and water in amounts ranging from 1 to 2 liters daily on average.

Stefansson and Andersen stayed in laboratory under close observation for several weeks, then resumed their ordinary activities while dietitians supervision their diets. The researchers tested the men's urine for ketones regularly and these tests confirmed that the men did not consume carbohydrates (plants) during the year under observation. Stefansson adhered to the strictly carnivorous diet for 375 days, and Andersen for 367 days.

During the first few days of this experiment, Stefansson ate only lean meat with no added fat, resulting in a diet supplying 45% of energy as protein and 53% as fat, similar to what some observers had reported as the normal diet of the Inuit, because the observing

---

19 Sinclair HM. The Diet of Canadian Indians and Eskimos. Proceedings of the Nutrition Society 1953 March;12(1):69-82. <https://www.cambridge.org/core/services/aop-cambridge-core/content/view/851C24CF59A1B9DBF29C0CC7E4811523/S0029665153000188a.pdf/diet_of_canadian_indians_and_eskimos.pdf>

physicians wanted to test his claim that a diet of lean meat alone would cause gastrointestinal disorder. As Stefansson predicted, on the second day eating this very high protein diet he developed nausea and diarrhea. On the third day he resumed eating added fat with the meat, reducing his protein proportion to about 25% and increasing his fat proportion to about 75%. On the fourth day he had no nausea or diarrhea.

The researchers reported:[20]

"There was no evidence, as judged by weight, that the meat diet was detrimental to nutrition."

"The meat diet did not cause any elevation in the blood pressure of these two men despite the popular view that meat is a definite factor in producing such a result."

"The two explorers who had live on similar diets before, exhibited no mental reserve while eating meat exclusively. When the proportions of foodstuffs were correct, they ate with relish and no disturbances occurred."

They tested the mens' response to muscular exertion (with a 2.5 mile run in 20 minutes) three times during the meat diet, and found no adverse effect. The men reported no increase in fatigue and "no unusual discomfort" during the hot summer months.

The men "were not troubled by constipation more than when eating mixed diets."

Despite no intake of fruits or vegetables, "No clinical evidence of vitamin deficiency was noted. The mild gingivitis which V.S. [Stefansson] had at the beginning cleared up entirely, after the meat diet was taken."

20 McClellan WS, DuBois EF. Clinical Calorimetry XLV. Prolonged meat diets with a study of kidney function and ketosis. J Bio Chem 1930 July 1;87:651-668. <http://www.jbc.org/content/87/3/651.full.pdf+html>

"The clinical tests carried out on two of our subjects (V.S. and K.A.) revealed no evidence of irritation to the kidneys nor of damage to the kidney function."

"No symptoms were noted, which could be attributed to the mild ketosis. There was no depression of mental faculties and no significant change in the carbon dioxide-combining power of the blood. We had no way of telling whether or not any changes had occurred in the walls of the blood vessels, but as far as clinical observations and special tests revealed, no injuries resulted from the prolonged mild ketosis."

Cholesterol levels varied from 200 to 800 mg/dL during the experiment. The variance belies the conventional assumption that cholesterol levels are more or less fixed according to one's diet. Since the liver produces more cholesterol daily than provided by a carnivorous diet, the majority of change in blood cholesterol levels must come from the liver. Presumably the liver produces cholesterol in response to peripheral tissue needs for cholesterol. The idea that cholesterol levels should be fixed at a specific (and low) level may be akin to the absurd idea that the heart rate should be fixed at a specific and low level, rather than responding to specific and variable needs of the organism.

Most likely, Stefansson's nausea and diarrhea were due to the initial very high protein intake (250-270 g per day) from lean meat without sufficient fat, causing acute protein poisoning. Although recent experiments have reported no adverse effects in people habituated to consuming 250-300 g of protein per day from supplements for extended periods of time,[21, 22, 23] we have a limited ability to absorb and metabolize protein from whole foods, such that intakes of protein above 200 g per day are likely to cause nausea, diarrhea, and excessive blood levels of amino acids and ammonia in most people.[24] (More on this in Chapter 8.)

In summary, McClellan and DuBois concluded: "In these trained subjects, the clinical observations and laboratory studies gave no evidence that any ill effects had occurred from the prolonged use of the exclusive meat diet."

In 1935 Stefansson wrote a two-part article for Harper's Monthly entitled "Eskimos Prove An All Meat Diet Provides Excellent Health." He also wrote *Not By Bread Alone* and *Cancer: Disease of Civilization*, in which he documented that cancer was rare or non-existent among 'primitive' people eating whole foods meat-based diets.

For some years after this experiment Stefansson did not adhere to the all-meat diet, and gradually became ten pounds overweight. In 1953 he suffered a mild cerebral thrombosis, and afterwards attempted, on his physician's advice, to lose the ten pounds while eating a mixed diet, using food restriction, will power and starvation. He did not

---

[21] Antonio J, Peacock CA, Ellerbroek A, Fromhoff B, Silver T. The effects of consuming a high protein diet (4.4 g/kg/d) on body composition in resistance-trained individuals. *Journal of the International Society of Sports Nutrition*. 2014;11:19. doi:10.1186/1550-2783-11-19.

[22] Antonio J, Ellerbroek A, Silver T, Vargas L, Peacock C. The effects of a high protein diet on indices of health and body composition – a crossover trial in resistance-trained men. *Journal of the International Society of Sports Nutrition*. 2016;13:3. doi:10.1186/s12970-016-0114-2.

[23] Antonio J, Ellerbroek A, Silver T, et al. A High Protein Diet Has No Harmful Effects: A One-Year Crossover Study in Resistance-Trained Males. *Journal of Nutrition and Metabolism*. 2016;2016:9104792. doi:10.1155/2016/9104792.

[24] Bilsborough S and Mann N: A Review of Issues of Dietary Protein Intake in Humans. Int J Sport Nutr and Ex Metab 2006;16:129-152.

succeed, so in 1955 he and his wife Emily returned to the stone age diet he learned from the Inuit.

His return to hypercarnivory produced what Emily called "startling improvements in health" after several weeks.

"He began to lose his overweight almost at once, and lost steadily, eating as much as he pleased and felling satisfied the while. He lost seventeen pounds, then his weight remained stationary, although the amount he ate was the same. From being slightly irritable and depressed, he became once more his old ebullient, optimistic self. By eating mutton he became a lamb.

"An unlooked-for and remarkable change was the disappearance of his arthritis, which had troubled him for years and which he though of as a natural result of aging. One of his knees was so stiff he walked up and down stairs a step at a time, and he always sat on the aisle in a theatre so he could extend his stiff leg comfortably.

"Several times a night he would be awakened by pain in his hips and shoulder when he lay too long on one side; they he had to turn over and lie on the other side. Without noticing the change at first, Stef was one day startled to find himself walking up and down stairs, using both legs equally. He stopped in the middle of our stairs; then walked down again and up again. He could not remember which knee had been stiff!"[25]

Nutrition and Physical Degeneration

In the early 20th century, the high number of Americans suffering from tooth decay (known as caries), crooked and crowded teeth, and deformities of the palate and face disturbed an American dentist, Dr. Weston Price. He noticed that many people with dental and facial

25 Stefansson E. Preface to: Mackarness R. Eat Fat and Grow Slim (Harvill Press, 1958).

deformities also suffered from other medical conditions, reduced or retarded intelligence, or moral delinquency.

He formed an aim to discover the cause for the prevalence and severity of dental, general, and social disease in North America.

Unable to find any Americans unaffected by dental disease, Dr. Price resolved to study native groups that explorers, anthropologists, and frontier physicians reported to live free of dental decay. He and his wife visited Swiss in isolated mountain villages, Gaelics in the Outer Hebrides, Eskimos, Indians of North and South America, Melanesians and Polynesians, many African tribes, Australian Aborigines, and New Zealand Maori. Dr. Price took thousands of photographs of people eating primitive diets, and of people of the same genetic stock who had switched to modern diets. He also recorded what they ate and analyzed many of their foods. In 1936, Dr. Price published his findings in a landmark book, *Nutrition and Physical Degeneration*.

Price examined many mouths looking for dental disorders and spoke with frontier physicians familiar with the natives' general health. He found numerous people isolated from modern influences that had handsome faces, straight, decay-free teeth, and robust physiques. They also had a high resistance to both infections and degenerative disease, and fine moral characters.

Price found the lowest rates of caries among the most carnivorous tribes. Some of these tribes had no tooth decay, and none had a rate greater than 1 percent.

The vast differences are remarkable:
- In tribes living entirely or largely by fishing, hunting, and gathering wild game, along with variable but generally very small amounts of vegetables, fruits, and nuts, less than one-half percent of teeth were attacked by decay. That means 1 tooth in 200, or about 1 person in 60, had tooth decay.
- Among pastoral people living more or less entirely on the milk and meat of domesticated animals – primarily cattle – with no

grains and little or no vegetables, fruits, or nuts, the rate of caries was again about one-half percent.

- Gaelics eating oats with fish had a dental decay rate 120 times that of the Maori fisher-hunter-gatherers who ate no grains. Modernized people had rates up to 58 times higher than the primitive Gaelics.
- The Loetschental Valley Swiss living on milk products, whole rye bread, vegetables, and fruits had a rate 460 times that of the Maori. Modernized people had rates 15 times that of the isolated Swiss.
- The dental decay rate of the largely vegetarian Kikuyu was 550 times that of the Maori, but even the Kikuyu had teeth immensely better than modernized people, who have decay rates up to 13 times higher than the Kikuyu. (See Table 1.1.)

Recent research has confirmed that ancient humans who lived by hunting had excellent dental health but when they adopted plant-based diets they suffered severe dental decay.

Pleistocene hunter-gatherers in North Africa who relied on starchy wild plants had dental caries rates similar to civilized people (about 50% of teeth suffering from decay).[26]

Mesolithic hunters living on a meat-based, grain-free diet had virtually no cavities nor gum disease-associated bacteria, but caries and periodontal disease increased dramatically when people adopted starchy agricultural diets and even more upon the adoption of diets rich in refined carbohydrates following the industrial revolution.[27]

---

[26] Humphrey LT, De Groote I, Morales J, et al. Earliest evidence for caries and exploitation of starchy plant foods in Pleistocene hunter-gatherers from Morocco. *Proceedings of the National Academy of Sciences of the United States of America.* 2014;111(3):954-959. doi:10.1073/pnas.1318176111.

[27] Adler CJ, Dobney K, Weyrich LS, et al.. Sequencing ancient calcified dental plaque shows changes in oral microbiota with dietary shifts of the Neolithic and Industrial revolutions. Nature Genetics 2013 April;45(4):450-55.

Table 1.1: Percent of teeth attacked by decay in different peoples studied by Dr. Weston Price, DDS.

	Primitive	Modernized
Fisher/hunter/gatherers		
Amazon Jungle Indians	0.00	40.0
Australian Aborigines	0.00	70.9
New Zealand Maori	0.01	55.3
Eskimos	0.09	13.0
Malays*	0.09	20.6
Northern Indians	0.16	21.5
Polynesians*	0.38	21.9
Melanesians*	0.38	29.0
Herdsmen		
Masai	0.4	n.a.
Neurs	0.5	n.a.
Grain farmers		
Gaelics (seafoods, oats, produce)	1.20	30.0
Swiss (milk products, rye, produce)	4.6	29.8
Kikuyu (chiefly vegetarians)	5.5	n.a.

*Although these groups cultivated some fruits and vegetables, their main livelihood was fishing-hunting.

Table adapted from Crawford M, Marsh D, *Nutrition and Evolution* (New Canaan, CT, Keats Pub. Inc., 1995), p. 209, and Price W, *Nutrition and Physical Degeneration* (New Canaan, CT, Keats Publishing, 1998).

People who eat a low-fat, high-carbohydrate diet have a high risk of periodontal disease, while people who eat a high fat diet have a low risk of the disease.[28]

Evidently Nature designed our teeth for an animal-based diet. We simply do not have the dental tolerance for plant foods had by other primates. Dental decay provides an early alarm warning from Nature that we have adopted a diet forbidden to us by Nature.

A diet that harms the teeth can not benefit the body. Without good dentition, in the absence of modern corrective dentistry one can't chew well, which in turn leads to malnutrition, degeneration and infertility. Corrective dentistry illustrates the ignorance of our 'intelligence' because it silences Nature's alarm, enabling people to continue to eat harmful foods and cause themselves further, deeper suffering. Extensive evidence has accumulated proving that high carbohydrate – that is, plant-based – diets harm the teeth *and* the body.[29]

Through his research, Price ascertained that fat-soluble vitamins present in animal fats play very important roles in dental, skeletal, and general health. He found that groups immune to dental decay, crooked teeth, and other oral disorders ate diets high in animal-source vitamins A, D and another substance he identified as 'activator X' which we now know as vitamin K2,[30] whereas groups having poor dental and skeletal health ate diets lacking these vitamins. Collectively these vitamins fortify innate immunity and

---

[28] Hamasaki T, Kitamura M, Kawashita Y, Ando Y, Saito T. Periodontal disease and percentage of calories from fat using national data. J Periodontal Res. 2017 Feb;52(1):114-121. doi: 10.1111/jre.12375. Epub 2016 Mar 29. PubMed PMID: 27028150.

[29] University of Washington. "Diets Bad For The Teeth Are Also Bad For The Body." ScienceDaily. ScienceDaily, 12 July 2009. <www.sciencedaily.com/releases/2009/07/090709170807.htm>.

[30] Masterjohn C. On the Trail of the Elusive X-Factor: A Sixty-Two-Year-Old Mystery Finally Solved. 2008 Feb 13.

regulate the utilization or minerals and development of bones and teeth.

2 DEFINING HEALTH

What is health? Many if not most civilized people have no idea nor experience of genuine health, because civilization itself has denied us access to it. Most of us have been more or less damaged or handicapped in some way by civilized ideologies, diets and lifestyles.

Moreover, these days people have been led to believe that health is best evaluated by blood tests. You can feel, look and function poorly, but if your blood tests show "normal" values, many doctors will pronounce you healthy. Conversely you can feel, look and perform like a champ, but if you have elevated total or LDL cholesterol, many doctors will pronounce you unhealthy and want you to stop eating red meat and animal fat, and start taking drugs.

In 1948, the World Health Organization of the United Nations (an attempt to centralize all political power in one agency) defined "health" as "a state of complete physical, mental, and social well-being and not merely the absence of disease or infirmity."

The word "health" is derived from the Old English word hælth. This in turn comes from Germanic roots including

- Old English hāl
- Dutch heel
- German heil
- English hail

These evolved into the modern English "whole." Thus, to heal is to make whole what has been divided, as when a cut heals.

"Heal" is also related to the word "holy." In fact, "holy" is simply the truncation of "whole-y" which is derived from

- Proto-Germanic hailagaz ("holy, bringing health")
- Proto-Germanic haliaz ("healthy, whole")
- Proto-Indo-European *kóh$_2$ilus ("healthy, whole")

Right and Wrong

To have a true concept of health, we also have to understand the meaning of the words "right" and "wrong." Modern people are very confused about right and wrong. Some people (vegans) claim that it is wrong to eat animal products. Thanks to indoctrination by "authorities" who profit from the people being ignorant of their own Conscience and the objective difference between right and wrong, some people believe that right and wrong are "relative," a position known as moral relativism. In Reality, for humans, moral right and wrong are as objective as true and false in mathematics, or health and disease in medicine.

Nature or Reality is present and possesses all known and likely many unknown powers. Nature has obviously produced all that exists, including Humans. We are parts of Nature; we are in Nature and Nature is in us (Human Nature). All of our own powers (including life, awareness and intelligence, etc.) are undeniably powers of (given by) Nature. Thus, I maintain that Nature is the omnipotent, ever Present Creator in which we live, move and have our presence (awareness) and existence (body).

You may have noticed that we use the word "right" as a synonym for both *true* and *moral*. The word is derived from the Latin *rectus* which means "straight, aligned, right." The word "true" has the same meanings. Most basically, "right" and "true" mean *aligned with Nature/Reality/The Creator*. Right action arises from *alignment with* Nature (Reality), which is good or moral because it promotes the life (survival, health, fitness, and reproduction) one has received from Nature. When one makes *right use* of gifts received from Nature (The Creator, Providence), one is *righteous*.

The word "wrong" comes from the Proto-Germanic *wrang* which means "crooked, wry, twisted." In other words, "wrong" means *not aligned with Nature/Reality/The Creator*. That's why it is a synonym for *false:* "2 + 2 = 3" is wrong because it is false. Wrong action arises from either ignorance of Nature/Reality/Natural Laws, or deliberate rebellion against Nature/Reality (refusal to accept and abide by Truth), which is bad or immoral because it undermines life (survival, health, fitness, and reproduction). I believe that is why our ancestors gave us the word *evil* – *live* spelled backwards – to signify something harmful, bad, and immoral.

Table 2.1: Right vs. Wrong

Right	Wrong
LATIN *rectus* "straight, aligned, right"	PROTO-GERMANIC *wrang* "crooked, wry, twisted"
ALIGNED WITH REALITY	*NOT* ALIGNED WITH REALITY
TRUE 2 + 2 = 4	FALSE 2 + 2 = 3
GOOD, MORAL	BAD, IMMORAL
LIVE	EVIL
PRO-HEALTH PRO-LIFE	ANTI-HEALTH ANTI-LIFE

Thus, for our ancestors, who had larger brains and therefore greater understanding than we do today, health meant physical, mental, and moral and spiritual alignment with the Order of Nature, also known as *Natural Law* in Europe, *Dharma* in India, and *Tao* in East Asia.

Simply: Behavior that aligns with Nature – including Human Nature – promotes physical, mental, social and ecological health, so it is right, good and moral. On the other hand, behavior that is not aligned with Nature or goes against Nature promotes disease and disorder, so it is wrong, bad and immoral. Conversely: If a behavior makes you healthy and strong, it is good and moral, and any behavior that produces physical, mental, social or moral weakness, disease or disorder is wrong, bad and immoral.

Just as Nature empowers the surfer or sailor who aligns with the Nature of the ocean or winds, Nature heals those who align with (obey) their own biological Nature. On the other hand, Nature delivers disease, disorder and destruction upon those who rebel against Natural Law, just as surely as Nature will destroy a surfer or sailor who does not align with the Natural Laws of the ocean or winds.

As I will show throughout this book, plant-based, vegetarian and vegan diets produce or increase the risk for weakness and physical, mental, social and ecological disease and disorder. Therefore such diets are wrong, bad and immoral.

Evolution of Health Awareness

Natural selection has given us the ability to evaluate our own health and that of others without the use of blood tests.

For millions of years our ancestors had to be able to evaluate their own health without having any idea of the levels of various chemicals in their blood. During these many generations, the ability to evaluate one's own health and that of others was critical to survival and reproductive success.

Individuals who had the ability to evaluate their own health and adjust their own behavior to acquire appropriate nutrition, maintain health or recover from illness would have had greater vitality and reproductive success than individuals who lacked this ability. Individuals who had the ability to identify a healthy mate by outer appearance alone (without knowing the chemical composition of the mate's blood) naturally had more and healthier offspring than those who lacked the ability to detect health and vitality.

Keep in mind that health means strength and illness means weakness. Individuals who could correctly identify vitality or vulnerability in animals or other humans were more successful as hunters and in picking allies or avoiding fatal fights. Less capable individuals would more likely chase the wrong prey, choose the wrong friends, and get into losing battles.

Thus, in the state of Nature, not many if any individuals incapable of correctly identifying the difference between health and illness would have survived and reproduced. Nature (natural selection) gave us the ability to identify health and disease, strength and weakness, with our common senses.

The entire modern cosmetics industry stands as witness to this. This industry is devoted to playing and preying on our innate ability to detect health and illness with our five senses. Cosmetics, deodorants, and perfumes are used to hide visible, smellable, and palpable signs of illness and project false signs of health. The whole purpose is to trick others into being attracted to someone who is not likely as healthy as advertised.

Therefore it is highly unlikely that one needs to know the chemical composition of the blood (via a blood test) in order to determine whether anyone is healthy or ill. You can use the common senses.

Those who want us to rely on blood tests to determine health and disease have vested interests in the process; they profit either from doing the tests, interpreting the tests, or "treating" the alleged chemical imbalances they urge you to find in your blood.

Hence, so long as you keep watch for cosmetics, you can be confident that your senses do not deceive you. No one who, in the absence of cosmetics, looks vibrantly healthy, fit and strong is actually unhealthy, fit and weak. Anyone who looks unhealthy, frail and weak is just that.

Health Standards

The human body is a Natural animal body. Therefore, our physical health, vigor and temper should be judged by the very same veterinary standards we would use for any other animal.

Physical Health

Appearance

Healthy hair grows well and is lustrous without any splitting or a need for 'products' to make it attractive.

Healthy skin is moist and lustrous without any rashes or lesions. The individual does not need lotions etc. to make her/his skin moist and attractive. The nails are strong, without ridging, splitting or cracking.

The muscles are well developed. The body fat is at a natural level for sex and race (neither too little nor too much). The waist circumference is not larger than one-half the standing height (greater indicates insulin resistance).

The eyes and complexion are clear and radiant.

Vigor

A healthy individual wants to live and enjoys living. Loss of the desire to live or joy in living indicates deep physical and mental illness.

He or she is alert to and aware of his or her surroundings, energetic, strong, agile and has quick reflexes. Absence of any of these characteristics indicates poor energy metabolism, especially in the neuromuscular system. This represents reliance on low energy carbohydrate for fuel, rather than high energy fats; as well as deficiencies of vitamins, minerals, and essential amino and fatty acids.

To thrive in life requires health and strength, so a healthy individual also strives for health and strength. He or she is highly selective and discriminating about what he or she will eat and like any wild animal (cats in particular) rejects anything that is unnatural and unpalatable.

Just as a healthy cat or dog enjoys playing games, wrestling, running and jumping, a healthy human enjoys engaging in physical activity, mild, moderate, and vigorous that tests or improves physical prowess. A healthy individual spontaneously engages in such activity as an expression of vigor and joy in living.

Although physical activity does improve health, fundamentally, good health causes a person to engage in physical activity. If you have no desire for physical activity, you need proper nutrition to restore your vigor. When it returns, you will by Nature get moving.

Senses

Nature gives us the senses to enable us to navigate in our habitat to obtain food to support vitality, health, strength and reproduction. Nature guides us to choose food that satisfies our aesthetic sense as well as our taste and hunger.

In healthy individuals, all five senses function fully without any artificial aids. If you have trouble with vision, hearing, smelling, tasting or feeling, your body is damaged. In the absence of direct trauma to the sense organs, malfunction or degeneration of the senses is due to malnutrition, either chronic lack of nutrients essential to structure and function of the sense organs, or damage due to consumption of toxins.

Depending on the degree of damage done by living an agricultural diet, you may never recover your potential. However, adopting a hypercarnivore diet may prevent further degeneration and if you still have the opportunity to have children, you can give them a chance at avoiding your own disability.

Mouth

A healthy person has 32 fully developed teeth (including wisdom teeth), all well aligned without any crowding, and without tooth decay or fillings. If you have had teeth extracted to prevent crowding, or you had orthodontic treatment, your head and jaw did not develop properly because you were fed improperly during your formative years.

If you have any tooth decay, you have consumed food incompatible with Human Nature. It either lacked vitamins and minerals necessary for dental health, or included carbohydrates – fiber, starch and sugar – which interfere with vitamin and mineral metabolism, and feed the growth of acid-producing bacteria that damage the teeth.

Healthy gums properly cover the roots of the teeth and are free of irritation or inflammation. The breath has no unpleasant odor. Receding gums and bad breath are caused by eating foods that feed acid-producing bacteria that inflame the gum tissues: various carbohydrates.

A healthy individual keeps his/her lips closed and mouth sealed except when eating or talking. The tongue rests on the roof of the mouth, lightly pressing against the upper palate and supporting the middle of the face.

If you have improper tongue posture, learn and start practicing proper tongue posture immediately. Keep your lips sealed, your teeth lightly held together, and your tongue pressed lightly against the roof of your mouth. Holding your tongue in the proper position can gradually, over a long period of time, improve the alignment of your teeth and development and attractiveness of your face and jaw.

Breathing

In a healthy human, breathing occurs as Nature intended, through the nose, not the mouth, especially when at rest or sleeping. Inability to breath through the nose results from incomplete development of the face or inflammation of the nasal passageways and sinuses. Poor facial development is a result of eating a soft, nutrient-deficient plant-based diet, and improper tongue posture (usually initiated by bottle feeding, pacifiers and thumb sucking during the first few years of life).

Appetite for Food

Since you need food to regenerate and reproduce yourself on a daily basis, the appetite for food represents a basic desire to continue living indefinitely into the future. Loss of appetite for or enjoyment of your food is an early indicator of malnutrition or impending sickness.

A healthy animal has a strong appetite for its natural food as a means and requirement to continue its individual life. Wild animals generally consume a very limited diet and never tire of their natural foods. You'll never see a natural carnivore tire of eating meat, nor a natural grazer tire of eating grass. Nor do these animals crave foods not part of their natural diets. If you eat what you are by Nature designed to eat, you will always have an appetite for that food and never have cravings for foods that you know do not promote health and strength.

Gut

Nature gives us pain to guide us away from harm. Through gut pain Nature gives you a signal that you have eaten something that is harmful. A healthy person has no stomach trouble after meals, no, acid indigestion, no abdominal bloating or cramping, and no trouble passing stools when the urge arises, nor any discomfort after passing the stools. If you have any chronic or recurrent gut discomfort, you are eating foods incompatible with your digestive tract.

Contrary to popular belief, there is no optimum frequency of bowel evacuation. Frequency of stools reflects the content of the diet.

The bowels naturally function to expel any material that is harmful to the gut. The more harmful the material in the gut, the more frequently the bowels move. In extreme, diarrhea develops as the gut works to eliminate the harmful material. Therefore, the more harmful material you eat, the more frequent and urgent your bowel movements. Contrariwise, the more digestible and nutritious your diet, the less frequently you will have bowel movements.

Constipation consists of difficulty passing stools, regardless of frequency of bowel elimination. A healthy, properly nourished individual easily passes stools.

Immunity

Every healthy mammal has an immune system that patrols the borders and ports of entry (gut, skin, etc.), rejects unwanted invaders (whether large or small), and quarantines expels or destroys foreign pathogens that do gain passage. If your immune system is unable to properly patrol and maintain your boundaries you will frequently suffer infections or have great difficulty recovering from them. Poor nutrition and lifestyle choices that deplete vitality impair the immune system. A healthy individual has good border control that maintains healthy boundaries, and takes care to keep expenditure and recovery in balance, so infrequently suffers infectious disease and quickly recovers when s/he does.

Sexual Appetite

A strong sex drive represents strong vitality. Loss of sexual appetite during prime reproductive years indicates a loss of vitality and poor health.

Personal conscious choices aside, evolutionarily speaking, in Nature the sex drive is a reproductive drive, representing a desire to extend oneself into the future through progeny. Loss of sexual appetite during reproductive years therefore represents a loss of a desire to extend your lineage into the future.

Of interest, never married men and women have substantially more disease, particularly heart disease, unhappiness, and shorter life expectancy than ever married men and women.[1, 2]

Raising biological children within a stable marriage tends to increase one's life expectancy.[3, 4, 5] Having one's children at an early age (before age of 25) increases the potential lifespan of those children.[6, 7] Evidently, Nature rewards those who create *healthy* new life with more life.

----

[1] BBC News. Marriage makes people live longer. Thursday, 10 August 2006. Accessed 16 October 2015 at <http://news.bbc.co.uk/2/hi/health/4779267.stm>

[2] Lynch JJ. The Broken Heart: The Medical Consequences of Loneliness. Basic Books, 1979.

[3] McArdle PF, Pollin TI, O'Connell JR, et al. Does having children extend life span? A genealogical study of parity and longevity in the Amish. J Gerontol A Biol Sci Med Sci. 2006 Feb;61(2):190-5. PubMed PMID: 16510865. <http://www.ncbi.nlm.nih.gov/pubmed/16510865>

[4] Sun F, Sebastiani P, Schupf N, et al. Extended maternal age at birth of last child and women's longevity in the Long Life Family Study. Menopause. 2015 Jan; 22(1):26-31. <http://www.ncbi.nlm.nih.gov/pubmed/24977462>

[5] Gavrilov LA, Gavrilova NS. Biodemography of Exceptional Longevity: Early-life and Mid-life predictors of Human Longevity. *Biodemography and Social Biology*. 2012;58(1):14-39. doi:10.1080/19485565.2012.666121.<http://www.ncbi.nlm.nih.gov/pmc/articles/PMC3354762/>

[6] Ibid., op. cit.

[7] Kemkes-Grottenthaler A, "Parental effects on offspring longevity--evidence from17th to 19th century reproductive histories," *Ann Hum Biol* 2004 Mar-Apr; 31(2):139-58. PubMed PMID: 15204358. <http://www.ncbi.nlm.nih.gov/pubmed/15204358/>

A healthy parent sees him or herself in his or her biological child. Therefore he or she protects, loves and nurtures biological children as much as self. Caregivers who are genetically unrelated to children have no biological incentive to invest resources in those children. Evolutionary theory predicts that adults who are genetically unrelated to a child lack a biological incentive to care for that child, because the unrelated child does not carry their genes into the future. Non-relatives actually have a perverse incentive to harm the children of other parents to free resources for themselves or their biological offspring. As this perspective predicts, statistically speaking, children raised by two biological parents maintaining a stable marriage run the lowest risk of physical, mental, or moral disorder, neglect, abuse or violence; are by far most likely to perform well in sports, social and academic development; and are healthier, happier, smarter, more capable, and more self-confident, as compared to any other caregiver arrangement.[8,9,10]

Monogamy evidently has a profoundly positive influence on child care and social order. It suppresses destructive intrasexual (male vs. male, and female vs. female) competition and reduces the size of the pool of unmarried men, which reduces crime rates, including rape, murder, assault, robbery and fraud, as well as decreasing personal abuses. "Normative monogamy also decreases the spousal age gap, fertility, and gender inequality. By shifting male efforts from seeking wives to paternal investment, normative monogamy increases savings, child investment and economic productivity. By increasing the relatedness within households, normative monogamy

---

[8] US Dept of Health and Human Services. Fourth National Incidence Study of Child Abuse and Neglect (NIS-4). Report to Congress. Section 5.3.1. <http://www.acf.hhs.gov/sites/default/files/opre/nis4_report_congress_full_pdf_jan2010.pdf>

[9] Sprigg P, Daily T. Getting It Straight. Family Research Council, 2004. <http://downloads.frc.org/EF/EF08L45.pdf>

[10] Sullins DP, "Emotional Problems among Children with Same-Sex Parents: Difference by Definition," *British Journal of Education, Society and Behavioural Science* 2015;7(2):99-120.

reduces intra-household conflict, leading to lower rates of child neglect, abuse, accidental death and homicide."[11]

Mental Health

Self-Respect

All healthy wild and domesticated animals groom and take care of themselves as needed. One of the first signs of physical or mental illness in any animal is an absence of self-cleaning and grooming, which is why our ancestors said that cleanliness is next to "godliness" i.e. holiness i.e. health.

No healthy wild or domesticated animal deliberately injures or disfigures itself. Only individuals suffering from some degree of unnatural stress, malnutrition or brain degeneration will engage in self-injury or self-mutilation. Animals confined to cages or overcrowded conditions and not able to eat a natural diet will develop self-destructive habits.

Focused Attention and Mental Quietude

Every healthy wild animal is able to spend long periods of time awake, alert and yet very quiet, simply engaged in Witnessing Creation. Every one can sit still and just watch Nature without boredom or needing special 'entertainment.'

This applies equally to us. A healthy human can sit still for long periods of time, awake, alert and Witnessing Creation without feeling bored.

---

[11] Henrich J, Boyd R, Richerson PJ, "The puzzle of monogamous marriage," *Philosophical Transactions of the Royal Society B, Biological Sciences* 2012 March 5;367(1589):DOI: 10.1098/rstb.2011.0290 <http://rstb.royalsocietypublishing.org/content/367/1589/657>

Joy and Equanimity

A mentally healthy person frequently enjoys life, and usually abides in equanimity. Depression, anxiety, neuroses and psychoses have a biological basis in malnutrition. If the brain is not properly nourished, or is exposed to toxins, it will malfunction, resulting in mental illness.

Curiosity and Creativity

The mind and hands are the two main tools gifted to us by Nature. In comparison to a human with functional hands and a healthy brain all other species are practically speaking disabled.

A healthy human enjoys these gifts. S/he has an insatiable curiosity and drive to learn, and also a love of creating various attractive and useful works of art or craft according to individual gift and inclination, including:

- Visual arts such as drawing and painting
- Crafts such as woodworking, leather working, pottery, sewing, knitting, etc.
- Musical arts including song and creating and playing musical instruments
- Literary arts such as prose and poetry

To name a few.

3 THE OMNIVORE MYTH

It bears repeating that no wild animal exhibits any confusion about what to eat. None needs doctors, dietitians, nutritionists, diet books or blood tests to help them decide what to eat. All of them simply follow Nature.

As long as they follow Nature, they live free of diet-related diseases. Only animals under the care of so-called "wise wise man"[1] suffer diet-related diseases.

Only humans are confused about what to eat, and, apparently, about what to feed the animals we have domesticated.

Zoologists classify animals according to their dietary habits, using the following categories:

- Herbivores, which make leaves of plants their primary or exclusive foods.
- Frugivores, which make fruits of plants their primary or exclusive foods.
- Insectivores, which make insects and worms their primary foods.
- Carnivores, which eat flesh of other animals, primarily herbivores.
- Omnivores, which consume both plants and animals.

To which of these categories do we belong?

Most people (including 'experts') classify humans as omnivores, because as a matter of fact, we find humans eating both plants and animals. However, the fact that humans as a matter of fact can and do eat both plants and animals does not prove that humans are biologically designed (or adapted) to eat both plants and animals in any proportion whatsoever. People as a matter of fact smoke tobacco, but this does not prove that people are biologically designed for or adapted to smoking tobacco.

---

[1] The literal meaning of the zoological name we have given ourselves: *Homo sapiens sapiens*.

It seems that most people also believe that we are designed for or adapted to primarily plant-based diets. Many laypeople and experts believe that although we can and do eat and perhaps even require animal products (to obtain certain nutrients not provided by plants), we by Nature need a so-called "balanced" diet composed primarily of a variety of plants.

In other words, most people believe that we are an *obligate omnivore*: an animal that *must* eat both plants and animals. People often support their belief that humans are by Nature plant-based obligate omnivores by noting that zoologists classify us as primates, and, besides sharing traits like binocular vision and opposable thumbs, all known non-human primates (with the possible exception of one species of monkey) eat both plants and animals.

The syllogism goes like this:

1. All non-human primates eat both plants and animals.
2. We are primates, and we as a matter of fact eat both plants and animals.
3. Therefore, we must *need* to eat both plants and animals.

Like some other popular advocates of so-called paleo diets, I believed that this syllogism is sound when I wrote the first seven chapters of *The Garden of Eating: A Produce-Dominated Diet and Cookbook*. In that book I argued that because we are primates we *must* eat *both* plants – specifically, fruits and vegetables – *and* meat in order to be healthy. 'Expert authorities' had convinced me that we need to eat plants to, at the very minimum, get vitamin C, adequate glucose, and alkaline bicarbonate compounds to 'balance' the acids provided by metabolism of meat.

I followed that produce-dominated pseudo-paleolithic diet for more than 10 years, hoping that by eating large amounts of the best of plants (fruits and vegetables) and meats, I would find relief from psoriasis. When that didn't happen, I reasoned that perhaps I was eating something incompatible with my biology.

Zoologists and paleoanthropologists allege that humans and chimps have a common ancestor that existed in the neighborhood of 6 million years ago. Consequently, they allege that we are genetically more closely related to chimpanzees than to any other primate. The genetic relationship is supposedly so close that some biologists claim that chimps should be classified as members of the human (*Homo*) genus, not a separate genus (*Pan*). According to these experts "We humans appear as only slightly remodeled chimpanzee-like apes," and we should classify chimps not as *Pan troglodytes*, but as *Homo troglodytes*.[2]

If one gets entranced by the spells (words) cast by these "authorities" (as I once did) and accepts the idea that humans are really "only *slightly*" different from chimps, then one is likely to conclude humans must be designed to eat very much like chimps. The chimps do eat some meat, but the amount is so small that a respected guide to caring for chimpanzees emphasizes their frugivory, and practically identifies their usual diet as 100 percent composed of plants only occasionally containing quite small amounts of animal products:

> "The chimpanzee diet consists mainly of fruit (48%), but they also eat leaves and leaf buds (25%), and around 27% of their diet consists of a mixture of seeds, blossoms, stems, pith, bark and resin. Chimpanzees are highly specialized frugivores and preferentially eat fruit, even when it is not abundant. They supplement their mainly vegetarian diet with insects, birds, birds' eggs, honey, soil, and small to medium-sized mammals (including other primates)."[3]

---

[2] Pickrell J. Chimps Belong on Human Branch of Family Tree, Study Says. National Geographic News 2003 May 20. Accessed online on Dec 6, 2017 at: <https://news.nationalgeographic.com/news/2003/05/0520_030520_chimpanzees.html>

[3] The Chimpanzee Species Survival Plan. Caring For Chimpanzees. http://www.lpzoosites.org/chimp-ssp/chimpanzees.htm

According to *The Pictorial Guide To The Living Primates*, wild chimps get 95 to 100 percent of their food from plants, primarily fruits; animal prey, including grubs, wasps, termites, ants, ten bird species, and mammals, composes zero to five percent of the diet.[4]

Moreover, field studies of chimpanzees indicate that well-fed adult males, who have the least nutritional need, are the primary consumers of animal flesh, and the low-ranking females and young, who have the greatest need for additional energy and macronutrients, eat "little or no flesh."[5]

That suggests that chimpanzees may have little or no nutritional requirement for animal flesh, protein, or fat, since not all chimps actually eat meat, and even among those who do eat some meat, their diet doesn't always contain it.

This illustrates very well the problem with classifying a species as an omnivore based only on the fact that some members as a matter of fact do eat both plant and animal matter. The fact that some chimps as a matter of fact do eat meat doesn't prove that all chimps *need* to eat meat or even that their meat-eating provides them any nutritional benefit.

Anyway, the idea that we are only slightly remodeled chimpanzee-like apes has led some biologists to assert that human ancestors "tended to mostly eat vegetable matter."[6]

When eating a grain- and legume-free, meat-based but fruit- and vegetable- rich pseudo-paleo (or *paleoid*) diet didn't provide me

---

[4] Rowe N. The Pictorial Guide to the Living Primates. Pogonias Press, 1996. 230.

[5] Gilby IC, Wrangham RW. **Risk-prone hunting by chimpanzees (Pan troglodytes schweinfurthii) increases during periods of high diet quality**. Behav Ecol Sociobiol (2007) 61:1771–1779.

[6] Dunn R. Human Ancestors Were Nearly All Vegetarians. Scientific American 2012 July 23. Accessed Dec 10, 2017 at: <**https://blogs.scientificamerican.com/ guest-blog/human-ancestors-were-nearly-all-vegetarians/**>

with relief from my psoriasis, or prevent my wife from gaining unwanted fat and developing fibrocystic breasts, I reasoned along these lines:

1. Many authorities assert that meat-eating probably causes or promotes various maladies – such as heart disease and cancer – in humans.
2. Chimps don't appear to have a nutritional *need* for meat.
3. We are only slightly remodeled chimpanzee-like apes.
4. We must eat plants to get adequate vitamin C, glucose, alkaline substances and who knows what else.
5. Therefore, we definitely *need* to eat plants but we may not *need* to eat meat, and meat-eating might be the cause of psoriasis.

Advocates of plant-based diets follow this line of reasoning. It led me to (once again) cut animal products out of my diet and experiment with various permutations of plant-based eating, in search of a cure for my psoriasis.

It also led me to write *Powered By Plants: Natural Selection and Human Nutrition*, in which I argued that although we are as a matter of fact omnivorous, we are not *obligate* omnivores. I believed and, I attempted to support with argument and evidence the proposition that we are by Nature (like chimps) obligate plant-eaters, unspecialized frugivores that have the ability to eat meat, but neither any specific heritable natural adaptation to nor any dietary requirement for meat. My argument was similar to but more extensive than that made in 2002 by Hladik and Pasquet in the journal *Human Evolution*, where they wrote:

> "In this paper, we discuss the hypothesis, proposed by some authors, that man is a habitual meat-eater. Gut measurements of primate species do not support the contention that human digestive tract is specialized for meat-eating, especially when taking into account allometric factors and their variations between folivore, frugivores and meat-eaters. The dietary status of the human species is that

of an unspecialized frugivore, having a flexible diet that includes seeds and meat (omnivorous diet)."[7]

So, for a little more than 5 years I adhered to a whole foods plant based diet, often emphasizing, like chimps and other primates, a high intake of fruits and greens, but also including tubers and/or seeds (including grain and legume seeds), as well as lots of leaves (folivory). I believed and hoped that by eating in alignment with my supposedly frugivorous, chimpanzee-like ape physiology, I would finally obtain relief from the psoriasis that had plagued me for more than 35 years.

Unfortunately, as time went on, the psoriasis did not improve. On the contrary, as time progressed, new lesions appeared and old lesions became more severe or re-emerged. In addition, I had daily bloating, flatulence, and loose stools, during all of those 5 years, and toward the end, I developed recurrent post meal acid reflux.

After five vegan years, a routine blood test showed that I had fasting glucose on the high side of the normal range, somewhat elevated triglycerides (compared to when I ate a meat-based higher fat diet), and my phosphorus and globulin level dropped below normal, indicating probable dietary phosphorus and protein deficiency, in spite of the fact that nutrient analysis of my diet consistently showed high intake of phosphorus and protein.

This experience led me to an embarrassing cognitive impasse. I had believed that we are obligate plant-eaters, regardless of whether we ate meat or not. I had gone all in and published *Powered by Plants*, in which I had argued that we had no evolved dietary requirement for meat. Now my experience had me eating my words.

---

[7] Hladik CM, Pasquet P. The human adaptations to meat eating: a reappraisal. Human Evolution, Springer Verlag 2002;17:199-206. Accessed online on Dec 6, 2017 from: <**https://hal-univ-diderot.archives-ouvertes.fr/hal-00545795/ document**>

At this point, I realized that if it was indeed necessary for me to eat some sort of plant-based diet in order to reduce my cardiovascular disease and cancer risk, then I would also have to accept that I would have to agree to continue to suffer with psoriasis and digestive discomfort, with no hope of relief.

At this impasse, to remedy the deficiencies that arose eating high phytate plant based diet, I initially added some meat back into my diet and cut out the plant foods highest in phytates, whole grains and legumes. I rationalized this approach as similar to the diet of some chimpanzees: predominantly plants, with a small amount of animal products to prevent nutrient deficiencies. I continued for several months eating this omnivorous, produce-dominated, more- or less-"paleo" (i.e. dairy-, grain- and legume-free) diet.

At this point I had no clear idea what I anything I could do for my psoriasis. I knew from previous experience that eating an omnivorous plant-based diet would not heal my skin, but I still believed that I had to eat lots of fruits and vegetables to gain or maintain health.

Then, one day, I came across a website called *ZeroCarbZen*, which had a posted testimonial by a woman named Candi Leftwich who had obtained almost complete relief from Crohn's disease and psoriasis by eating only meat, fat and water for 3 months.[8] As I recounted in the Introduction, I had years before (during my first paleo diet phase) come across another website promoting an animal-only diet, *ZeroingInOnHealth*, but I had been unable to accept the idea that a diet containing little or no plants could benefit health. This time, as a result of my own experiences and studies, my mind was more open to testing the idea that over-eating fruits and vegetables might be causing or contributing to my condition.

What if my disease was caused by eating too many plants and not enough animal products? I had briefly tried a very low carbohydrate

---

[8] Leftwich C. My First 30 Days on Zero Carb. <**https://zerocarbzen.com/ 2015/04/02/my-first-30-days-on-zero-carb-by-candi-leftwich/**>

animal-based diet in the past, but I included a substantial amount of nuts, and I had experienced muscle cramps and sluggish elimination. During that trial I had limited my intake of egg yolks, animal fats, and salt, and took no mineral supplements.

I would have to try severely limiting or eliminating even nuts, fruits and vegetables to find out if they were causing my condition, and I would also have to figure out how to break my dependence on fiber-rich plants to have regular healthy bowel movements. I would have to set aside all my beliefs in the potential toxicity of animal protein and fat, and eat these in whatever proportion most appealed to me, without limiting protein, fat or cholesterol intake.

So that's what I did.

I cut my plant food intake dramatically. Within days I went from more than 300 grams of carbohydrate daily to 50-75 g on most days.

I knew from experience that eating high fat meals could induce bowel movements by stimulating bile flow. I also knew that magnesium improves bile flow and intestinal motility, and draws water into the bowel to keep the stool soft.

To break my apparent dependence on plant fibers for defecation, I increased my animal fat intake to at least 65% of calories, and also started taking 300 mg of magnesium once or twice daily. After just one week of keeping my plant food intake low enough to limit carbohydrate intake to 50-75 g per day on most days, my gut was far more comfortable, and my skin was in better condition than in years. After two weeks it was even better.

As I followed this path, I found that I preferred less and less plant foods, but seemed to have no difficulty with some carbohydrate from dairy products. I was limiting plant foods even more, on many days consuming only animal products, or having plant foods only as garnishes. During those months my gut comfort and elimination improved bit by bit. After 6 months I still had some psoriasis lesions but they had improved dramatically, I no longer had more or less continuous gas, bloating and flatulence, and my bowel elimination was far less frequent but far more comfortable than I could ever remember it being on any plant-based diet.

My experience and study led me to question whether we really are obligate omnivores who, like other primates, *need* to eat plants.

Two Kinds of "Omnivores"

Since the equipment required for successful acquisition, digestion, and metabolism of plants and their major components differs so markedly from the equipment required to capture, digest, and metabolize animals, it should not surprise anyone if we found that very few if any species have native physical equipment equally well-suited to processing plant foods and animals.

Based on behavior, people have classified pigs, chimps, wolves, dogs, and bears as omnivores, yet the wild feeding behavior, anatomy, and physiology of the former two differs markedly, and in a similar fashion, from the latter two. Classifying bears, dogs, and pigs all as omnivores obscures very important physical and behavioral differences between them.

Although they will eat some animal flesh, wild pigs primarily consume roots, fruits, leaves, grasses, and flowers, and they have specialized dentition and guts clearly adapted to a plant-based diet, including a hindgut specialized for fermentation of plant fibers. Wild pigs innately forage for plant foods, and only consume animal flesh opportunistically. Commercially raised pigs develop and grow very well on diets composed entirely of plants, indicating that pigs require little or no animal food.

In contrast to pigs, bears and wolves clearly have physiological and innate behavioral adaptations to a meat-based diet (claws, teeth, guts, predatory behavior), neither one having any gut features specialized for processing plant foods. That's largely why they are classified as members of the order *Carnivora*.

Table 3.1: Some behavioral omnivores, their gut features and primary foods

Species	Order	Gut features	Diet
Badgers	Carnivora	Shearing teeth, short simple gut	Mainly animals, some roots and fruits
Bears	Carnivora	Sharp pointed incisors and large shearing canines, short simple gut	Animal-based when possible; mainly botanical fruits[1] (acorns, nuts, berries, drupes) when plant-based
Coatis	Carnivora	Shearing teeth, short simple gut	Mainly animals, some fruits
Canines (wolves, dogs)	Carnivora	Shearing teeth, short simple gut	Mainly (~80%) animals, some fruits
Raccoons	Carnivora	Shearing teeth, short simple gut	Mainly animals, some fruits and nuts
Skunk	Carnivora	Shearing teeth, short simple gut	Mainly animals, some fruits, nuts, fungi, leaves
Opossums	Didelphimorph (marsupial)	Shearing teeth, short simple gut	Mainly animals, supplemented by fruits
Hedgehogs	Erinaceomorpha (previously Insectivora)	Shearing teeth, short simple gut	Mainly animals, some fruits, roots, fungi
Sloth	Pilosa (Folivora)	Grinding teeth, long complex gut	Mainly buds, shoots, and leaves
Chimpanzee	Primates	Grinding teeth, long complex gut	Mainly fruits[1] and leaves
Spider monkey	Primates	Grinding teeth, long complex gut	Mainly (up to 90%) fruits[1]
Chipmunks	Rodentia	Grinding teeth, long complex gut	Mainly fruits, seeds and grains
Mice	Rodentia	Grinding teeth, long complex gut	Mainly seeds, grains, fruits[1]
Rats	Rodentia	Grinding teeth, long complex gut	Mainly seeds and grains
Pigs	Artiodactyla	Grinding teeth, long complex gut	Mainly fruits, roots, and leaves
Squirrels	Rodentia	Grinding teeth, long complex gut	Mainly nuts and seeds

1. Botanical fruits include fleshy fruits, berries, and nuts, all characterized by a relatively low fiber content coupled with high contents of enzymatically digestible sugars, starches, proteins, or fats.

Some authors have questioned the historically-firm classification of dogs and wolves as carnivores based on the fact that canines, unlike cats, have a very limited ability to taste the sweet flavor, and lack some of the unique metabolic pathways found in felines. However, vegetal matter forms no more than 3% of the total weight of food a wild wolf consumes and contributes negligible energy and micronutrients, so "wolves can be considered true carnivores in their nature."[9]

Wild wolves probably have evolved sweet taste receptors because they will sometimes eat fruits or nuts – including blucberries, strawberries, raspberries, juniper berries, wolfberry, walnuts, and others.[10] The fact that wolves and dogs lack the highly specialized metabolic pathways found in cats does not make them obligate omnivores. It simply means they have a different evolutionary lineage.

In fact, the word "carnivore" means "meat-eater." It specifies only what is eaten, not what is not eaten. Any animal that routinely eats meat is a carnivore.

Biologists have further classified carnivores into hypocarnivores, which get less than 30% of their total food energy from animal matter; mesocarnivores, which get 50-70% of their total food energy from animal matter; and hypercarnivores, which get at least 70% of their total food energy from animal matter. This division of carnivores into three groups appears to have originated about 40 million years ago.[11]

Some examples of non-human hypercarnivores include: crocodiles, alligators, owls, shrikes, eagles, cats, dolphins, snakes, marlin, polar bears, spiders, scorpions, an most sharks.

---

[9] Bosch G, Hagen-Plantinga EA, Hendriks WH. Dietary nutrient profiles of wild wolves: insights for optimal dog nutrition? Br J Nutr 2015;113:S40-S54.

[10] Ibid.

[11] Van Valkenburgh B. **Déjà vu: the evolution of feeding morphologies in the Carnivora**. Integrative and Comparative Biology 47(1): 147-163.

Some examples of non-human mesocarnivores include: canines (coyotes, foxes), civets, martens, ring-tailed cat, raccoon, skunks, and some mongooses.

Some examples of non-human hypocarnivores include: black bears, binturong, and kiknajou.

Wolves are not the only hypercarnivores that consume some plant matter. Even cats, polar bears and crocodilians may eat some plant foods on occasion,[12] but this would not justify classifying these creatures as omnivores. The mere fact that a creature swallows some plant food under some circumstances does not make it an unspecialized omnivore rather than an animal specialized for eating meat that happens to sometimes eat some plants.

The pertinent questions are:

1. Is this creature specialized for eating meat, or for eating plants?
2. In its natural habitat, can this creature thrive without eating meat?

If a creature is specialized for eating meat, and in its natural habitat, must eat meat to thrive, then it is an obligate carnivore, regardless of how much meat it manages to eat in various circumstances.

Thus, the idea that only animals who only eat meat should be called carnivores lacks logical or evidential basis. In fact, almost all carnivores ingest some plants; and likewise almost all natural herbivores are omnivores to some extent.

As we can see from Table 3.1, many and I venture most likely all mammalian, terrestrial "omnivores" fall into one of two groups:

1. Animals such as the bear, wolf, coatis, raccoon, etc., which have shearing teeth and a short, simple gut *lacking significant fiber fermentation vats*. These creatures have *no dietary requirement for fiber or other carbohydrates* and *can thrive without ever eating*

---

[12] Ibid.

any plant foods, typical of a physiology specifically adapted to hunting and meat-eating. Whenever possible these animals eat animal-based diets, but they may eat variable amounts of fruits or nuts, or nutritionally similar plant parts when in certain circumstances. Most *but not all* of these are so specialized for animal-based diets that they belong to the order Carnivora.

2. Animals such as rodents, primates, and pigs, which have the grinding molars and long, complex guts typical of evolved herbivores. These species are either hindgut or foregut fermenters and they depend on fiber fermentation for such a significant proportion ($\geq 10\%$) of their energy that they can't thrive without eating plant matter. Whenever possible they primarily consume plant-based diets rich in fruits or nutritionally similar plant parts (e.g. tubers), and containing plenty of fiber, but they will consume animal flesh opportunistically or out of necessity (e.g. starvation).

Since the ancestors of extant meso- and hyper- carnivores *always* pursued meat as their primary food, natural selection favored among them the survival of individuals having a nutritional dependence upon certain substances present only in flesh. However, they have no nutritional dependence on direct consumption of plants; they can live their entire lives in excellent health without ever consuming plant foods.

Frugivores have the ability to enzymatically digest botanical fruits and their seeds, some of which (e.g. peas, coconuts, avocados, almonds, sunflower seeds) contain large amounts of protein or fat. Therefore, the carnivore and frugivore gut physiologies display some similarities (exemplifying convergent evolution), and the frugivore's digestive physiology allows it to digest animal flesh. However, since frugivores descended from a lineage that for millennia specialized in acquisition, digestion, and metabolism of fruit and vegetables, natural selection favored among them the reproduction of individuals having a nutritional dependence, not on flesh, but on the primary constituents of fruits and vegetables: fibers and other fermentable carbohydrates.

For example, the so-called omnivorous primates have guts highly adapted to hindgut fermentation so are primarily adapted to high fiber leaves and fruits, not to carnivory. This is why chimpanzees spend the vast majority – 95-100% – of their time collecting plant foods, not hunting animals.

Indeed, Jane Goodall reported evidence that chimpanzees can't efficiently digest the meat that they do eat.

> "During the year when chimpanzee feces were regularly examined, we could tell immediately when chimpanzees had been eating meat, as the samples were full of hair, bones, even lumps of flesh. One sample yielded a monkey finger, another an ear, and a third an incredible five inches of tail, bone, and all! One morning, after Mike had been eating bushbuck meat, he picked pieces of flesh out of his own dung and ate them."[13]

This drives home a very important point: although *some* chimps eat flesh, they don't digest it very well. In short, chimpanzees have an ability to *ingest* meat, but can't really *digest* meat, which explains why they all focus on gathering plants, not on hunting, when they have low supplies of high-quality fruits.[14] Chimpanzees thus aptly illustrate the fact that an animal may as a matter of fact eat both plants and animals, but as a matter of survival it will have to focus on eating the foods that it can by Nature best digest.

Gorillas consume an almost exclusively plant-based diet. They obtain about 60-75% of their total energy requirements from saturated fats produced by hindgut bacterial fermentation of fiber.[15]

---

[13] Goodall J. The Chimpanzees of Gombe. Harvard University Press, 1986. 298.

[14] Gilby IC, Wrangham RW. **Risk-prone hunting by chimpanzees (Pan troglodytes schweinfurthii) increases during periods of high diet quality**. Behav Ecol Sociobiol (2007) 61:1771–1779.

[15] Popovich DG, Jenkins DJA, Kendall CWC, et al. The Western Lowland Gorilla Diet Has Implications for the Health of Humans and other Hominoids. J Nutr 1997 Oct 1;127(10):2000-2005. **<http://jn.nutrition.org/content/127/10/2000.full>**

A gorilla can't survive without consuming fiber, or without his colon, wherein the fiber is fermented and converted to fats. Therefore, a gorilla is, like a chimpanzee, an obligate plant-eater.

Now the question is, what is our specialization?

Nature Is Simple

To reiterate, zoologists classify animals according to their dietary habits, using the following categories:

- Herbivores, also known as folivores, which make leaves of plants (herbage, foliage) their primary or exclusive foods.
- Frugivores, which make fruits of plants their primary or exclusive foods.
- Insectivores, which make insects and worms their primary foods.
- Carnivores, which eat other animals, primarily herbivores.
- Omnivores, which consume both plants and animals.

As I have just demonstrated, probably every so-called omnivore belongs to one of the following two groups:

1. Obligate plant-eaters, including herbivores and frugivores, that have a gut specialized for processing plant foods and in their natural habitat have a dietary requirement for fiber or other plant constituents, but can live without deliberate acquisition of animal protein and fat. For simplicity, I will henceforth refer to all of these as obligate plantivores, or plantivores for short.[16]
2. Obligate animal-eaters, including insectivores and carnivores,[17] that have guts specialized for processing animal foods. These animals have no dietary requirement for fiber or other primary plant constituents, but do have a dietary requirement for animal protein, animal fats, or other nutrients found exclusively or

---

[16] From the Latin words planta (sprout, cutting), plantare (fix in place, plant) and vorare, -vorus (devour).

[17] From the Latin carnivorus, caro/carn- (flesh) and vorare/-vorus (devour).

virtually exclusively in animal tissues. These creatures can thrive without ever eating plant matter, but can't thrive without at least a minimum of animal products. Zoologists also call these faunivores, but henceforth I will refer to all faunivores as carnivores, because the word "carnivore," literally meaning "flesh-eater, meat-eater" is very accurate and more widely understood than the word "faunivore."

So, are we natural plantivores or natural carnivores? And, if we are carnivores, are we designed by Nature for a hypocarnivore diet ($\leq$30% animal matter), a mesocarnivore diet (50-70% animal matter), or a hypercarnivore diet ($\geq$70% animal matter)?

Should we eat lots of plant matter and very little animal matter, or lots of animal matter and little if any plant matter?

The answer lies in our guts.

4 HOMO CARNIVORUS

> You may drive out Nature with a pitchfork, but she will ever hurry back, to triumph in stealth over your foolish contempt.
>
> Horace
> 'Epistles,' Book I, X, 24

As mentioned in the last chapter, some biologists have claimed that we humans are just "slightly remodeled chimpanzee-like apes," designed for a plantivorous – or mainly frugivorous – diet. *Scientific American* published an editorial by such an authority – a biologist named Rob Dunn– who claimed:

> "Our guts are remarkably similar to those of chimpanzees and orangutans--gorillas are a bit special--which are, in turn, not so very different from those of most monkeys. If you were to sketch and then consider the guts of different monkeys, apes and humans you would stop before you were finished, unable to remember which ones you had drawn and which ones you had not."[1]

Unfortunately, many 'authorities' believe – or pretend to believe – this, and try to get the rest of us to accept it as well. In this chapter I will show that any 'authorities' who make this claim either lack knowledge of the many differences between our guts and those of other primates, or, if they do not lack this knowledge, they conceal the truth and deliberately lie.

As you learn, keep this question in mind: Why do they want you to believe that you are an ape and should eat like one?

---

[1] Dunn R. Human Ancestors Were Nearly All Vegetarians. Scientific American 2012 July 23. Accessed Dec 10, 2017 at: <**https://blogs.scientificamerican.com/ guest-blog/human-ancestors-were-nearly-all-vegetarians/**>

The Key Difference

As already mentioned, animals adapted to plant-based diet have guts designed for extracting energy from fiber, the primary constituent of all plant parts, while obligate carnivores have guts designed for extracting energy from flesh composed of animal protein and fat. In their natural habitats, obligate plantivores have a dietary requirement for fiber, but may have none for animal protein and fat, while obligate carnivores have a dietary requirement for animal protein and fat, but none for fiber.

An herbivore can consume, digest and thrive on grass and other leaves. A frugivore can thrive on the highly fibrous fruits provided by Nature. Herbivorous and frugivorous animals fall into two categories: hindgut fermenters and foregut fermenters. Pigs, horses, chimpanzees, gorillas and other 'omnivorous' primates are hindgut fermenters; they have special fermentation vats called cecums in their lower intestines. Cows, sheep, and goats are examples of foregut fermenters; they have multiple stomachs that act as fermentation vats, and they chew the cud, meaning they regurgitate the partially fermented plant matter from their first stomach and chew it a second time.

The fermentation compartments of either herbivores and frugivores are populated with predominantly fermentative microbes. When these microbes (including bacteria, yeasts, molds and fungi) ferment fiber and other carbohydrates, they produce gas (carbon dioxide), alcohol, and acids, principally acetic acid (vinegar), propionic acid, and butyric acid. (Take careful note of this, as we will return to it in a later chapter.)

In contrast, the gut of a natural carnivore eating nothing but its native diet of animal protein and fat contains virtually no fermentative bacteria, because fermentative microbes can't effectively process protein and fat. Instead, the carnivore digestive tract harbors proteolytic bacteria – also known as putrefactive bacteria – that thrive on meat and fat and enzymatically reduce them to fatty acids, glycerine, and amino acid complexes called proteoses and peptides.

How We Differ From Apes

From mouth to anus, the human digestive tract differs markedly from that of the chimpanzee or any other ape.

Mouth

Starting in the mouth, the chimpanzees differ from both ourselves and Miocene apes in incisor/molar proportions, molar wear gradient, dentine penetrance into molars, molar enamel thickness, molar occlusal basins, canine crowns, and diastema (spaces between teeth).[2] Chimpanzees have incisor/molar proportions so different from what we find in ourselves and our known ancestors that it is highly unlikely that any common ancestor of humans and chimps had teeth like chimps.[3] (See Table 4.1)

In addition, our teeth are sharper and have a much greater shear than found in chimpanzees, although somewhat less than found in gorillas. Carnivores and folivores have shearing teeth to process tough foods (meat and leaves, respectively). Anyone who has bitten his/her own tongue or cheek and eaten a cabbage salad knows that human teeth can slice raw meat as well as raw green leaves.

---

[2] Pickford M. Orrorin and the African ape/hominid dichotomy. In: Reynolds SC, Gallagher A (eds.). African Genesis:Perspectives on Hominin Evolution. Cambridge University Press, 2012. 110.

[3] Ibid., 116.

Table 4.1: Summary of derived features of chimpanzees (genus Pan) suggesting that they are not a good model for the last common ancestor of hominids and African apes.

Morphology	Miocene apes	Pan	Homo
Incisor/molar proportions	within hominoid variation	outside hominoid variation	within hominoid variation
Molar wear gradient	marked	weak	marked
Dentine penetrance in molars	low	high	low
Molar enamel thickness	thick	thin	thick
Molar occlusal basins	small	capacious	small
Canine crowns	low	high (in males)	low
Diastema	absent	present	absent

Source: Pickford M. Orrorin and the African ape/hominid dichotomy. In: Reynolds SC, Gallagher A (eds.). African Genesis: Perspectives on Hominin Evolution. Cambridge University Press, 2012. 110.

Advocates of plant-based diets often claim that humans can't chew raw meat, hence can't be natural carnivores. Evidently these people have never tried eating raw meat themselves. Raw meat is not too tough for human dentition. Many native people eat raw meat on a regular basis. I can easily eat a pound of raw meat in 15-20 minutes.

If Nature designed us to eat a diet rich in vegetables, she would have also given us a natural love for vegetables. However, most children intensely dislike raw and green leafy vegetables, but like and readily accept meat, fish, poultry, cheese, butter, yogurt, and cream.[4] This dislike of foods has a genetic basis.[5]

Children reject raw green vegetables and some fruits because they taste bitter, sour or astringent. These tastes come from natural but toxic phytochemicals to be discussed in the next chapter. Nature provided us with bitter taste receptors to guide us to reject foods that can harm us. Unless fooled by processing and cooking that makes edible things that are by Nature inedible to us (e.g., grains, potatoes and cane grass), children obey Nature and reject what tastes bad, including green leafy vegetables or other bitter foods, before adults have programmed them to believe that things that taste bad are actually good to eat.

Hence, Nature provided us with sharp teeth for eating meat, not greens.

---

[4] Fildes A, van Jaarsveld CHM, Llewellyn CH, et al.. Nature and nurture in children's food preferences. Am J Clin Nutr 2014 April; 99(4):911-917. <http://ajcn.nutrition.org/content/99/4/911.long> This study also found that children like cooked starches and sweets, but Nature does not provide us these foods. Children can eat them only because adults have ignored Nature's warnings and used fire (cooking) and other processes to make them edible and digestible.

[5] Fildes A, van Jaarsveld CH, Cooke L, Wardle J, Llewellyn CH. Common genetic architecture underlying young children's food fussiness and liking for vegetables and fruit. *The American Journal of Clinical Nutrition*. 2016;103(4):1099-1104. doi:10.3945/ajcn.115.122945. <https://www.ncbi.nlm.nih.gov/pmc/articles/PMC4807704/#b6>

Saliva

Humans have more copies of the gene AMY1 that codes for production of salivary α-amylase than other primates. Although humans show a wide variation in copy number of this gene, since amylase can function to digest starches, some authors have argued that at least some modern humans have a genetic adaptation to starch-based diets.[6] Some authors have gone further to suggest that the evolution of greater salivary α-amylase levels was necessary for evolution of the unusually large human brain.[7]

Fernández and Wiley have highlighted a number of facts that cast doubt on these hypotheses.[8]

First, a 2016 analysis of a world-wide sample of genetic variations surrounding the amylase locus concluded that preagricultural populations already carried multiple copies of the AMY1 gene.[9] Evidently the amplification of AMY1 copy number occurred in the late Middle Pleistocene, *after* the emergence of the largest human brains and adoption of cooking. Moreover, Neanderthals had larger brains than modern man, but only two AMY1 copies per diploid genome, and the increase in AMY1 copy number in non-Neanderthal

---

[6] Perry GH, Dominy NJ, Claw KG, et al. Diet and the evolution of human amylase gene copy number variation. *Nature genetics*. 2007;39(10):1256-1260. doi: 10.1038/ng2123. <https://www.ncbi.nlm.nih.gov/pmc/articles/PMC2377015/>

[7] Hardy K, Brand-Miller J, Brown KD, Thomas MG, Copeland L. THE IMPORTANCE OF DIETARY CARBOHYDRATE IN HUMAN EVOLUTION. Q Rev Biol. 2015 Sep;90(3):251-68. Review. PubMed PMID: 26591850.

[8] Fernández, C., & Wiley, A. (2017). Rethinking the starch digestion hypothesis for AMY1 copy number variation in humans. American Journal of Physical Anthropology, 163(4), 645-657.

[9] Inchley CE, Larbey CDA, Shwan NAA, et al.: Selective sweep on human amylase genes postdates the split with Neanderthals. Nature Scientific Reports 2016 Nov 17; 6:37198. DOI:10.1038/srep37198 <https://core.ac.uk/download/pdf/74228453.pdf>

humans occurred after the split between Neanderthal and African human lineages. Therefore, amplification of AMY1 and salivary α-amylase could not have played any role in the evolution of the large brain and since it occurred millennia prior to the adoption of agriculture, agriculture played no role in the amplification of brain size, AMY1 or salivary α-amylase.

Second, salivary α-amylase plays little role in and is unnecessary for starch digestion. In the mouth amylase can at most reduce starch into maltose, trisaccharides, and larger starch fragments, none of which is directly absorbable and all of which require further digestion in the small intestine. Thus, if salivary amylase was significant in oral digestion of starch, it would increase the requirement for various glucosidases in the small intestine, but we have no evidence that people with high AMY1 copy numbers also have higher expression of the enzymes required downstream in the intestine. Moreover, it has recently been shown that α-amylase hydrolysis is not even required for starch digestion and the rate of starch digestion depends almost entirely on the small intestine brush border enzymes and maltase-glucoamylase (MGAM). Therefore, α-amylase does not materially increase glucose availability to the brain and therefore could not have played any role in evolution of our large brain.

Upon being swallowed into the stomach, salivary α-amylase itself is rapidly inactivated and degraded by stomach acid. The pancreas also produces α-amylase which performs the same functions as salivary α-amylase, indicating that salivary α-amylase is not essential for starch digestion. Some have proposed that greater salivary α-amylase activity would contribute to a starchy food preference by improving palatability of starches, but a 2015 study found no association between salivary amylase activity and starch consumption or preference.[10]

Fernández and Wiley further identify four more key challenges to the hypothesis that higher AMY1 copy number and variation reflect adaptation to starch-rich diets. These include:

1. We currently encounter considerable methodological difficulties in exactly quantifying AMY1 copy numbers. Studies have shown that current methods cannot determine exact absolute copy numbers for complex variations as in the case of AMY1 and AMY2.
2. Higher copy numbers of AMY1 has an unknown biological significance and weak correlation with phenotypic expression (i.e. higher salivary amylase). The mean difference in AMY copies between alleged high-starch and low-starch populations was only 1.28 copies, which results in only small differences in actual salivary amylase concentration and thus has dubious biological significance.
3. Advocates of the hypothesis that AMY1 copy number amplification is an adaptation to starch consumption have characterized various populations as "high starch" or "low starch" consumers. However, they have failed to substantiate these classifications or prove that these differences in starch intake had occurred during time-frames that could have acted as selection for AMY1 copy numbers. They did not use standardized dietary intake assessments to prove that either "high" or "low" starch groups were in fact so. Fernández and Wiley note that data on prehistoric diets of most of the populations claimed to support the hypothesis does not exist, no one knows whether any specific pattern of starch consumption has occurred for long enough to

---

[10] "Amylolysis was positively associated with both total ($\beta = 0.20$, 95% CI = 0.01; 0.38) and simple carbohydrate intake ($\beta = 0.21$, 95% CI = 0.01; 0.39), but not with complex carbohydrate intake ($P = 0.77$)." Méjean C, Morzel M, Neyraud E, Issanchou S, Martin C, Bozonnet S, et al. (2015) Salivary Composition Is Associated with Liking and Usual Nutrient Intake. PLoS ONE 10(9): e0137473. https://doi.org/10.1371/journal.pone.0137473

result in genetic selection. Moreover, only small numbers of individuals from each population have been studied, and no controls for inbreeding and admixture have been applied, so no one knows how much these have contributed to the observed differences in AMY1 copy number.

4. Existing studies have almost universally reported that high AMY1 copy number is associated with a higher post-meal insulin levels and lower post-meal glucose levels, but reduced risk of insulin resistance, obesity, diabetes, and metabolic syndrome in contemporary populations. Therefore, the hypothesis that selection for high AMY1 copy number in humans is due to more efficient starch digestion and energy availability and storage appears at odds with evidence that AMY1 copy number is associated with *reduced* energy stores.

Fernández and Wiley point out that amylase is produced not only in saliva and the pancreas, but also in the liver, nervous system tissue, mammary tissue, uterus, and testes, among other locations. Since there is no starch in human milk, some authors have proposed that amylase is antibacterial via hydrolyzing the polysaccharides in bacterial cell walls. Some investigators have reported that uterine amylase activity was significantly lower among infertile than parous women, suggesting that amylase may play a role in fertility. Others have shown that sperm function was significantly enhanced by amylase treatment in infertile men.[8]

In their conclusion, Fernández and Wiley note:

> "It could also be that higher AMY1 copies play no adaptive role, but have waxed and waned in copy number without strong selection favoring or disfavoring them. In this regard, Iskow and colleagues (2012) indicate that although several examples of CNV [copy number variation] at coding regions show signals of positive selection, it remains unclear whether these examples present a pattern for CNV in humans. Alternatively, it is suggested that most CNVs across the human genome may have evolved under neutrality due tot he existence of 'hotspots' for CNV

(Cooper, Nikerson, & Eichler, 2007; Perry et al., 2006) and the fact that CNV in the genome of healthy individuals contain thousands of these variant with weak or no phenotypically significant effect (Cooper et al., 2007). More research is necessary to understand the evolutionary significance of high CN [copy number] and CNV in AMY1 in human populations."[8]

Thus, we must conclude that at present "there is insufficient evidence supporting enhanced starch digestion as the primary adaptive function for high AMY1 CN in humans."[8]

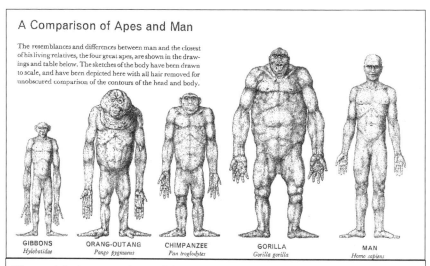

A Comparison of Apes and Man

The resemblances and differences between man and the closest of his living relatives, the four great apes, are shown in the drawings and table below. The sketches of the body have been drawn to scale, and have been depicted here with all hair removed for unobscured comparison of the contours of the head and body.

| GIBBONS | ORANG-OUTANG | CHIMPANZEE | GORILLA | MAN |
| *Hylobatidae* | *Pongo pygmaeus* | *Pan troglodytes* | *Gorilla gorilla* | *Homo sapiens* |

Figure 4.1: A comparison of the body proportions of apes and man.
Source: Moore RE, *Evolution* (New York, Time Incorporated, 1962).

Gut Mass and Proportions

Figure 4.1 provides a visual comparison of the gut sizes of the gibbon, orangutang, chimpanzee, gorilla, and human. All of the apes are plantivores. Those depicted are frugivores. Gibbons eat a 60-75% ripe fruit diet, the orangutans' diet consist of nearly 90% fruit, chimpanzees eat about 48% fruit, and gorillas get about 67% of their diet from fruit. Compared to the apes, we have much smaller guts.

The three apes that have a body length in the human range (orangutan, chimpanzee, and gorilla) have much larger guts than humans. Our gastro-intestinal tract has a total mass (on average, 781 g) about 900 g less than expected, only about 60% of what we would find in an ape having a similar total body mass.[11] This demonstrates

---

[11] Aiello LC. Brains and guts in human evolution: The Expensive Tissue Hypothesis. Brazilian J Genetics 1997 March;20(1). Accessed online on Dec 10, 2017 at: <**http://www.scielo.br/scielo.php?**
script=sci_arttext&pid=S0100-84551997000100023>

that a Natural frugivore has a much more capacious digestive system than we do.

Across nature, carnivores have small gut masses compared to plantivores. This rule applies to primates.

Primarily carnivorous primates (the insect eaters) have simple, globular stomachs; convoluted small intestines; a short, conical caecum; and a simple, smooth-walled colon.[12] Most primate species that rely primarily or largely on insects have relatively small bodies (smaller than chimpanzees).[13] Small-bodied primates weighing less than 500 grams (1.1 pounds) can capture enough insects to supply a majority portion of their energy requirements, but large-bodied non-human primates weighing more than 500 grams can not and must rely primarily on fruits or leaves.[14]

Primarily frugivorous primates have simple stomachs; long, convoluted small intestines; a reduced caecum; and a relatively compact, but haustrated (pouch-walled) colon.[15]

Carnivores have relatively small guts because they specialize in consuming meat and fat, which have a low mass/nutrient ratio. Plantivores generally need larger guts because they specialize in consuming plant foods that have a high mass/nutrient ratio. However, similar to carnivores, primarily frugivorous species can have smaller guts than folivorous plantivores because fruits have a lower bulk/nutrient ratio than leaves and herbage.

Besides having much less total gut mass than an ape, we also have markedly different proportions of the gut devoted to each compartment (Table 4.2). We have the largest proportion of our gut

[12] McNab B. The Physiological Ecology of Vertebrates: A View from Energetics. Cornell University Press, 2002. 399.

[13] Fleagle JG. Primate Adaptation and Evolution. Academic Press, 1998. 286-288.

[14] Ibid.

[15] McNab, op. cit., 399.

mass in our small intestine, where we enzymatically digest foods and assimilate nutrients. The apes have the largest proportion of their gut masses in their colons, where they harbor large populations of microbes that ferment fiber to produce saturated fats (short-chain fatty acids, or SCFAs).

Table 4.2: Stomach, small intestine, cecum and colon proportions in five primate species

Species	Stomach	Small Intestine	Cecum	Colon
Spider monkey[1]	13	62	8	18
Orangutan	17	28	3	54
Gorilla[2]	25	14	7	53
Chimpanzee[2]	20	23	5	52
Human[2]	17	62	Vestigial Appendix	20

1. Milton K. Food choice and digestive strategies of two sympatric primate species. The American Naturalist, April 1981; 117 (4): 496-505.
2. Milton K. Primate diets and gut morphology: Implications for Hominid Evolution. In Harris M (ed.), Food And Evolution: Toward a Theory of Human Food Habits, Temple University Press, 1989. 93-116.

Our guts are similar to those of the carnivores and frugivores. So far, this indicates that we have a gut specialized for consuming meat, fruits, or some combination of meat and fruits.

As shown in Table 4.2, we have gut *proportions* similar to those of the "extremely frugivorous"[16] spider monkey, which eats a diet that

[16] Milton K. Food choice and digestive strategies of two sympatric primate species. The American Naturalist, April 1981; 117 (4): 496-505.
<nature.berkeley.edu/miltonlab/pdfs/foodchoice.pdf>

averages about 75 percent fruit and at times consists of 90 percent fruit and nuts. From this one might be led to conclude that we have a gut adapted to frugivory. Indeed, as I have already noted, anthropologists Hladik and Pasquet have argued that "The dietary status of the human species is that of an unspecialized frugivore, having a flexible diet that includes seeds and meat (omnivorous diet)."[17]

In *Powered By Plants* I agreed with this line of reasoning. However, I have concluded I was wrong to do so. Here's why:

Besides the spider monkeys, the New World capuchin monkeys also have relative gut proportions similar to ours.[18] These monkeys routinely devote 40-50 percent of their daily foraging time to acquiring animal protein and fat.[19]

These two monkeys differ in total gut mass and brain size.[20] The frugivorous spider monkeys (*Ateles* sp.) have a more complex gut than the capuchins (*Cebus* sp.), and the former have a greater relative gut mass and much smaller relative brain size than the latter.

The crude brain:body mass ratio of the spider monkey is 1.4% and that of the capuchin is 2.6%. Further, the relative brain mass of the

---

[17] Hladik CM, Pasquet P. The human adaptations to meat eating: a reappraisal. Human Evolution, Springer Verlag 2002;17:199-206. Accessed online on Dec 6, 2017 from: <**https://hal-univ-diderot.archives-ouvertes.fr/hal-00545795/document**>

[18] Milton K. Primate diets and gut morphology: Implications for Hominid Evolution. In Harris M (ed.), Food And Evolution: Toward a Theory of Human Food Habits, Temple University Press, 1989. 93-116.

[19] Ibid.

[20] Hartwig W, Rosenberger AL, Norconk MA, Owl MY. Relative Brain Size, Gut Size, and Evolution in New World Monkeys. The Anatomical Record 2011 Dec; 294:12:2207-2221. <**http://onlinelibrary.wiley.com/doi/10.1002/ar.21515/full**>

capuchins is more than 4 times that of the spider monkey.[21] The spider monkey's brain:body mass ratio is less than ours, and the capuchin's ratio is greater than ours (~2%).

When you consider relative brain and gut size, we're built like the more carnivorous capuchin, not like the frugivorous spider monkey. Because of the large energy demands of the brain and the low energy density of wild fruits, in Nature (absent agriculture) a large animal such as the human can maintain a brain:body mass ratio of 2% or greater only by eating an animal-based, fat-rich diet.

The frugivores need a large gut mass to extract energy from the low energy-density fruits. These large guts consume large amounts of energy. Consequently a large-bodied frugivore – such as the chimpanzee, gorilla, or orangutan – simply can't build a large brain. Meat and especially its associated animal fat have a much higher energy density than fruit, so only carnivores can obtain sufficient energy from meat to support a large brain with a relatively small gut mass.

Some people think humans are designed or adapted to a diet consisting primarily of whole grains and legumes, that is, a seed-based diet. Like other plantivores, seed-eating primates also have complex guts and relatively small brains.[22] Evidently, a primate can't evolve or maintain a large brain and small simple gut eating any type of plant-based diet.

The plantivorous monkeys and apes have massive guts adapted to extracting energy from low energy density, high bulk fruits and vegetables. Such guts and diets simply can not support large brains. Like wolves (or dogs), capuchins and humans have relatively small guts adapted to extracting energy from high energy density, low bulk

---

[21] Ibid. Tables 1 and 3.

[22] Hartwig W, Rosenberger AL, Norconk MA, Owl MY. Relative Brain Size, Gut Size, and Evolution in New World Monkeys. The Anatomical Record 2011 Dec; 294:12:2207-2221. <**http://onlinelibrary.wiley.com/doi/10.1002/ar.21515/full**>

food such as fruits (e.g. nuts) and meat. Nature has awarded large brains only to animals that have compact, simple, energy efficient guts and a highly carnivorous diet.

Stomach

High stomach acidity is energetically expensive to maintain. Also, it is maladaptive to a plantivore because plantivores depend on microbes to fermentatively digest the fiber they consume, and an extremely acid stomach kills those bacteria.

We have a much more acidic stomach than the apes. We produce an extremely low pH of 1.5 in our stomach. Our stomach is more acidic than any other primate, considerably more acidic than most carnivores and "omnivores," and most similar to carrion feeders,[23] probably because our early ancestors could not thrive without eating scavenged raw meat (see Table 4.3)

Table 4.3: Stomach pH of various species

Common name	Diet/digestion type	Stomach pH
Colobus monkey	plantivore/foregut	6.3
Sheep	plantivore/hindgut	4.7
Dog	scavenger	4.5
Ox	herbivore/foregut	4.2
Horse	herbivore/hindgut	4.4
Cat	carnivore	3.6
Baboon	omnivore	3.7
Crab-eating macaque	omnivore	3.6

23 Beasley DE, Koltz AM, Lambert JE, et al., "The Evolution of Stomach Acidity and Its Relevance to the Human Microbiome," PLOS One 2015 July 29. <**http://journals.plos.org/plosone/article?id=10.1371/journal.pone.0134116**>

Common name	Diet/digestion type	Stomach pH
Skyes monkey	omnivore	3.4
Snowy owl	carnivore	2.5
Bottlenose dolpin	carnivore	2.3
Cynomolgus monkey	omnivore	2.1
Rabbit	plantivore/hindgut; eats feces	1.9
Grey falcon	scavenger	1.8
Peregrine falcon	scavenger	1.8
American bittern	scavenger	1.7
Red tailed hawk	scavenger	1.8
Swanson's hawk	scavenger	1.8
Human	**carnivore**	**1.5**
Ferret	carnivore	1.5
Wandering albatross	scavenger	1.5
Possum	scavenger	1.5

Source: Beasley DE, Koltz AM, Lambert JE, et al., "The Evolution of Stomach Acidity and Its Relevance to the Human Microbiome," PLOS One 2015 July 29.

Small Intestine and Pancreas

The small intestine comprises the majority (62%) of the mass of our gastro-intestinal tract, whereas it comprises only 23% of the mass of the chimpanzee's gut. By proportion alone, we have 2.7 times more gut mass devoted to the small intestine than the chimp does, and 4.4 times more than the gorilla does.

We digest our food in the small intestine using enzymes secreted by our pancreas and bile coming from our liver by route of the gall bladder. The pancreas produces enzymes for digesting protein, fat, sugars and starches, but no enzyme for digesting fiber.

We derive all necessary nutrients from enzymatic digestion of foods in and assimilation through the small intestine. We can't live without it.

Among our protein-digesting enzymes, we have some devoted to digesting proteins that only meat provides. For example, our pancreas produces elastase, an enzyme specifically adapted to digesting proteins found only in meat.[24, 25] Pancreatic elastase specifically digests elastin, a component of connective tissue that holds organs together. Thus we have pancreatic enzymes that could have no purpose other than to digest connective tissue in meat.

Carnitine and carnosine are peptides found only in meat. We produce two specific transporters for absorption of carnitine – OCTN2 and ATP$^{0,+}$ – and loss of function mutations in OCTN2 may be linked to inflammatory bowel disease, suggesting that consumption of carnitine is necessary for maintaining intestinal health.[26] We also produce a specific intestinal transporter for uptake of carnosine – PEPT1 – and it appears that carnosine has a protective

[24] Largman C, Brodrick JW, Geokas MC. Purification and characterization of two human pancreatic elastases. Biochemistry. 1976 Jun 1;15(11):2491-500. PubMed PMID: 819031. Abstract.

[25] Ohlsson K, Olsson AS. Purification and partial characterization of human pancreatic elastase. Hoppe Seylers Z Physiol Chem. 1976 Aug;357(8):1153-61. PubMed PMID: 824194. Abstract.

[26] Srinivas SR, Prasad PD, Umapathy NS, Ganapathy V, Shekhawat PS. Transport of butyryl-L-carnitine, a potential prodrug, via the carnitine transporter OCTN2 and the amino acid transporter ATB$^{0,+}$. *American journal of physiology Gastrointestinal and liver physiology*. 2007;293(5):G1046-G1053. doi:10.1152/ajpgi.00233.2007. <https://www.ncbi.nlm.nih.gov/pmc/articles/PMC3583010/>

effect against oxidative stress in intestinal epithelial cells.[27] Thus our intestines are specifically adapted to (or designed for) absorbing peptides that only meat provides.

We also have specific mechanisms for the absorption of cholesterol.[28]

Although we do produce enzymes that digest sugars and starches, we have a somewhat limited ability to digest and assimilate this carbohydrate, as demonstrated by the fact that some undigested starch and sugar reaches the colon to feed intestinal flora, which convert the carbohydrates into fats, acids and gas. This is why we get bloating after meals rich in carbohydrate but never from meals consisting of only protein and fat (unless bile flow is impaired resulting in fat indigestion). In fact, it is not uncommon for people to find whole plant foods – such as corn or peas – passing through the gut and deposited with feces wholly undigested. This strongly indicates that our gut is not primarily adapted to processing whole plant foods.

Gall Bladder

The gall bladder temporarily stores bile made by the liver. It empties itself into the small intestine in response to a high fat meal. Bile plays a very important role in digestion of fats: it breaks large globs of fat into smaller globs, so that fat-digesting enzymes can attack it and reduce it to molecules the small intestine can absorb. Bile flow stimulated by fat intake also stimulates intestinal peristalsis or "mass movement" to evacuate the intestines.

---

[27] Son DO, Satsu H, Kiso Y, Shimizu M. Characterization of carnosine uptake and its physiological function in human intestinal epithelial Caco-2 cells. Biofactors. 2004;21(1-4):395-8. PubMed PMID: 15630234.

[28] Cohen DE. Balancing Cholesterol Synthesis and Absorption in the Gastrointestinal Tract. *Journal of clinical lipidology*. 2008;2(2):S1-S3. doi: 10.1016/j.jacl.2008.01.004. **<https://www.ncbi.nlm.nih.gov/pmc/articles/PMC2390860/>**

Since carnivores eat intermittent meals rich in fat, with very few exceptions Nature has provided them with very well-developed gall bladders. This enables them to efficiently digest their naturally high-fat diet, and to have regular bowel movements.

A fruit-based diet would be low in fat in comparison to a meat-based diet. If we eat a low fat diet, the gall bladder does not completely empty, giving rise to gall stone formation and constipation.[29, 30]

A fruit-based diet would be high in carbohydrates. Plant-based diets high in carbohydrates increase the risk for gall bladder stones.[31]

This evidence indicates that Nature designed our gall bladder for a fat-rich, not a carbohydrate-rich, diet. In Nature, only an animal-based diet regularly provides a high fat intake, and only a plant-based diet can provide a high carbohydrate, low fat intake.

In contrast, the apes eat a naturally low-fat diet but do not suffer either gall stone formation or constipation as a result. This indicates that Nature designed the ape gall bladder for a low-fat intake, as Nature provides them through fruit and leaves.

---

[29] Festi D, Colecchia A, Larocca A, Villanova N, Mazzella G, Petroni ML, RomanoF, Roda E. Review: low caloric intake and gall-bladder motor function. Aliment Pharmacol Ther. 2000 May;14 Suppl 2:51-3. Review. PubMed PMID: 10903004.

[30] Stokes CS, Gluud LL, Casper M, Lammert F. Ursodeoxycholic Acid and Diets Higher in Fat Prevent Gallbladder Stones During Weight Loss: A Meta-analysis of Randomized Controlled Trials. Clin Gastroenter and Hepat 2014;12:1090-1100. <http://www.cghjournal.org/article/S1542-3565(13)01837-5/pdf>

[31] Tsai C-J, Leitzmann MF, Willett WC, Giovannucci EL. Dietary carbohydrates and glycaemic load and the incidence of symptomatic gall stone disease in men. Gut. 2005;54(6):823-828. doi:10.1136/gut.2003.031435. <https://www.ncbi.nlm.nih.gov/pmc/articles/PMC1774557/>

Cecum and Colon

In the apes, the cecum is well-developed and the colon and cecum together comprise the majority of the mass of the gut, for chimps 57% and for gorillas 60% (Table 4.2). In the apes both the cecum and colon perform the vital function of serving as fermentation vats wherein microbes convert plant fiber into saturated fatty acids upon which these animals depend for the majority of their metabolic fuel.

For example, saturated fats (not unsaturated fats) obtained from microbial fermentation of fiber provide about 57% of the gorilla's daily energy requirement.[32] Microbial fermentation also liberates amino acids from green leaves, thereby providing apes with the constituents of animal protein.

The apes thus obtain protein and saturated fat from those microbes, greatly reducing their need to eat meat (some insects will suffice). However, because of their near complete dependence on this microbial fermentation, these animals must have both cecum and colon intact in order to survive in their natural habitats.

In contrast, our colon forms only 20% of the total mass of our gut, and we have an insignificant cecum – better known as the appendix – which performs no vital digestive function. Surgeons perform thousands of appendectomies and colostomies on humans every year, and the patients live for many years afterwards, proving that a human can obtain enough energy and protein from food to survive and reproduce without an appendix or colon.

Microbes that enzymatically digest protein and fat – known as putrefactive microbes – naturally predominate in a carnivore's colon when his/her diet consists of meat and fat. However, when carnivores consume carbohydrates, undigested starches, sugars, and fiber reach the colon, and this will disturb the normal gut flora

---

[32]Popovich DG, Jenkins DJA, Kendall CWC, et al. The Western Lowland Gorilla Diet Has Implications for the Health of Humans and other Hominoids. J Nutr 1997 Oct 1;127(10):2000-2005. <**http://jn.nutrition.org/content/127/10/2000.full**>

populations, causing fermentative flora to flourish. These flora convert fiber to short-chain fatty acids (SCFAs) that, hypothetically, the colon can absorb and use as an energy source.

Consequently, some authors hypothetically estimate that obligately carnivorous dogs[33] and even cats can derive about 7 percent of energy requirements from microbial fermentation when chronically fed carbohydrates.[34] Similarly, some authors have hypothetically estimated that we obtain 5 to 10% of energy requirements (mean, 7.5%) from fermentation of fiber.[35]

In my previous book *Powered By Plants* I accepted this estimate as legitimate for prediction of energy yields from very high fiber intakes.[36] However, I now do not give it much credence, for two reasons. First, it did not come from direct observation of people consuming high fiber diets, but was calculated from the theoretical short chain fatty acid yield from fiber fermentation, with the unsupported assumption that as fiber intakes increase, human gut flora will linearly increase SCFA production, and the colon will absorb all of the SCFA produced. Second, humans on very high fiber fruit and vegetable diets (fiber 150 g/d) excrete large amounts of SCFA in their feces, proving that our colons – unlike those of apes dependent on this energy source – do not efficiently absorb all of the fats produced from fiber fermentation.[37]

---

[33] Dogs are obligate carnivores in the most important sense: in their natural habitat, without human assistance, they must eat animal meat and fat to survive.

[34] Subcommittee on Dog and Cat Nutrition, Committee on Animal Nutrition, National Research Council. **Nutrient Requirements of Dogs and Cats**. National Academies Press, 2006. 62.

[35] McNeil NI. **The contribution of the large intestine to energy supplies in man**. Am J Clin Nutr 1984 Feb;39(2):338-342.

[36] Matesz D. Powered By Plants: Natural Selection and Human Nutrition. CreateSpace, 2013.

[37] Jenkins et al.. **Effect of a Very-High-Fiber Vegetable, Fruit, and Nut Diet on Serum Lipids and Colonic Function.** Metabolism 2001 April;50(4):494-503.

People who have had surgical removal of the colon on average weigh about 4 kg (8.8 lb.) less than age- and height- matched controls who have a similar food energy intake; "the loss of both the large intestine and the ability to conserve energy may be a major factor contributing to this difference."[38] Dogs and cats fed conventional pet foods containing carbohydrates also weigh more than dogs and cats eating only meat and fat. Given that the average individual is at least 10 pounds overweight, this suggests that colonic fermentation of carbohydrates, though limited, may contribute enough excess energy to colonic energy needs to produce overweight in carnivores, including humans.

In any case, to reiterate, we can, unlike the apes, live and reproduce without the colon, as demonstrated by the many people who have had surgical removal of the colon.

Clearly, the apes require both the colon and dietary fiber from plants in order to survive, while we do not require either the colon or dietary fiber from plants in order to survive. Therefore, the apes are in Nature obligate plantivores, and we are not.

---

[38] McNeil NI. **The contribution of the large intestine to energy supplies in man.** Am J Clin Nutr 1984 Feb;39(2):338-342.

Gut Flora Dependence

The great apes can't survive without the fermentative microbes in their hindguts. These microbes digest the fiber the apes consume and convert it to saturated fats – short-chain fatty acids – that provide those animals with the majority of their energy requirements. If you were to kill all the microbes in their guts with antibiotics, they would be unable to obtain adequate nutrition from their food intake.

Healthy carnivores have predominantly putrefactive gut flora which, like our own pancreatic juices, decompose meat and fat to release amino acids and fatty acids. However, meat and fat are virtually 100 percent digested by stomach acid, pepsin, and pancreatic enzymes in the small intestine, so very little or nothing of ingested meat or fat reaches the colon of a healthy carnivore. Consequently, carnivores do not need these microbes in order to survive. If you give them antibiotics that kill all gut flora, they will still be able to digest and obtain adequate nutrition from meat and fat. The flora that do inhabit their colons survive on the cells and mucus sloughed off the inner lining of the colon.

Like carnivores, we can take antibiotics that kill off any microbes inhabiting our guts, yet retain the ability to digest and obtain adequate energy and nutrients from meat and fat.

If given carbohydrates, the putrefactive microbes that typically inhabit the guts of carnivores can decompose those carbohydrates, but this process will produce gas and acid that are not produced when decomposing protein and fat. This gas will cause bloating and the acid will irritate the bowel, generally causing either diarrhea or constipation.

Protein Requirements

In order to obtain adequate protein from plants, a plantivore must have a digestive system capable of liberating plant protein from raw plant matter, in which fiber tightly binds the plant proteins.

Fruits are poor sources of protein, and primates do not produce enzymes that digest fiber, so the apes primarily rely upon colonic microbial fermentation of green leaves to digest plant protein and meet their amino acid and energy requirements. If we could do this, impoverished people and individuals lost in the wilderness would never suffer from protein or energy deficiencies, because green leaves are abundant.

Green leaves provide a high proportion of their macronutrients as protein, but they have a very low protein density by weight. For example, about 50% of the energy supplied by spinach comes from protein.[39] However, spinach provides only 2.9 g of protein per 100 g fresh weight. A man weighing 150 pounds (68 kg) would need to eat 2 kg (4.4 lb.) of spinach daily – that's about 6 bunches – to meet the recommended daily intake of protein of 0.8 g/kg, which would only provide 460 kcalories – only about one-sixth his energy requirements.

This assumes that we could extract 100% of the protein from spinach. Our enzymatic digestive system has no enzymes for digestion of fiber, so in reality we would extract less than 60% of the protein from green leaves. Unlike apes, we can't process enough green leaves and fruit in a day to acquire adequate protein and calories, and we do not obtain any of our protein requirements from colonic fermentation of plant matter. Even if microbes in our colon liberated amino acids from plant matter, our colon can't absorb them. Unlike ape colons, ours does not take up nutrients and deliver them to the general circulation.

Cooking plant matter makes plant protein somewhat more digestible, but even with this recent invention that played no role in Nature's design of our gut, we have difficulty obtaining from plants adequate amounts of total protein and the proper proportions of amino acids we require for tissue maintenance or growth.

---

[39] Burned in a bomb calorimeter, very different from the human gut.

Pregnant women who have high intakes of carbohydrates (hence plant proteins) and low intakes of animal protein have an increased risk of bearing infants having low birth weights.[40] Children of women who consumed less than 50 g of animal protein daily in late pregnancy had an increased risk of adult hypertension.[41]

Children raised exclusively on plant proteins often fail to grow as well as children who eat animal protein, despite having plant protein intakes exceeding the RDA, probably because of the low bioavailability and poor amino acid profiles of plant proteins.[42] Elderly people rapidly lose body protein (from muscles and organs) if not consuming high quality proteins. Experiments with elders have shown that diets rich in animal proteins promote greater protein synthesis (hence repair and growth) than plant proteins.[43, 44]

[40] Godfrey K, Robinson S, Barker DJ, Osmond C, Cox V. Maternal nutrition in early and late pregnancy in relation to placental and fetal growth. *BMJ: British Medical Journal.* 1996;312(7028):410-414. <**https://www.ncbi.nlm.nih.gov/pmc/articles/PMC2350090/**>

[41] Campbell DM, Hall MH, Barker DJ, Cross J, Shiell AW, Godfrey KM. Diet in pregnancy and the offspring's blood pressure 40 years later. Br J Obstet Gynaecol. 1996 Mar;103(3):273-80. PubMed PMID: 8630314. Abstract.

[42] Acosta PB. Availability of essential amino acids and nitrogen in vegan diets. Am J Clin Nutr. 1988 Sep;48(3 Suppl):868-74. Review. PubMed PMID: 3046316.

[43] Pannemans DL, Wagenmakers AJ, Westerterp KR, Schaafsma G, Halliday D. Effect of protein source and quantity on protein metabolism in elderly women. Am J Clin Nutr. 1998 Dec;68(6):1228-35. PubMed PMID: 9846851.

[44] Campbell WW, Barton ML Jr, Cyr-Campbell D, Davey SL, Beard JL, Parise G, Evans WJ. Effects of an omnivorous diet compared with a lactoovovegetarian diet on resistance-training-induced changes in body composition and skeletal muscle in older men. Am J Clin Nutr. 1999 Dec;70(6):1032-9. PubMed PMID: 10584048.

People eating diets high in animal protein have a higher bone density than those eating predominantly plant proteins.[45] We have evidence that we require animal protein, vitamin B12 and perhaps other meat-based nutrients to maintain healthy bones.[46] Evidence has accumulated indicating that dietary animal protein improves calcium absorption, increases muscle mass, suppresses parathyroid hormone levels, and increases IGF-1 levels, all of which improve bone mass.[47]

Unlike animal proteins, plant proteins do not have the balance of amino acids that we require (this is why plant proteins are said to be incomplete, whereas animal proteins are said to be complete). Plant

---

[45] Hoffman JR, Falvo MJ. Protein – Which is Best? *Journal of Sports Science & Medicine*. 2004;3(3):118-130. <**https://www.ncbi.nlm.nih.gov/pmc/articles/PMC3905294/#ref12**>

46 Herrmann W, Obeid R, Schorr H, et al., "Enhanced bone metabolism in vegetarians--the role of vitamin B12 deficiency," Clin Chem Lab Med 2009;47(11):1381-7. doi: 10.1515/CCLM.2009.302. PubMed PMID: 19817650.

[47] Mangano KM, Sahni S, Kerstetter JE. Dietary protein is beneficial to bone health under conditions of adequate calcium intake: an update on clinical research. *Current opinion in clinical nutrition and metabolic care*. 2014;17(1):69-74. doi: 10.1097/MCO.0000000000000013. <**https://www.ncbi.nlm.nih.gov/pmc/articles/PMC4180248/**>

proteins do not contain the amino acid taurine, for which we probably have a dietary requirement.[48, 49, 50, 51, 52]

We may also require animal protein to obtain adequate amounts of the amino acid methionine; a 2000 study found low methionine levels in typical vegans and vegetarians.[53] Low methionine intake has several harmful or accelerated aging effects, including:

- reduced levels of sulfur, which impairs detoxification and connective tissue repair[54]
- reduced levels of glutathione, compromising antioxidant defenses and promoting inflammation[55]

48 Laidlaw SA et al., "Plasma and urine taurine levels in vegans," Am J Clin Nutr 1988 Apr;47(4):660-3.

49 Eishorbagy A et al., "Amino acid changes during transition to a vegan diet supplemented with fish in healthy humans," Eur J Nut 2016 Jun. <http://link.springer.com/article/10.1007%2Fs00394-016-1237-6>

50 Rana SK, Sanders TA, "Taurine concentrations in the diet, plasma, urine and breast milk of vegans compared with omnivores," Br J Nutr 1986 Jul;56(1):17-27.

51 Naismith DJ, Rana SK, Emery PW, "Metabolism of taurine during reproduction in women," Hum Nutr Clin Nutr 1987 Jan;41(1):37-45.

52 McCarty MF, "Sub-optimal taurine status may promote platelet hyperaggregability in vegetarians," Med Hypotheses 2004;63(3):426-33.

53 Krajcovicová-Kudláčková M, Blazícek P, Kopcová J, Béderová A, Babinská K, "Homocysteine levels in vegetarians versus omnivores," Ann Nutr Metab 2000;44(3):135-8. PubMed PMID: 11053901.

54 Nimni ME, Han B, Cordoba F. Are we getting enough sulfur in our diet? *Nutrition & Metabolism*. 2007;4:24. doi:10.1186/1743-7075-4-24. <https://www.ncbi.nlm.nih.gov/pmc/articles/PMC2198910/>

55 Ibid.

- inflammation and deterioration of gut structure[56]
- impaired immune function and recovery from injury[57]
- greying of hair; methionine depletion leads to a buildup of hydrogen peroxide in hair follicles which causes loss of hair color[58, 59]
- increased risk for venous thrombosis[60]
- increased risk of infertility[61]

[56] Ruth MR, Field CJ. The immune modifying effects of amino acids on gut-associated lymphoid tissue. J Animal Sci and Biotech 2013;4:27. **<https://jasbsci.biomedcentral.com/articles/10.1186/2049-1891-4-27>**

[57] Grimble RF. The Effects of Sulfur Amino Acid Intake on Immune Function in Humans. J Nutr 2006 June;136(6):1660S-1665S. **<https://doi.org/10.1093/jn/136.6.1660S>**

[58] Wood JM, Decker H, Hartmann H, et al. Senile hair graying: H2O2-mediated oxidative stress affects human hair color by blunting methionine sulfoxide repair. FASEB J. 2009 Jul;23(7):2065-75. doi: 10.1096/fj.08-125435. Epub 2009 Feb 23. PubMed PMID: 19237503.

[59] Schallreuter KU, Salem MM, Hasse S, Rokos H. The redox--biochemistry of human hair pigmentation. Pigment Cell Melanoma Res. 2011 Feb;24(1):51-62. doi: 10.1111/j.1755-148X.2010.00794.x. Epub 2010 Dec 1. PubMed PMID: 20958953.

[60] Keijzer MB, den Heijer M, Borm GF, et al. Low fasting methionine concentration as a novel risk factor for recurrent venous thrombosis. Thromb Haemost. 2006 Oct;96(4):492-7. PubMed PMID: 17003928.

[61] Grandison RC, Piper MDW, Partridge L. Amino acid imbalance explains extension of lifespan by dietary restriction in *Drosophila*. *Nature* 2009;462(7276): 1061-1064. doi:10.1038/nature08619.

Limiting meat intake also limits intake of highly bioavailable iron, zinc, selenium, and B-complex vitamins.[62, 63]

Advances in measuring protein needs suggest that the current RDA underestimates protein requirements by as much as 50%, and high protein diets have been found beneficial for reducing excess energy (calorie) intake and cardiovascular risk factors.[64]

We also have evidence that very high protein, low carbohydrate diets may limit cancer initiation and growth.[65, 66] Individuals have stalled or reversed cancer consuming a paleolithic ketogenic diet with a 2:1 fat:protein weight ratio, based on fatty red meats and offal and excluding plant foods for 6 months then allowing selected fruits and

[62] D.K. Layman, A. Arne Astrup, P.M. Clifton, H.J. Leidy, D. Paddon-Jones, S.M. Phillips, "The contrived association of dietary protein with mortality," Comments submitted to Cell Metabolism April 2, 2014 (2014) (Available at: **http://www.cell.com/cell-metabolism/comments/S1550-4131(14)00062-X**. Accessed March 29, 2017).

[63] Binnie MA, Barlow K, Johnson V, Harrison C, "Red meats: Time for a paradigm shift in dietary advice," Meat Science 2014 Nov;98(3):445-51. <**http://www.sciencedirect.com/science/article/pii/S0309174014001922**>

[64] Ibid.

[65] Ho VW, Leung K, Hsu A, Luk B, et al., "A Low Carbohydrate, High Protein Diet Slows Tumor Growth and Prevents Cancer Initiation," Cancer Research 2011 July;71(13): DOI: 10.1158/0008-5472.CAN-10-3973 <**http://cancerres.aacrjournals.org/content/71/13/4484.full-text.pdf**>

[66] Ho VW, et al. "A Low Carbohydrate, High Protein Diet Combined with Celecoxib Markedly Reduces Metastasis." Carcinogenesis 35.10 (2014): 2291–2299. PMC. Web. 29 Mar. 2017. <**https://www.ncbi.nlm.nih.gov/pmc/articles/PMC4178469/**>

vegetables constituting no more than 30% of the volume of the diet.[67, 68]

A Taste For Fat

With few exceptions, plant foods have low fat contents. Although chimpanzees eat some palm nuts, their natural diet contains very little fat, estimated at 2.5% of the dry weight. In contrast, humans in their various natural habitats (hunter-gatherers) eat meat-based diets containing on average 38% to 49% fat, i.e. about 20 times as much fat as chimpanzees.[69]

Across cultures, humans have a preference for high fat foods,[70, 71] and hunter-gatherers not influenced by modern dietary ideologies ate all parts of wild game, including high-fat marrow and storage fat,

---

[67] Toth C, Schimmer M, Clemens Z. Complete Cessation of Recurrent Cervical Intraepithelial Neoplasia (CIN) by the Paleolithic Ketogenic Diet: A Case Report. J Cancer Res and Treat 2018;6(1):1.5.

[68] Toth C, Clemens Z. Halted Progression of Soft Palate Cancer in a Patient Treated with the Paleolithic Ketogenic Diet Alone: A 20-months Follow-up. American J Med Case Rep 2016;4(8):288-292.

[69] Finch CE and Stanford CB. **Meat-Adaptive Genes and the Evolution of Slower Aging in Humans**. The Quarterly Review of Biology 2004 Mar;79(1): 3-50.

70 Manabe Y, Matsumura S, Fushiki T. Preference for High-Fat Food in Animals. In: Montmayeur JP, le Coutre J, editors. Fat Detection: Taste, Texture, and Post Ingestive Effects. Boca Raton (FL): CRC Press/Taylor & Francis; 2010. Chapter 10. Available from: https://www.ncbi.nlm.nih.gov/books/NBK53543/

71 Drewnowski A, Almiron-Roig E. Human Perceptions and Preferences for Fat-Rich Foods. In: Montmayeur JP, le Coutre J, editors. Fat Detection: Taste, Texture, and Post Ingestive Effects. Boca Raton (FL): CRC Press/Taylor & Francis; 2010. Chapter 11. Available from: https://www.ncbi.nlm.nih.gov/books/NBK53528/

when possible and palatable.[72] Ancestral Europeans were hunters of fat animals, because they could not have survived in Europe without making animal fat their main energy source.[73]

Micronutrient Requirements

Archaeological evidence of iron and vitamin B12 deficiency diseases in the bones of a 2 year-old child dated to 1.5 million years ago indicates that by that time humans in their natural habitat (our ancestors) already had a dietary requirement for meat from grass-eating animals to prevent childhood iron and vitamin B12 deficiency diseases.[74]

This requirement remains with us today. Impoverished children in developing countries who do not get adequate animal source foods (meat, eggs, milk) in their diets suffer from micronutrient malnutrition that causes growth stunting, lower intelligence, lethargy, poor attention, and greater rates and severity of infections.[75] Children raised in Europe on unsupplemented vegan diets have a high risk of deficiencies of vitamins B12 and D with consequences

---

72 Abrams HL. The Preference for Animal Protein and Fat: A Cross-Cultural Survey. In: Harris M and Ross EB, eds. Food and Evolution. Philadelphia, PA: Temple University Press, 1987: 207.

73 Ben-Dor M, Gopher A, Hershkovitz I, Barkai R, "Man the Fat Hunter," PLOS One 2011;6(12): e28689. doi:10.1371/journal.pone.0028689. <http://journals.plos.org/plosone/article?id=10.1371/journal.pone.0028689>

74 Domínguez-Rodrigo M, Pickering TR, Diez-Martín F, Mabulla A, Musiba C, Trancho G, et al. (2012) Earliest Porotic Hyperostosis on a 1.5-Million-Year-Old Hominin, Olduvai Gorge, Tanzania. PLoS ONE 7(10): e46414. doi:10.1371/journal.pone.0046414 **<https://www.ncbi.nlm.nih.gov/pmc/articles/PMC3463614/>**

75 Demmet MW, Young MM, Sensenig RL. Animal Source Foods to Improve Micronutrient Nutrition and Human Function in Developing Countries. Providing Micronutrients through Food-Based Solutions: A Key to Human and National Development. J Nutr 2003;133:3879S-3885S. Accessed online on Dec 12, 2017 from: **<http://jn.nutrition.org/content/133/11/3879S.full.pdf>**

including stunted growth, rickets, and impaired cognitive capacity, with the latter persisting despite subsequent diet enrichment.[76, 77]

People who avoid animal protein develop vitamin B12 deficiency even if they use typical vitamin B12 supplements; vitamin B12 deficiency and elevated plasma homocysteine have been found to be the "normal" state for vegans.[78] Vitamin supplements contain a form of B12 that Nature does not provide in plants, microbes or animal tissues, so they can't replace animal foods.[79]

Feeding Habits

Since plants have a very low energy density, natural plantivores must eat plants more or less continuously in order to obtain adequate energy intake. On the other hand, since meat and fat have a high energy density, natural carnivores eat intermittently, in discrete meals.

---

[76] Di Genova T, Guyda H. Infants and children consuming atypical diets: Vegetarianism and macrobiotics. *Paediatrics & Child Health*. 2007;12(3):185-188. <https://www.ncbi.nlm.nih.gov/pmc/articles/PMC2528709/>

[77] Roberts IF, West RJ, Ogilvie D, Dillon MJ. Malnutrition in infants receiving cult diets: a form of child abuse. *British Medical Journal*. 1979;1(6159):296-298. <https://www.ncbi.nlm.nih.gov/pmc/articles/PMC1597704/?page=1>

[78] Obersby D, Chappell DC, Dunnett A, Tsiami AA. Plasma total homocysteine status of vegetarians compared with omnivores: a systematic review and meta-analysis. Brit J Nutr 2013 Mar 14;109(5):785-94. <https://www.cambridge.org/core/journals/british-journal-of-nutrition/article/div-classtitleplasma-total-homocysteine-status-of-vegetarians-compared-with-omnivores-a-systematic-review-and-meta-analysisdiv/1754320C613E6CD7F9AED4EE60C421B5/core-reader>

[79] Kelly G. The Coenzyme Forms of Vitamin B12: Toward an Understanding of their Therapeutic Potential. Alternative Medicine Review 1997;2(6):459-471. Accessed Dec 12, 2017 from: <http://www.anaturalhealingcenter.com/documents/Thorne/articles/CoEnzymeB12.pdf>

This means that carnivores are adapted to long periods of fasting, whereas plantivores are not. Plantivores are more or less continuous grazers, whereas carnivores eat distinct meals.

Apes in their natural habitat eat more or less continuously from the time they awaken in the morning to the time they retire in the evening. They fit the plantivore pattern.

In contrast, humans in their natural habitat – hunters – eat intermittently, generally having only one or two meals daily, based on meat and fat.[80]

Many studies indicate that human metabolism malfunctions when we eat frequently, and improves when we eat infrequently and have longer daily periods of fasting.[81]

Thus, in and by Nature we feed infrequently, like carnivores, not frequently, like plantivores.

Physique

All of the apes have torsos and arms longer than legs, whereas we have relatively long legs and short arms in comparison. Nature designed the former type of physique for natural frugivores: long arms are essential for success in climbing trees and reaching out to harvest fruits.

In contrast, our long legs make us capable of highly efficient long-distance travel on the ground, necessary for tracking and chasing

---

[80] Mattson MP, Allison DB, Fontana L, et al. Meal frequency and timing in health and disease. *Proceedings of the National Academy of Sciences of the United States of America.* 2014;111(47):16647-16653. doi:10.1073/pnas.1413965111. <**https://www.ncbi.nlm.nih.gov/pmc/articles/PMC4250148/**>

[81] Ibid.

prey animals.[82] Our relatively short arms make us capable of forcefully launching projectiles with our hands.

We love chasing and throwing things with great accuracy so much that we make these the main actions in some of our favorite games: baseball, basketball, American football, rugby, polo, and lacrosse to name a few.

Aging Rate and Life Expectancy

Relative to humans, chimpanzees have a 30-year shorter potential life span, which means that chimpanzees age much faster than we do. At the age of 15, a wild chimpanzee has only 15 years left to live. In contrast, wild human hunter-gatherers at the age of 15 have an average life expectancy of 40 more years. Chimpanzees reach old age about 20 years earlier than wild human hunter-gatherers.[83]

The wild chimpanzee diet consists of very low-fat foods. Fat constitutes only about 2.5% of the dry weight of foods consumed by chimps. In contrast, fat, primarily from wild game, constitutes 38-49% of the dry weight of foods consumed by wild hunter-gatherers. In other words, wild humans eat diets containing 15-20 times as much fat as wild chimpanzees.[84]

Although chimpanzees eat more meat than any other ape, they consume far less meat than wild humans. Meat constitutes less than 5% of the wild chimpanzee diet. In contrast, most (73%) of hunter-gatherer tribes obtain 55-65% of their total energy from animal meat

---

[82] Steudel-Numbers KL. The energetic cost of locomotion: humans and primates compared to generalized endotherms. Journal of Human Evolution 2003;44: 255–262.

[83] Finch CE and Stanford CB. **Meat-Adaptive Genes and the Evolution of Slower Aging in Humans**. The Quarterly Review of Biology 2004 Mar;79(1): 3-50.

[84] Ibid.

and fat.[85] In other words, wild humans typically consume about 12 times as much meat as wild chimpanzees (as a proportion of total dietary energy).

Some people seem to think that the idea that meat shortens lifespan is logically compatible with the above data. I disagree. I submit that the logical hypothesis to draw from the evidence is that meat-eating (generally, eating animal products) with concomitant restriction of plant foods has probably played an important role in extending human lifespan beyond that of the vegetarian great apes. Greater meat-eating may promote longevity by providing large intake of highly bioavailable nutrients required for maintaining body tissues – such as protein, various fats (including essential fatty acids), cholesterol, vitamins and minerals – which would delay physical degeneration. Reducing consumption of plants may promote longevity by reducing exposure to toxic sugars and phytochemicals.

Some evidence suggests that restriction of carbohydrate intake and consequent reduction of chronic insulin exposure increases lifespan. Glucose restriction (i.e. reduced carbohydrate metabolism) shifts cell metabolism to fatty acid oxidation, which increases mitochondrial respiration and oxidative stress, which in turn stimulates an increase in stress defense responses with a marked increase in lifespan.[86, 87] On the other hand, glucose feeding increases insulin exposure and IGF-1 activity and shortens life span in worms and likely mammals

---

[85] Cordain L, Miller JB, Eaton SB, Mann N, Holt SHA, Speth JD. Plant-animal subsistence ratios and macronutrient energy estimations in worldwide hunter-gatherer diets. *Am J Clin Nutr* 2000;71:682-92.

[86] Schulz T, Karse K, Voigt A, et al.. Glucose restriction extends Caenorhabditis elegans life span by inducing mitochondrial respiration and increasing oxidative stress. Cell Metabolism 2007 Oct 3;6(4):280-293. **<http://www.sciencedirect.com/science/article/pii/S1550413107002562>**

[87] Kenyon C, Chang J, Gensch E, et al. A C. elegans mutant that lives twice as lone as wild type. Nature 1993;366:461-464.

because the insulin-signaling pathway is evolutionarily well conserved from worms to mammals.[88]

Cholesterol, Meat & Longevity

Elders who have higher blood cholesterol levels have lower mortality rates than those with low cholesterol. In one study, elders with a total cholesterol level under 170 mg/dL had a 36% higher risk of all-cause mortality than those with higher cholesterol; elders with a total cholesterol greater than 200 mg/dL had a 24% reduced all-cause mortality risk.[89] High LDL was also associated with reduced mortality risk. The authors reported that "Low TC [total cholesterol] is related to nutritional deficiencies and general poor health, which could justify this poor prognostic."

In another similar study, elders with high total cholesterol concentrations were found to live longer than those with low cholesterol.[90] Each 1 mmol/L increase in total cholesterol corresponded to a 15% decrease in all-cause mortality risk. Risk of death from cardiovascular disease was similar in people with high and low cholesterol, but those with high cholesterol had significantly lower rates of death from cancer and infections, which was the main reason for their lower total mortality.

---

[88] Lee S, Murphy CT, Kenyon C. Glucose shortens the life span of C. elegans by downregulating DAF-16/FOXO activity and aquaporin gene expression. Cell metabolism 2009 Nov 4;10(5):379-391.<**http://www.sciencedirect.com/science/article/pii/S1550413109003027**>

[89] Cabrera MAS, de Andrade SM, Dip RM. Lipids and All-Cause Mortality among Older Adults: A 12-Year Follow-Up Study. The Scientific World Journal. Volume 2012, Article ID 930139, 5 pages. doi:10.1100/2012/930139.

[90] Wecerling-Rijnsburger AW, Blauw GJ, Lagaay AM, et al. Total cholesterol and risk of mortality in the oldest old. Lancet 1997 Oct 18;350(9085):1119-23. Abstract.

Shibata et al found that Japanese centenarians ate more animal protein than average Japanese, and that high intakes of eggs, milk, fish, meat and fat were associated with longer life span.[91]

In 2018, the people of Hong Kong had the longest life expectancies in the world: 81.3 years for men, and 87.3 years for women.[92] In 2014, annual per capita meat (including fish and seafood) consumption in Hong Kong was 144 kg (317 pounds).[93] That is 0.87 pound of animal flesh per person per day; since that includes children, this likely means adults consume more than a pound daily.

In comparison, U.S. annual per capita meat consumption reached 222.2 pounds in 2018.[94] In 2015, the U.S. ranked 43 for healthy life expectancy: 78.88 years for both sexes, 76.47 for men, and 81.25 for women.[93] The Chinese in Hong Kong are on average physically smaller people than the people of European descent in the U.S.A., yet they eat more meat.

According to the U.N. Department of Economic and Social Affairs, in 2015 the top 10 nations for healthy life expectancy, in order from 1-10 were: Japan, Italy, Switzerland, Singapore, Israel, Iceland,

---

[91] Shibata H, Nagai H, Haga H, et al. Nutrition for the Japanese elderly. Nutr Health 1992;8(2-3):165-75.

[92] Senthilingam M. This urban population is leading the world in life expectancy. CNN online, March 2, 2018. <https://www.cnn.com/2018/03/02/health/hong-kong-world-longest-life-expectancy-longevity-intl/index.html>

[93] Friend E. Meat consumption trends in Asia Pacific, and what they mean for foodservice strategy. Euromonitor International 2015 Aug 15. <https://blog.euromonitor.com/2015/08/meat-consumption-trends-in-asia-pacific-and-what-they-mean-for-foodservice-strategy.html>

[94] Durisin M and Singh SD. Americans' meat consumption to hit a record in 2018. Seattle Times online 2018 January 2. <https://www.seattletimes.com/business/americans-meat-consumption-set-to-hit-a-record-in-2018/>

Spain, Australia, Hong Kong and Sweden.[95] (Hong Kong has since ascended to first rank.[90]) All consume meat and fish liberally (Table 4.4).

Table 4.4: Per capita annual meat and fish consumption in 2011 in the top eleven most long-lived nations of 2015

Nation	Life expectancy (y)	Meat kg (2011)	Fish kg (2011)	Total kg
Japan	83.74	49	54	103
Italy	83.31	87	25	112
Switzerland	82.84	75	17	92
Singapore	82.66	Not avail.	Not avail.	90
Israel	82.64	102	20	122
Iceland	82.30	87	90	177
Spain	82.28	93	42	135
Australia	83.42	121	26	147
Hong Kong	82.07	154	71	225
Sweden	81.93	82	31	113
France	81.85	89	35	124

Sources: References 90, 91, 93
Meat and fish consumption 2011: Helgi Library: Meat consumption per capita by country. <https://www.helgilibrary.com/indicators/meat-consumption-per-capita/>; Helgi Library. Fish consumption per capita by country. <https://www.helgilibrary.com/indicators/fish-consumption-per-capita/>

---

[95] UN DESA: World Population Prospects, The 2015 Revision. United Nations, 2015. <https://esa.un.org/unpd/wpp/Publications/Files/WPP2015_Volume-I_Comprehensive-Tables.pdf>

As noted, as of 2018 Hong Kong has ascended to the first rank for longevity.[90] It is therefore of interest to note that in 2015 they had the highest per capita meat+fish consumption of the top eleven most long-lived populations (Table 4.4).

In Japan between 1970 and 2007 deaths from coronary heart disease decline while the people increased their meat and fat consumption and their mean total serum cholesterol.[96] During this time Japan rose to the top of the ranks for healthy life expectancy. This is called the Japanese Paradox.

Similarly, in Spain, between 1966 and 1990 intakes of meat, dairy, fish, fat, saturated fat, and fruit increased while intakes of olive oil, sugar and all foods rich in carbohydrates decreased, and rates of death from death from cardiovascular disease, coronary heart disease, and stroke all decreased.[97] This is called the Spanish Paradox.

The French eat diets high in saturated fat, dairy and meat – more than in the U.S. – and yet have low risk of cardiovascular disease.[98] In 2015 they also ranked 11 in the world for life expectancy, way ahead of the U.S.. This is called the French paradox.

In comparison, in India in 2014 annual per capita meat consumption was only about 11 kg and vegetarians made up 30-40% of the population.[91] In 2015 India ranked 143 for healthy life expectancy: only 67.47 years overall, 66.13 for men and 68.93 for women.[93]

---

[96] Ueshima H. Explanation for the Japanese paradox: prevention of increase in coronary heart disease and reduction in stroke. J Atheroscler Thromb. 2007 Dec;14(6):278-86. Epub 2007 Dec 17. Review. PubMed PMID: 18174657.

[97] Serra-Majem L, Ribas L, Tresserras R, et al.: How could changes in diet explain changes in coronary heart disease mortality in Spain? The Spanish paradox. Am J Clin Nutr 1995 June 1;61(6):1351S-1359S. https://doi.org/10.1093/ajcn/61.6.1351S

[98] Ferrières J. The French paradox: lessons for other countries. *Heart*. 2004;90(1): 107-111. <https://www.ncbi.nlm.nih.gov/pmc/articles/PMC1768013/>

These findings seem paradoxical only if you believe that humans are designed to eat a plant-based diet. The fact that so many of these paradoxes exist tells us that the underlying assumption that we are adapted to a plant based diet is erroneous. If you accept that we are apex predators – hypercarnivores – highly adapted to eating animal protein and fat, these paradoxes evaporate. Of course a meat-based diet is going to promote health and longevity of a carnivorous animal.

Cholesterol, Muscular Strength & Longevity

Muscular strength "has an independent role in the prevention of chronic diseases whereas muscular weakness is strongly related to functional limitations and physical disability."[99] Muscular strength reduces the risk of premature death from cancer and all causes in men,[100] and women.[101] High midlife grip strength dramatically increases the probability of extreme longevity; centenarians belonged 2.5 times more often to the highest third of grip strength in midlife.[102] Muscular weakness in middle-aged and older individuals

---

[99] Volaklis KA, Halle M, Meisinger C. Muscular strength as a strong predictor of mortality: A narrative review. Eur J Intern Med 2015 June;26(5):303-10.

[100] Ruiz JR, Sui X, Lobelo F, et al. Association between muscular strength and mortality in men: prospective cohort study. BMJ: British Medical Journal. 2008;337(7661):92-95. doi:10.1136/bmj.a439. <**http://www.ncbi.nlm.nih.gov/pmc/articles/PMC2453303/**>

[101] Rantanen T, Vopato S, Ferrucci L, et al. Handgrip strength and cause-specific and total mortality in older disabled women: Exploring the mechanism. J Am Geriatrics Soc 2003 April 29;51(5):636-41.

[102] Rantanen T, Masaki K, He Q, et al.: Midlife muscle strength and human longevity up to age 100 years: a 44-year prospective study among a decedent cohort. Age (Dordr) 2012 jun;34(3): 563-570. <https://www.ncbi.nlm.nih.gov/pmc/articles/PMC3337929/>

is strongly related to functional limitations and physical disability, including fatal falls and bone fractures.[103]

Strength training is the only physical training method proven to retard and even reverse aging of muscles.[104] Therefore, the best diet for longevity would likely be that which best supports muscular strength and recovery from strength training.

Cholesterol is an intrinsic part of muscle cell membranes and therefore very important for muscle health and strength. Heavy resistance exercise depletes blood cholesterol needed for muscle cell membrane repair while supplementing cholesterol accelerates recovery from such exercise.[105]

Riechman et al found a dose-response relationship between dietary and serum cholesterol and gains in lean mass among men and women 60- to 69- years of age (the more cholesterol they consumed, the more lean mass they gained).[106] A placebo-controlled study found greater strength gains among subjects supplemented with 800

---

[103] Strasser B, Volaklis K, Fuchs D, Burtscher M: Role of dietary protein and muscular fitness on longevity and aging. Aging Dis. 2018 Feb;9(1):119-132. <https://www.ncbi.nlm.nih.gov/pmc/articles/PMC5772850/>

[104] Melov S, Tarnopolsky MA, Beckman K, et al.. Resistance Exercise Reverses Aging in Human Skeletal Muscle. PLOS 23 May 2007. **<http://journals.plos.org/plosone/article?id=10.1371/journal.pone.0000465>**

[105] Riechman SE, Woock Lee C, Chikani G, et al. Cholesterol and Skeletal Muscle Health. World Review of nutrition and dietetics 2009 Feb;100:71-9.

[106] Riechman SE, Andrews RD, Maclean DA, et al. Statins and dietary and serum cholesterol are associated with increased lean mass following resistance training. J Gerontol A Biol Sci Med Sci 2007 Oct;62(10):1164-71. https://www.ncbi.nlm.nih.gov/pubmed/17921432

mg/d (3 egg yolks) of cholesterol compared to 400 or 200 mg/d.[107] Another study found that subjects assigned to eating a high cholesterol diet containing 3 eggs daily gained more muscle mass and strength than those who consumed 0 or 1 egg daily.[108] A final study found that healthy, young (20-28 y) adults who consumed 800 mg/d cholesterol had nearly 3 times greater post-resistance training myofibrillar protein synthesis rate 22 h after training than the low cholesterol group – heralding increased muscle growth.[109]

Older individuals need 1.2 to 2.0 g protein per kg body mass to maintain and regain muscle and bone mass, and animal proteins are more effective at promoting muscle protein synthesis after resistance training, perhaps due to their higher proportion of the amino acid • leucine.[110]

Physical Regeneration and Longevity

Longevity is based on *reproduction* of cells to regenerate body tissues. Reproduction of cells and regeneration of tissues requires

---

[107] Riechman SE, Woock Lee C, Gasier HG, Chikani G. Dietary Cholesterol and Skeletal Muscle Hypertrophy with Resistance Training: A Randomized Placebo-Controlled Trial. The FASEB Journal 2008 March;22:962.13.<http://www.fasebj.org/cgi/content/meeting_abstract/22/1_MeetingAbstracts/962.13>

[108] Riechman SE, Gasier HG. Effect of Dietary Cholesterol on Muscle Hypertrophy with Resistance Training: Randomized Double Blind Placebo-Controlled Trial. Med Sci Sports Exer 2007 May;39(5):S291-S292. http://journals.lww.com/acsm-msse/Fulltext/2007/05001/Effect_of_Dietary_Cholesterol_on_Muscle.1949.aspx

[109] Lee CW, Lee TV, Chen VCW, et al. Dietary Cholesterol Affects Skeletal Muscle Protein Synthesis Following Acute Resistance Exercise. FASEB J 2011 April;25(1):Supplement lb 563. http://www.fasebj.org/content/25/1_Supplement/lb563.short

[110] Strasser B, Volaklis K, Fuchs D, Burtscher M: Role of dietary protein and muscular fitness on longevity and aging. Aging Dis. 2018 Feb;9(1):119-132. <https://www.ncbi.nlm.nih.gov/pmc/articles/PMC5772850/>

nutrients obtained from food. Aside from water, the main constituents of our cells and vital body tissues (muscles, bones, organs, brain) are animal protein, fat, cholesterol and minerals (calcium, phosphorus, sulfur, magnesium).

By shifting from a plant-based diet to increased meat-eating, human ancestors would have reduced carbohydrate intake and insulin exposure, factors which appear to shorten lifespan. They also would have had increased their supply of cholesterol, protein, essential fatty acids, minerals, fat-soluble vitamins (see Chapter 7 for the role of retinol vitamin A in promoting life extension), and other animal-based nutrients which the body can use to repair and regenerate itself.

Thus, the shift from a plant-based subsistence to animal-based subsistence (meat or milk) provided material, nutritional support for the dramatic increase in human lifespan compared to the primarily vegetarian great apes.

Heart Disease

Although heart disease is a leading cause of death in captive chimpanzees, responsible for about 36% of chimpanzee deaths, chimps who die of heart disease do not have gross coronary atherosclerosis, and, of interest, they develop the disease despite being fed diets providing less than 5% of energy from fats.[111] In contrast human hunter-gatherers rarely or never develop atherosclerosis or coronary heart disease despite consuming meat-based diets.[112] This makes us similar to dogs and cats, both of which

---

[111] Varki N, Anderson D, Herndon JG, et al. Heart disease is common in humans and chimpanzees, but is caused by different pathological processes. *Evolutionary Applications*. 2009;2(1):101-112. doi:10.1111/j.1752-4571.2008.00064.x <**https://www.ncbi.nlm.nih.gov/pmc/articles/PMC3352420/**>

112 Cordain L, Eaton SB, Brand-Miller J, et al., "The paradoxical nature of hunter-gatherer diets: meat-based, yet non-atherogenic," Eur J Clin Nutr 2002;56(1):542-552. DOI:101.1038/sj/ejcn/1601353. <**http://www.nature.com/ejcn/journal/v56/n1s/pdf/1601353a.pdf**>

exhibit a high resistance to atherosclerosis when fed their natural, meat-based diets.

General Cholesterol Metabolism

Carnivores consume large amounts of cholesterol, whereas plantivores do not. Consequently, carnivores have mechanisms for maintaining normal body levels of cholesterol in the face of high meat, fat and cholesterol intake, whereas plantivores do not.

When carnivores consume cholesterol, they produce less themselves.[113] In modern humans, consumption of dietary cholesterol suppresses endogenous cholesterol synthesis.[114, 115] Inuit hunters eating carnivorous diets supplying 60-80% energy from animal fats, and African herdsmen eating diets rich in saturated fats from dairy, have *on average* low normal cholesterol levels (mean 141 and 135-166 mg/dL, respectively).[116]

---

[113] Pertsemlidis D, Kirchman EH, Ahrens EH. **Regulation of Cholesterol Metabolism in the Dog.** J Clin Invest 1973 Sept;52(9):2353-2367. PMCID: PMC333040.

114 Jones PJH, Pappu AS, Hatcher L, et al., "Dietary Cholesterol Feeding Suppresses Human Cholesterol Synthesis Measured by Deuterium Incorporation and Urinary Mevalonic Acid Levels," Arteriosclerosis, Thrombosis, and Vascular Biology 1996;16:1222-1228. **<http://atvb.ahajournals.org/content/16/10/1222>**

[115] Cohen DE. Balancing Cholesterol Synthesis and Absorption in the Gastrointestinal Tract. *Journal of clinical lipidology*. 2008;2(2):S1-S3. doi: 10.1016/j.jacl.2008.01.004. **<https://www.ncbi.nlm.nih.gov/pmc/articles/PMC2390860/>**

[116] Eaton SB, Konner M, Shostak M. Stone Agers in the Fast Lane: Chronic Degenerative Diseases in Evolutionary Perspective. Am J Med 1988 April; 84:739-747.

In contrast, chimpanzees fed diets containing as little as 5% fat from palm oil develop cholesterol levels greater than 200 mg/dL.[117] Evidently chimpanzees are much more sensitive to dietary saturated fat than humans.[118]

Contrary to popular belief, elevated total or LDL cholesterol evidently does not in and of itself have harmful effects in humans. If triglycerides are low and HDL high, which typically occurs on a low carbohydrate hypercarnivore diet, then the LDL will generally be primarily composed of a low number of large fluffy lipoproteins which evidence indicates are less or non- atherogenic and possibly even protective against coronary artery disease.[119, 120, 121, 122]

The Framingham Study found that individuals who had an LDL of 130 mg/dL (so-called high LDL) or greater but high HDL and

---

[117] Finch CE and Stanford CB. **Meat-Adaptive Genes and the Evolution of Slower Aging in Humans**. The Quarterly Review of Biology 2004 Mar;79(1): 3-50.4.

[118] Ibid.

[119] McNamara JR, Jenner JL, Wilson PW, Schaefer EJ. Change in LDL particle size is associated with change in plasma triglyceride concentration. Art Thromb Vasc Biol 1992;12:1284-90.

[120] Tchernof A, Lamarche B, Prud'Homme D, Nadeau A, Moorjani S, Labrie F, Lupien PJ, Després JP. The dense LDL phenotype. Association with plasma lipoprotein levels, visceral obesity, and hyperinsulinemia in men. Diabetes Care. 1996 Jun;19(6):629-37. PubMed PMID: 8725863.

[121] Cromwell WC, Otvos JD, Keyes MJ, et al. LDL Particle Number and Risk of Future Cardiovascular Disease in the Framingham Offspring Study – Implications for LDL Management. *Journal of clinical lipidology*. 2007;1(6):583-592. doi: 10.1016/j.jacl.2007.10.001. https://www.ncbi.nlm.nih.gov/pmc/articles/PMC2720529/

[122] Lamarche B, Lemiex I, Després JP. The small, dense LDL phenotype and the risk of coronary heart disease: epidemiology, patho-physiology and therapeutic aspects. Diabetes Metab 1999 Sep;25(3):199-211.

triglycerides less than 100 mg/dL had a low cardiovascular disease risk ratio similar to individuals with high HDL and both triglycerides and LDL below 100 mg/dL.[123] Elevated LDL increased cardiovascular disease risk only if accompanied with low HDL or triglycerides greater than 100 mg/dL.

Elevated fasting serum insulin level is a risk factor for coronary artery disease, hypertension and stroke.[124, 125, 126]

The USDA has stated that cholesterol "is not a nutrient of concern for overconsumption" because "available evidence shows no appreciable relationship between consumption of dietary cholesterol and serum cholesterol."[127]

Critical reviews of some of the key studies commonly claimed to support the need for dietary or serum cholesterol reduction have shown that these studies do not support the conclusion. For

---

[123] Bartlett J, Predazzi IM, Williams SM, et al. Is Isolated Low HDL-C a CVD Risk Factor?: New Insights from the Framingham Offspring Study. *Circulation Cardiovascular quality and outcomes*. 2016;9(3):206-212. doi:10.1161/CIRCOUTCOMES.115.002436. <https://www.ncbi.nlm.nih.gov/pmc/articles/PMC4871717/>

[124] Lamarche B, Tchernof A, Mauriège P, et al. Fasting Insulin and Apolipoprotein B Levels and Low-Density Lipoprotein Particle Size as Risk Factors for Ischemic Heart Disease. *JAMA*. 1998;279(24):1955–1961. doi:10.1001/jama.279.24.1955 <https://jamanetwork.com/journals/jama/fullarticle/187669>

[125] Ginsberg HN. Insulin resistance and cardiovascular disease. *Journal of Clinical Investigation*. 2000;106(4):453-458.

[126] Xun P, Wu Y, He Q, He K. Fasting insulin concentrations and incidence of hypertension, stroke, and coronary heart disease: a meta-analysis of prospective cohort studies. *The American Journal of Clinical Nutrition*. 2013;98(6): 1543-1554. doi:10.3945/ajcn.113.065565.

[127] USDA. <https://health.gov/dietaryguidelines/2015-scientific-report/06-chapter-1/d1-2.asp>

example, in 2016 the BMJ published a re-evaluation of the traditional diet-heart hypothesis through analysis of recovered data from the Minnesota Coronary Experiment of 1968-73, which found that *reducing* serum cholesterol *increased* the risk of death by 22% for each 30 mg/dL drop:

> "The intervention group had significant reduction in serum cholesterol compared with controls (mean change from baseline −13.8% v −1.0%; P<0.001). Kaplan Meier graphs showed no mortality benefit for the intervention group in the full randomized cohort or for any prespecified subgroup. There was a 22% higher risk of death for each 30 mg/dL (0.78 mmol/L) reduction in serum cholesterol in covariate adjusted Cox regression models (hazard ratio 1.22, 95% confidence interval 1.14 to 1.32; P<0.001). **There was no evidence of benefit in the intervention group for coronary atherosclerosis or myocardial infarcts**. Systematic review identified five randomized controlled trials for inclusion (n=10 808). In meta-analyses, **these cholesterol lowering interventions showed no evidence of benefit on mortality from coronary heart disease** (1.13, 0.83 to 1.54) or all cause mortality (1.07, 0.90 to 1.27)." [128, bold added]

In people aged at least 60 years, high LDL and total cholesterol is inversely associated with mortality; elderly people with high cholesterol live as long or longer than those with low LDL.[129]

---

[128] Ramsden Christopher E, Zamora Daisy, Majchrzak-Hong Sharon, Faurot Keturah R, Broste Steven K, Frantz Robert P et al. Re-evaluation of the traditional diet-heart hypothesis: analysis of recovered data from Minnesota Coronary Experiment (1968-73) BMJ 2016; 353 :i1246 <http://www.bmj.com/content/353/bmj.i1246>

[129] Ravnskov U, Diamond DM, Hama R, *et al*. Lack of an association or an inverse association between low-density-lipoprotein cholesterol and mortality in the elderly: a systematic review. *BMJ Open* 2016;**6**:e010401. doi: 10.1136/bmjopen-2015-010401 <http://bmjopen.bmj.com/content/6/6/e010401>

A study of Yugoslavian males aged 35-62 years found that those with a lower cholesterol level experienced a higher mortality than those with a higher cholesterol.[130]

Some studies that identify total cholesterol as a risk factor for coronary mortality have also found that "having a low cholesterol level does not prolong survival in the elderly; on the contrary, low cholesterol predicts neoplastic [cancer] mortality in women and any other noncardiovascular mortality in both genders."[131]

Reduced concentrations on LDL and total cholesterol have been associated with increased mortality from cancer, severe respiratory diseases and inflammatory diseases.[132]

Remnant cholesterol, defined as total lipoprotein cholesterol minus LDL and HDL [TC - (LDL + HDL)] appears to have a stronger

---

[130] Kozarevic D, McGee D, Vojvodic N, et al. Serum cholesterol and mortality: the Yugoslavia Cardiovascular Disease Study. Am J Epidemiol 1981 Jul;114(1): 21-8. PMID:7246527

[131] Casiglia E, Mazza A, Tikhonoff V, Scarpa R, Schiavon L, Pessina AC. Total cholesterol and mortality in the elderly. J Intern Med. 2003 Oct;254(4):353-62. PubMed PMID: 12974874.

[132] Varbo A, Freiberg JJ, Nordestgaard BG. Extreme Nonfasting Remnant Cholesterol vs Extreme LDL Cholesterol as Contributors to Cardiovascular Disease and All-Cause Mortality in 90000 Individuals from the General Population. Clin Chem 2015;61(3):533-543. <http://clinchem.aaccjnls.org/content/clinchem/61/3/533.full.pdf>

relationship to cardiovascular disease risk than LDL or total cholesterol.[133, 134]

A nonfasting remnant cholesterol increase of 39 mg/dl was found associated with a 2.8-fold causal risk for ischemic heart disease, independent of reduced HDL cholesterol.[110] Remnant cholesterol was highly correlated with non-fasting triglyceride levels, inversely related to HDL levels, and "less correlated with LDL cholesterol levels." Increasing remnant cholesterol and decreasing HDL levels were more strongly predictive of ischemic heart disease than increasing LDL levels.

Remnant cholesterol was found to cause arterial wall inflammation and a multilevel cellular immune response in humans.[135]

People with ischemic heart disease and remnant cholesterol greater than 39 mg/dL were found to have a higher risk of all-cause mortality than those with less than 39 mg/dl, whereas people with ischemic heart disease and an LDL greater than 116 mg/dL did not

[133] McPherson R. Remnant Cholesterol: "Non-(HDL-C + LDL-C)" as a Coronary Artery Disease Risk Factor. J Am Coll Card 2013 Jan 29:61(4):437-439. <https://www.sciencedirect.com/science/article/pii/S0735109712055210?via%3Dihub>

[134] Varbo A, Benn M, Tybjaerg-Hansen A, et al. Remnant Cholesterol as a Causal Risk Factor for Ischemic Heart Disease. J Am Coll Card 2013 Jan 29;61(4): 427-36. <https://www.sciencedirect.com/science/article/pii/S0735109712055222>

[135] Moens SJB, Verweij SL, Schnitzler JG, et al. Remnant Cholesterol Elicits Arterial Wall Inflammation and a Multilevel Cellular Immune Response in Humans. Arterioscler Thromb Vasc Biol. 2017;37: <http://atvb.ahajournals.org/content/atvbaha/early/2017/03/23/ATVBAHA.116.308834.full.pdf>

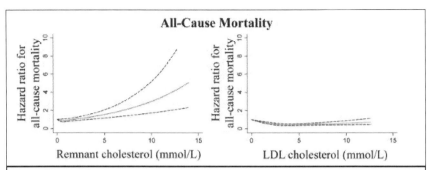

All-Cause Mortality

Remnant cholesterol (mmol/L)

LDL cholesterol (mmol/L)

Figure 4.2: Nonfasting remnant and LDL cholesterol and all-cause mortality risk. Solid lines represent hazard ratios, dotted lines represent 95% confidence intervals. Source: Reference 136.

have a higher all-cause mortality than those will LDL less than 116 mg/dL (Figure 4.2).[136]

Elevated nonfasting remnant cholesterol was found causally associated with low-grade inflammation (measured by C-reactive protein) and ischemic heart disease (IHD), with each 39 mg/dL increase associated with a 3-fold greater risk for IHD, compared to only 1.8-fold increased risk for a 39 mg/dL increase in LDL.[137]

Nonfasting remnant cholesterol concentrations were associated stepwise with all-cause mortality, whereas LDL cholesterol concentrations were associated with decreased all-cause mortality

[136] Jepsen AK, Langsted A, Varbo A, et al. Increased Remnant Cholesterol Explains Part of Residual Risk of All-Cause Mortality in 5414 Patients with Ischemic Heart Disease. Clin Chem 2016 April;62(4): 593-604. DOI: 10.1373/ clinchem.2015.253757 <clinchem.aaccjnls.org/content/62/4/593>

[137] Varbo A, Benn M, Tybjaerg-Hansen A, et al. Elevated Remnant Cholesterol Causes Both Low-Grade Inflammation and Ischemic Heart Disease, Whereas Elevated Low-Density Lipoprotein Cholesterol Causes Ischemic Heart Disease Without Inflammation. Circulation 2013;128:1298-1309. <http:// circ.ahajournals.org/content/128/12/1298? ijkey=1ad0cc939e185b2369f6fcf0323ea07aa961f345&keytype2=tf_ipsecsha >

risk in a U-shaped pattern.[138] Remnant cholesterol was the best predictor of all-cause mortality (Figure 4.2). Diets low in carbohydrates (plants) typically minimize remnant cholesterol.

In 2018, the REGARDS study authors reported that coronary heart disease, stroke and all cause mortality risks were lowest in people with an LDL between 70 mg/dL and 200 mg/dL and a CRP below 2. Subjects with an LDL between 125 and 150 mg/dL had the lowest all-cause mortality risk.[139]

Dietary Cholesterol Requirement for Reproduction

We have some evidence suggesting that we need dietary fat and cholesterol – in other words, animal products – to maintain healthy levels of reproductive hormones and fertility.
In men, HDL cholesterol and testosterone levels are positively related.[140, 141] Eating egg yolks and saturated animal fat raises HDL

---

[138] Varbo A, Freiberg JJ, Nordestgaard BG. Extreme Nonfasting Remnant Cholesterol vs Extreme LDL Cholesterol as Contributors to Cardiovascular Disease and All-Cause Mortality in 90000 Individuals from the General Population. Clin Chem 2015;61(3):533-543. <http://clinchem.aaccjnls.org/content/clinchem/61/3/533.full.pdf>

[139] Penson PE, Long DL, Howard G, et al.: Associations between very low concentrations of low density lipoprotein cholesterol, high sensitivity C-reactive protein, and health outcomes in the Reasons for Geographical and Racial Differences in Stroke (REGARDS) study. Eur Heart J 218;0:1-13. doi:10.1093/eurheartj/ehy533.

140 Freedman DS, O'Brien TR, Flanders WD, et al., "Relation of serum testosterone level to high density lipoprotein cholesterol and other characteristics in men," Arterioscler Throm Vas Bio 1991 Mar-Apr;11(2):307-15. <http://atvb.ahajournals.org/content/11/2/307.long>

141 Stanworth RD, Kapoor D, Channer KS, Jones TH, "Testosterone levels correlate positively with HDL cholesterol levels in men with Type 2 diabetes," Endocrine Abstracts 2007;14:P628.

levels.[142, 143, 144, 145, 146] A low-fat high-fiber diet decreases testosterone in healthy Caucasian males age 50-60 years,[147] and lowers estrogen levels by up to 30 percent and lengthens menstrual

[142] Mutungi G, Ratliff G, Publisi M, et al. Dietary Cholsterol from Eggs Increases Plasma HDL Cholesterol in Overweight Men Consuming a Carbohydrate-Restricted Diet. J Nutr 2008 Feb;138(2):272-76. <http://jn.nutrition.org/content/138/2/272.full?cited-by=yes&legid=nutrition;138/2/272#cited-by>

[143] Schnohr P, Thomsen OO, Riis Hansen P, Boberg-Ans G, Lawaetz H, Weeke T. Egg consumption and high-density-lipoprotein cholesterol. J Intern Med. 1994 Mar;235(3):249-51. PubMed PMID: 8120521.

[144] Mayurasakorn K, Srisura W, Sitphahul P, Hongto PO. High-density lipoprotein cholesterol changes after continuous egg consumption in healthy adults. J Med Assoc Thai. 2008 Mar;91(3):400-7. PubMed PMID: 18575296.

[145] Hayek T, Ito Y, Azrolan N, et al. Dietary fat increases high density lipoprotein (HDL) levels both by increasing the transport rates and decreasing the fractional catabolic rates of HDL cholesterol ester and apolipoprotein (Apo) A-I. Presentation of a new animal model and mechanistic studies in human Apo A-I transgenic and control mice. *Journal of Clinical Investigation*. 1993;91(4): 1665-1671.

[146] Wolf G. High-fat, high-cholesterol diet raises plasma HDL cholesterol: studies on the mechanism of this effect. Nutr Rev. 1996 Jan;54(1 Pt 1):34-5. Review. PubMed PMID: 8919697.

147 Wang C, Catlin DH, Starcevic B, et al., "Low-fat high-fiber diet decreased serum and urine androgens in men," J Clin Endocrinol Metab 2005 Jun;90(6): 3550-9.

cycle in premenopausal women.[148, 149, 150] Reducing fat intake from 40 to 25 percent of calories and cholesterol from 400 mg to 200 mg per day produced a 36% decrease in serum estrogen levels in premenopausal women.[151]

Premenopausal women eating vegetarian, low cholesterol diets (Seventh Day Adventists) were found to have a 5 times increased incidence of menstrual irregularities, indicating that women may need dietary cholesterol intake to maintain adequate estrogen levels and fertility.[152]

Some studies show that, compared to meat-eaters, vegetarians in modernized nations have lower rates of marriage and child-bearing,

148 Gann PH, Chatterton RT, Gapstur SM, et al., "The effects of a low-fat/high-fiber diet on sex hormone levels and menstrual cycling in premenopausal women," Cancer 2003 Nov 1;98(9):1870-1879. ,http://onlinelibrary.wiley.com/doi/10.1002/cncr.11735/full>

149 Goldin BR, Woods MN, Spiegelman DL, et al., "The effect of dietary fat and fiber on serum estrogen concentrations in premenopausal women under controlled dietary conditions," Cancer 1994 Aug 1;74(S3):1125-1131. <http://onlinelibrary.wiley.com/doi/10.1002/1097-0142(19940801)74:3%2B%3C1125::AID-CNCR2820741521%3E3.0.CO;2-5/pdf>

150 Bagga D, Ashley JM, Geffrey SP, et al., "Effects of a Very Low Fat, High Fiber Diet on Serum Hormones and Menstrual Function," Cancer 1995;76:2491-6. <http://onlinelibrary.wiley.com/doi/10.1002/1097-0142(19951215)76:12%3C2491::AID-CNCR2820761213%3E3.0.CO;2-R/pdf>

151 Woods MN, Gorbach SL, Longcope C, et al., "Low-fat, high-fiber diet and serum estrone sulfate in premenopausal women," Am J Clin Nutr 1989 Jun;49(6): 1179-83.

152 Pedersen AB et al.,"Menstrual differences due to vegetarian and nonvegetarian diets," Am J Clin Nutr 1991;53:879-85.

providing further evidence that vegetarian diets may reduce sexual attractiveness, libido and/or fertility.[153]

Whereas the great apes have good fertility on their natural plant-based diets containing little or no meat, we have evidence that meat-free vegetarian and especially vegan diets reduce both female and male fertility.[154, 155, 156]

Brain Size

As a general rule, relative to body mass, carnivores need and have larger brains than herbivores. An herbivore does not require much cognitive power to obtain its food. No one needs a plan or strategy to successfully graze grass or collect fruit. In contrast, a predator must outwit his prey with a winning strategy; therefore the predator must have more cognitive power than his prey.

The nervous system including brain is largely composed of lipids including fat and cholesterol. The myelin sheath surrounding all nerves is 78-81% lipids; white matter is 49-66% lipids; and gray matter is 36-40% lipids. Cholesterol forms 19-22% of myelin, 7-8%

153 Appleby, Paul N et al. "Mortality in Vegetarians and Comparable Nonvegetarians in the United Kingdom." The American Journal of Clinical Nutrition 103.1 (2016): 218–230. PMC. Web. 8 Mar. 2017.

154 Pedersen AB, Bartholomew MJ, Dolence LA, et al., "Menstrual differences due to vegetarian and nonvegetarian diets," Am J Clin Nutr 1991;53:879-85.

155 Orzylowska EM, Jacobson JD, Ko EY, et al., "Decreased sperm concentration and motility in a subpopulation of vegetarian males at a designated Blue Zone geographic region," <http://www.fertstert.org/article/S0015-0282(14)01556-8/pdf>

156 Orzylowska EM, Jacobson JD, Bareh GM, Ko EY, Corselli JU, Chan PJ. Food intake diet and sperm characteristics in a blue zone: a Loma Linda Study. Eur J Obstet Gynecol Reprod Biol. 2016 Aug;203:112-5. doi: 10.1016/j.ejogrb.2016.05.043. PubMed PMID: 27280539.

of gray matter, and 12-15% of white matter.[157] Literally we are all fat heads.

The chimpanzees have brains in the general range of 262-500 cm³. In contrast, we have brains about 3 times larger, with an average volume of about 1330 cm³.

The earliest known members of our genus had brains about 1.5 to 2.0 times the size of chimpanzees. They hunted large animals using ambush methods as early as 2.5 million years ago, and by 2.0 million years ago our ancestors were certainly persistently eating meat from grazing herbivores.[158, 159, 160, 161]

Over the course of the past 2.5 million years, human brain size increased so long as our ancestors sustained animal-based diets. Neanderthal and Cro-Magnon people had the largest brains, 1736 cm³ and 1600 cm³ respectively. Our ancestors' bones contain nitrogen isotopes that reveal their predominant protein sources. From 100,000 to 28,000 years ago, Neanderthals had top-level

---

[157] O'Brien JS and Sampson EL. Lipid composition of the normal human brain: gray matter, white matter, and myelin. J Lipid Research 1965;6:536-544.

158 Ferraro JV, Plummer TW, Pobiner BL, Oliver JS, Bishop LC, Braun DR, et al. (2013) Earliest Archaeological Evidence of Persistent Hominin Carnivory. PLoS ONE 8(4): e62174. doi:10.1371/journal.pone.0062174 <https://www.ncbi.nlm.nih.gov/pmc/articles/PMC3636145/>

159 McKie R. Humans hunted for meat 2 million years ago. The Guardian 2012 Sep 22. Accessed Dec 1, 2017 at: <https://www.theguardian.com/science/2012/sep/23/human-hunting-evolution-2million-years>

160 Bunn HT, Gurtov AN. Prey mortality profiles indicate that Early Pleistocene Homo at Olduvai was an ambush predator. Quaternary International 2014 Feb 16;322-23:44-53.

161 Pobiner B. Meat-Eating Among the Earliest Humans. American Scientist 2016 Mar-Apr;104(2):110. Accessed online Dec 5, 2017 at: <https://www.americanscientist.org/article/meat-eating-among-the-earliest-humans>

carnivore diets, no more than 20% plant foods.[162] People living in Eurasia 30,000 to 20,000 years ago also ate animal-based diets, perhaps including more aquatic animals than the Neanderthals, and upper Paleolithic Europeans living in southern England 13,000 years ago also ate an animal-based diet, and most likely composed primarily of herbivore flesh.[163]

Since that time we have collectively shifted to plant-based diets and we now have smaller brains (as well as less brawn) than our ancestors.[164]

Evidently, our shift to a plant-based diet caused the brain atrophy. Animal foods provide nutrients critical to brain development that plant foods do not provide, including vitamin B12, the omega-6 fatty acid arachidonic acid (AA), the omega-3 essential fatty acid DHA.

Human infants need both AA and DHA for proper development and function of the retina and central nervous system. DHA and AA together form 20 percent of the dry weight of the brain, and the brain consumes about 17.8 mg daily of AA. Supplementation with AA has improved cognitive functions in autistic children and in elderly individuals.[165]

---

162 Richards MP, "A review of the archaeological evidence for Paleolithic and Neolithic subsistence," Eur J Clin Nutr 2002;56. doi:10.1038/sj.ejcn.1601646 <http://www.nature.com/ejcn/journal/v56/n12/full/1601646a.html>

163 Ibid.

164 Choi CQ, "Humans Still Evolving as Our Brains Shrink," LiveScience 2009 Nov 13.

165 Tallima H, El Ridi R. Arachidonic acid: Physiological roles and potential health benefits – A review. J Adv Res 2017. <https://doi.org/10.1016/j.jare.2017.11.004>

People with lower red blood cell contents of DHA showed progressive brain atrophy over 8 years compared to those who had higher DHA levels from animal food intake.[166]

Elders with lower vitamin B12 intakes and status were found to have an increased risk of progressive brain atrophy over the course of five years of observation.[167] As already noted, vegans and some vegetarians typically have lower B12 levels than found in these elders.[168]

Compared to plant foods animal foods are also richer sources of several brain-specific minerals: iron, zinc, iodide, copper, and selenium. I discuss this in detail in Chapter 12.

Cognition and Emotion

The Framingham Study found a significant positive linear association between total cholesterol and measures of verbal fluency, attention/concentration, abstract reasoning, and a composite score

[166] Pottala JV, Yaffe K, Robinson JG, Espeland MA, Wallace R, Harris WS. Higher RBC EPA + DHA corresponds with larger total brain and hippocampal volumes: WHIMS-MRI Study. *Neurology*. 2014;82(5):435-442. doi:10.1212/WNL. 0000000000000080. <**https://www.ncbi.nlm.nih.gov/pmc/articles/ PMC3917688/**>

[167] Vogiatzoglou A, Refsum H, Johnston C, et al.. Vitamin B12 status and rate of brain volume loss in community-dwelling elderly. Neurology 2008;71:826-832. Accessed Dec 12, 2017 from: <**http://citeseerx.ist.psu.edu/viewdoc/download? doi=10.1.1.509.9234&rep=rep1&type=pdf**>

[168] Obersby D, Chappell DC, Dunnett A, Tsiami AA. Plasma total homocysteine status of vegetarians compared with omnivores: a systematic review and meta-analysis. Brit J Nutr 2013 Mar 14;109(5):785-94. <**https://www.cambridge.org/ core/journals/british-journal-of-nutrition/article/div-classtitleplasma-total-homocysteine-status-of-vegetarians-compared-with-omnivores-a-systematic-review-and-meta-analysisdiv/1754320C613E6CD7F9AED4EE60C421B5/core-reader**>

measuring multiple cognitive domains.[169] Subjects with "desirable" TC levels (<200 mg/dL) performed less well than participants with borderline-high TC levels (200-239 mg/dL) and participants with high TC levels (>240 mg/dL). The authors concluded that "lower naturally occurring TC levels are associated with poorer performance on cognitive measures, which place high demands on abstract reasoning, attention/concentration, word fluency, and executive functioning."

Ingestion of fat reduces behavioral and neural responses to sad emotion, even when subjects are unaware that they are ingesting fat.[170] Increased meat, poultry and game consumption has been associated with a reduced risk of depression,[171, 172] and some studies report higher incidence of anxiety and depression among meat

---

[169] Elias PK, Elias MF, D'Agostino RB, Sullivan LM, Wolf PA. Serum cholesterol and cognitive performance in the Framingham heart study. Psychosomatic Medicine 2005;67:24-30.

[170] Van Oudenhove, Lukas et al. "Fatty Acid–induced Gut-Brain Signaling Attenuates Neural and Behavioral Effects of Sad Emotion in Humans." The Journal of Clinical Investigation 121.8 (2011): 3094–3099. PMC. Web. 27 Apr. 2017.

[171] Meyer BJ, Kolanu N, Griffiths DA, Grounds B, Howe PR, Kreis IA. Food groups and fatty acids associated with self-reported depression: an analysis from the Australian National Nutrition and Health Surveys. Nutrition. 2013 Jul-Aug; 29(7-8):1042-7. doi: 10.1016/j.nut.2013.02.006. PubMed PMID: 23759265.

[172] Mikolajczyk, Rafael T, Walid El Ansari, and Annette E Maxwell. "Food Consumption Frequency and Perceived Stress and Depressive Symptoms among Students in Three European Countries." Nutrition Journal 8 (2009): 31. PMC. Web. 27 Apr. 2017.

avoiders.[173] Low meat or fish intake has also been found to be characteristic of adults who had ever attempted suicide.[174]

In addition, several studies have linked low cholesterol to increased risk of suicide, parasuicide, propensity to violence, and antisocial personality (sociopathy or psychopathy).

Relatives of people who carry the Smith-Lemli-Opitz syndrome which produces a deficiency of the enzyme that catalyzes the last step in cholesterol biosynthesis attempt or complete suicide more often than non-carriers, and also have increased rates of intellectual disability, autism, attention deficits, obsessive compulsive disorders, sleep disorders, anxiety symptoms and self-injury.[175, 176] Men with a cholesterol less than 4.78 mmol/L (185 mg/dL) and declining cholesterol levels had a three-fold greater risk of suicide compared to those having greater cholesterol levels.[177] Serum cholesterol below

173 Burkert, Nathalie T. et al. "Nutrition and Health – The Association between Eating Behavior and Various Health Parameters: A Matched Sample Study." Ed. Olga Y. Gorlova. PLoS ONE 9.2 (2014): e88278. PMC. Web. 27 Apr. 2017.

174 Li Y, Zhang J, McKeown RE. Cross-sectional assessment of diet quality in individuals with a lifetime history of attempted suicide. Psychiatry Res. 2009 Jan 30;165(1-2):111-9. doi: 10.1016/j.psychres.2007.09.004. Epub 2008 Nov 30. PubMed PMID: 19046606.

175 Lalovic A, Merkens L, Russell L, Arsenault-Lapierre G, Nowaczyk MJ, Porter FD, Steiner RD, Turecki G. Cholesterol metabolism and suicidality in Smith-Lemli-Opitz syndrome carriers. Am J Psychiatry. 2004 Nov;161(11):2123-6. PubMed PMID: 15514417.

176 Diaz-Stransky A, Tierney E. Cognitive and Behavioral Aspects of Smith-Lemli-Opitz Syndrome. Am J Med Gen Part C (Seminars in Medical Genetics) 2012;160C: 295-300.

177 Zureik M, Courbon D, Ducimetiere P. Serum cholesterol concentration and death from suicide in men. Paris prospective study I. BMJ 1996 Sept 14;313:649-51. <https://www.ncbi.nlm.nih.gov/pmc/articles/PMC2351965/>

165 mg/dL has been linked to a doubled risk of death from suicide, homicide and accidents.[178]

Subjects who had committed parasuicide were found to have significantly lower total serum cholesterol levels than controls.[179] Subjects with antisocial personality disorders (sociopathy or psychopathy) were found to have a clearly lower mean level of serum cholesterol than subjects with other personality disorders.[180] A literature review found that many types of studies show a significant association between low or lowered cholesterol levels and violence, and that the data conform to criteria for a causal association.[181]

Women who had low serum cholesterol after giving birth were found to be more likely to have anxiety, anger, hostility and depression as measured by standardized psychological inventories.[182]

Evidently cholesterol deprivation has a harmful affect on not only cognition, but also emotion, in at least some people. Given the importance of cholesterol to the structure and function of the nervous system, this is not a surprising finding.

Based on this evidence and more, I believe that almost all civilized people are suffering from more or less brain degeneration or brain

---

[178] Boscarino, J., Erlich, P., & Hoffman, S. (2009). Low serum cholesterol and external-cause mortality: Potential implications for research and surveillance. Journal of Psychiatric Research, 43(9), 848-854.

[179] Gallerani M, Manfredini R, Caracciolo S, et al. Serum cholesterol concentrations in parasuicide. BMJ 1995 June 24;310:1632-6.

[180] Virkkunen M. Serum cholesterol in antisocial personality. Neuropsychobiology. 1979;5(1):27-30. PubMed PMID: 431794.

[181] Golomb BA. Cholesterol and Violence: Is There a Connection. Ann Intern Med 1998;128(6):478-487.

[182] Troisi A, Moles A, Panepuccia L, et al.: Serum cholesterol levels and mood symptoms in the postpartum period. Psychiatry Research 2002;109:213-219.

damage and consequent dementia compared to our ancestors. The degeneration, damage and dementia is greatest among those with diets most limited in animal products.

Time To and Type of Weaning

Human time to weaning is much reduced compared to the highly plant-based great-apes, and most like that of carnivores that obtain at least 20 percent of their calories from meat.[183]

Infants weaned onto meat (an ancestral food) have a lower incidence of zinc deficiency and larger head circumference (portending a greater IQ) than infants weaned onto iron-enriched cereals (an evolutionarily novel and artificial food).[184]

Other Features

We have some other physical, mental and behavioral features and abilities that appear to indicate specific adaptation to hunting, fishing, and animal food consumption including:

- Enjoyment of smell of cooking meat
- Ability to track and covertly stalk prey
- Ability to run or rapidly walk long distances chasing prey
- Ability to outsmart and trap prey animals
- Ability to create animal trapping devices including fishing hooks and nets
- Ability to produce hunting weapons, including knives, spears, and projectiles

---

183 Psouni E, Janke A, Garwicz M (2012) Impact of Carnivory on Human Development and Evolution Revealed by a New Unifying Model of Weaning in Mammals. PLoS ONE 7(4): e32452. doi:10.1371/journal.pone.0032452 **<https://www.ncbi.nlm.nih.gov/pmc/articles/PMC3329511/>**

184 Krebs NF, Westcott JE, Butler N, et al. Meat as a First Complementary Food for Breastfed Infants: Feasibility and Impact on Zinc Intake and Status. J Ped Gastroenterology and Nutrition 2006 Feb;42(2):207-14.

- Hand-eye coordination that facilitates accurate throwing of projectiles
- Shoulder girdle capable of throwing projectiles at high speed with great accuracy

Our Biological Drive To Eat Meat

All ancient *human* ancestors were hunters who, whenever possible, lived exclusively or very largely on animal flesh, organs, eggs and fats.[185, 186, 187, 188]

Across contemporary cultures, people prefer eating animal protein and fat to eating plant foods.[189]

Research shows that while 3% of U.S. citizens self-identify as vegetarians, 66% of these people report eating red meat, poultry, and fish on follow-up challenges; only 0.9% of the total study population both self-defined as vegetarian and provided dietary recalls that

---

[185] Meaning ancestors belonging to the human (*Homo*) genus.

[186] McKie R. Humans hunted for meat 2 million years ago. Anthropology, The Observer, The Guardian 2012 Sep 22. <https://www.theguardian.com/science/2012/sep/23/human-hunting-evolution-2million-years>

[187] Holzman D. Meat eating is an old human habit. New Scientist 2003 Sep 7. <https://www.newscientist.com/article/dn4122-meat-eating-is-an-old-human-habit/>

[188] Cordain L, Miller JB, Eaton SB, Mann N, Holt SHA, Speth JD. Plant-animal subsistence ratios and macronutrient energy estimations in worldwide hunter-gatherer diets. *Am J Clin Nutr* 2000;71:682-92.

[189] Abrams HL. The Preference for Animal Protein and Fat: A Cross-Cultural Survey. In: Harris M and Ross EB, eds. *Food and Evolution*. Philadelphia, PA: Temple University Press, 1987: 207.

included no animal flesh.[190] In addition, at least 84% of people who adopt a vegetarian or vegan diet eventually return to meat-eating.[191]

These facts indicate that only very few humans even attempt to adopt meat-free diets and even fewer succeed in adhering to them for any length of time.

Thus, it appears that we have an innate biological drive and need to eat meat.

HUMANS, DOGS AND SHEEP

In 1975, Walter L. Voegtlin, a practicing gastroenterologist, published *The Stone Age Diet, Based on In-depth Studies of Human Ecology and the Diet of Man*.[192] In this book, Voegtlin extensively reviewed archaeological, historical and zoological evidence showing that humans are by Nature carnivores specifically adapted to a high fat, high protein animal-based diet, and incapable of properly digesting plant foods or their constituent carbohydrates.

In his medical practice, Voegtlin discovered and repeatedly confirmed that either a lack of animal protein and fat or an excess of dietary carbohydrates will cause us many diseases, starting with disorders of hunger and the digestive tract, and including malnutrition, mental retardation (birth and developmental defects), fatty liver, gallstones, peptic ulcer, celiac, ulcerative colitis, enteritis, obesity, dental caries, and parasite infections.

---

190 Haddad EH, Tanzman JS, "What do vegetarians in the United States eat?," Am J Clin Nutr 2003;78(3):626S-632S. <http://ajcn.nutrition.org/content/78/3/626S.long>

191 Herzog H, "84% of Vegetarians and Vegans Return to Meat. Why?" Psychology Today 2014 Dec 2. <https://www.psychologytoday.com/blog/animals-and-us/201412/84-vegetarians-and-vegans-return-meat-why>

192 Voegtlin WL. The Stone Age Diet. Vantage Press, 1975.

He found that dietary carbohydrates, including fiber, cause both constipation and diarrhea in humans. Undigested carbohydrates feed fermentative bacteria that produce acids and gas that irritate and poison the intestines, which causes cramps, bloating and either diarrhea – as the intestines flood with water to dilute and expel the acids – or constipation – when the acid accumulation poisons and disables the intestinal smooth muscle. The excess bulk provided by fiber also makes stools too large to pass comfortably through the intestines and rectum. Voegtlin's findings have received confirmation by experiments showing that stopping or reducing fiber intake reduces constipation and its associated symptoms of bloating, abdominal pain and flatulence.[193]

Voegtlin, an expert in digestive tracts, provided a detailed comparison of our guts with those of the naturally carnivorous dog (same as the wolf) and the herbivorous sheep. This comparison, summarized in Table 4.5, provides further evidence that we are Natural carnivores.

Since plant foods primarily consist of fiber, and fiber causes gut dysfunction in humans, we must conclude that the human gut is by Nature adapted to those natural foods which – like human mothers' milk – contain no fiber, namely animal meat and fat.

---

[193] Ho K-S, Tan CYM, Mohd Daud MA, Seow-Choen F. Stopping or reducing dietary fiber intake reduces constipation and its associated symptoms. *World Journal of Gastroenterology: WJG*. 2012;18(33):4593-4596. doi:10.3748/wjg.v18.i33.4593. <https://www.ncbi.nlm.nih.gov/pmc/articles/PMC3435786/>

Table 4.5: Comparison of the digestive tracts of humans, dogs, and sheep.

	MAN	DOG	SHEEP
TEETH			
incisors	both jaws	both jaws	lower jaw only
molars	ridged and shearing	ridged and shearing	flat
canines	small	large	absent
JAW			
movements	vertical	vertical	rotary
function	tearing-crushing	tearing-crushing	grinding
mastication	unimportant	unimportant	vital function
rumination	never	never	vital function
STOMACH			
capacity	2 quarts	2 quarts	8.5 gallons
emptying time	3 hours	3 hours	never empties
interdigestive rest	yes	yes	no
bacteria present	no	no	yes
protozoa present	no	no	yes
gastric acidity	very strong	very strong	weak
plant fiber digestion	none	none	70% - vital
digestive activity	weak	weak	vital
food absorption	no	n	vital function

Table 4.5: Comparison of the digestive tracts of humans, dogs, and sheep.

	MAN	DOG	SHEEP
COLON AND CECUM			
colon size	short-small	short-small	long-capacious
cecum size	tiny	tiny	long-capacious
cecum function	none	none	vital function
appendix	vestigial	absent	cecum
rectum	small	small	capacious
digestive activity	none	none	30% - vital
plant fiber digestion	unimportant	unimportant	vital function
bacterial flora	putrefactive	putrefactive	fermentative
food absorption	none	none	vital function
fecal volume	small, firm	small, firm	voluminous
gross food in feces	rare	rare	large amount
GALLBALDDER			
size	well-developed	well-developed	often absent
function	strong	strong	weak or absent
DIGESTIVE ACTIVITY			
from pancreas	solely	solely	partial
from bacteria	none	none	partial
from protozoa	none	none	partial
efficiency	100%	100%	50% or less

Table 4.5: Comparison of the digestive tracts of humans, dogs, and sheep.

	MAN	DOG	SHEEP
FEEDING HABITS			
frequency	intermittent	intermittent	continuous
SURVIVAL WITHOUT			
stomach	possible	possible	impossible
colon and rectum	possible	possible	impossible
gut microbes	possible	possible	impossible
plant foods	possible	possible	impossible
animal foods	impossible in Nature	impossible	possible
RATIO OF BODY LENGTH TO			
entire digestive tract	1:5	1:7	1:27
small intestine	1:4	1:6	1:25

Carnivore Classifications

It bears repeating that the word "carnivore," derived from the Latin words for "flesh/meat" (caro) and "to devour" (vorare), means "flesh-eater" or "meat-eater." Therefore, by original definition any animal that eats meat is a carnivore, regardless of whether or not the animal eats some plant matter. The word specifies only what the animal does eat – meat – and does not tell us what the animal does not eat.

As already noted, biologists classify carnivores by their relative dependence upon animal flesh. A hypercarnivore (e.g. lion) consumes a diet consisting of more than 70 percent flesh, a mesocarnivore (e.g. coyote) 50 to 70 percent, and a hypocarnivore (e.g. black bear) less than 30 percent.[194] Biologists believe that the earliest members of the order Carnivora had mesocarnivorous diets.[195]

A a simple matter of fact, the vast majority of modern humans are carnivores to some extent, and some – e.g. the Inuit, Plains Indians, Laplanders – have been hypercarnivores for many generations. Further, humans have been carnivores for millions of years, and European ancestors – including Neanderthals and Cro-Magnon– were hypercarnivores who ate more animal flesh than consumed by the arctic foxes in their habitats.[196]

Many non-human apex predators consume some plant matter. Wolves, polar bears, crocodiles and even the iconic felines have all been observed to deliberately consume some plant matter in their natural habits.[197, 198] If total exclusion of plant matter is required for an animal to be classified as a carnivore, we can't call these animals carnivores, which is ridiculous.

---

[194] Van Valkenburgh B. **Déjà vu: the evolution of feeding morphologies in the Carnivora**. Integrative and Comparative Biology 47(1): 147-163.

[195] Ibid.

196 Richards MP, "A review of the archaeological evidence for Paleolithic and Neolithic subsistence," Eur J Clin Nutr 2002;56. doi:10.1038/sj.ejcn.1601646 <http://www.nature.com/ejcn/journal/v56/n12/full/1601646a.html>

[197] Bosch G, Hagen-Plantinga EA, Hendriks WH. Dietary nutrient profiles of wild wolves: insights for optimal dog nutrition? Br J Nutr 2015;113:S40-S54.

[198] Plantinga EA, Bosch G, Hendriks WH. Estimation of the dietary nutrient profile of free-roaming feral cats: possible implications for nutrition of domestic cats. Br J Nutr 2011 Oct 12;106(51):535-548. <**https://www.cambridge.org/core/journals/british-journal-of-nutrition/article/estimation-of-the-dietary-nutrient-profile-of-freeroaming-feral-cats-possible-implications-for-nutrition-of-domestic-cats/2E0E827469FFC1AF51387E045C06759A/core-reader**>

Therefore, to refer to an animal that only eats meat we would need some word other than just "carnivore." I suggest that people who make it a practice to avoid all plant foods choose for themselves an appropriate designation other than carnivore. They could call themselves strict carnivores, exclusive carnivores, plantavoiders, or vegavoiders.

Body Typing Nonsense

Some people believe that some people are natural carnivores, and others natural plantivores (vegetarians). They have imagined that people with different body or blood types are designed or adapted to different types of diets.

Frankly, this is ridiculous, and not supported by any evidence. Every member of any given species has a body designed for the same foods as all other members of that species.

For example, every rabbit has a body designed for a diet of grass and seeds. Although rabbits can sometimes be found eating animals, it never happens that some rabbits can *specialize* in hunting game and eating an animal-based diet. The same applies to all plantivores, including all the great apes; although they may eat animals now and then, they don't specialize in carnivory.

Similarly, although wolves sometimes eat fruits (such as wolfberry, *Lycium barbarum*), every wolf is physically specialized for carnivory. No wolf can survive in the wild on a plant-based diet. No primarily plantivorous wolf has ever existed, and none ever will exist. All wolves are born from other wolves, all of which are carnivores by Nature. Hence, no wolf couple can produce a plantivorous offspring.

Although humans have domesticated wolves to produce dogs, and we can feed dogs artificial plant-based diets, no dog can survive on wild plant foods because all dogs are carnivores by Nature. There exists a wide difference in external physical appearance of various breeds of dogs, yet all dogs have the same basic gut and metabolism.

All humans have the same basic digestive and metabolic systems. Neither blood type, bone structure, somatotype, or any other external physical difference between humans signals a difference in the structure or function of your stomach or intestines, the way you digest food, or the nutritional requirements of your brain, organs, muscles or bones. Since all humans have inherited a carnivore-type gut, the offspring of any two humans will also have a carnivore-type gut.

The biologically distinct human races exist by virtue of each subspecies having evolved in a distinctly different habitat imposing different demands. For example, compared to Asians and Africans, contemporary Europeans have as many as three times more Neanderthal gene variants involved in lipid metabolism,[199] indicating that Europeans are probably genetically well-adapted to higher fat diets, whereas Asians and Africans may be better adapted to somewhat lower fat diets.[200] Probably Europeans have this characteristic because only people who could metabolize diets very high in animal fat could have survived during the Ice Ages in Europe.

Salt tolerance or requirements also vary by ancestry. Europeans and Asians generally have a high tolerance for dietary salt, and may have a requirement for it, inherited from ancestors who had to use salt to preserve foods for long winters. Among Europeans, sodium intake below 3 g per day has been associated with higher mortality from cardiovascular disease.[201] Research suggests that at least for

---

199 People of pure African descent have no Neanderthal ancestors or DNA.

200 Max-Planck-Gesellschaft. "Europeans have three times more Neanderthal genes for lipid catabolism than Asians or Africans." ScienceDaily. ScienceDaily, 2 April 2014. <www.sciencedaily.com/releases/2014/04/140402100056.htm>.

201 Stolarz-Skrzypek K, Kuznetsova T, Thijs L, et al. Fatal and Nonfatal Outcomes, Incidence of Hypertension, and Blood Pressure Changes in Relation to Urinary Sodium Excretion. *JAMA*. 2011;305(17):1777-1785. <http://jama.jamanetwork.com/article.aspx?articleid=899663>

Europeans and Asians the sweet spot for *sodium* intake probably lies in the range of 3 to 7 g per day, which equates to 1.5 to 3 level domestic teaspoons daily of salt.[202, 203] People of African descent are genetically more likely to be salt sensitive hypertensives,[204] perhaps because their ancestors did not need to use salt for food preservation through long winters.

Nature gave Europeans light skin because one needs light skin to produce adequate vitamin D in the darker northern latitudes,[205] and for camouflage in an environment that has many light and gray colors (e.g. tree trunks) and snow cover for 4-8 months every year (many northern species have white or gray coloration for this purpose). Nature gave Africans dark skin to protect them from the intense solar radiation encountered in the tropics. European skin is vulnerable to burning and at a greatly increased risk for skin cancer when Europeans live in the tropics, rather than their Natural

---

[202] O'Donnell MJ, Yusuf S, Mente A, et al. Urinary Sodium and Potassium Excretion and Risk of Cardiovascular Events. *JAMA*. 2011;306(20):2229-2238. **<http://jama.jamanetwork.com/article.aspx?articleid=1105553>**

[203] McMaster University. "Low-salt diets may not be beneficial for all, study suggests: Salt reduction only important in some people with high blood pressure." ScienceDaily. ScienceDaily, 21 May 2016. **<www.sciencedaily.com/releases/2016/05/160521071410.htm>**

[204] American Heart Association. "Hold The Salt: Gene May Explain African Americans' Extra Sensitivity To Salt, Leading To High Blood Pressure." ScienceDaily. ScienceDaily, 26 March 1999. **<www.sciencedaily.com/releases/1999/03/990326061953.htm>**.

[205] Europeans need dietary vitamin D in addition to food source vitamin D to obtain adequate amounts to maintain health. Africans and other dark skinned people can't get adequate vitamin D from diet alone if they live in a dark northern region.

habitat.[206] Without dietary supplements, Africans and dark-skinned Asians are vulnerable to vitamin D deficiency when they live in Europe, rather than their natural habitats.[121, 207] European light skin is not adapted to the tropics, dark African or Asian skin is not adapted to temperate regions.

Europeans have specific adaptations for tolerance of the cold and moist climate characteristic of their homelands, while Africans have specific adaptations for tolerating the hot and dry climate characteristic of their homeland.[208]

Compared to Europeans, Africans have greater bone and skeletal muscle mass but smaller mass of the most metabolically active organs (liver, spleen, kidneys, heart, and brain), resulting in a lower total resting energy expenditure.[209] A lower resting energy expenditure is an advantage in a warmer climate that provides game animals having a lower body fat percentage (i.e. equatorial Africa), but a disadvantage in a colder, more humid climate that provides

[206] Jablonski NG, Chaplin G. Human skin pigmentation, migration and disease susceptibility. *Philosophical Transactions of the Royal Society B: Biological Sciences*. 2012;367(1590):785-792. doi:10.1098/rstb.2011.0308. <https://www.ncbi.nlm.nih.gov/pmc/articles/PMC3267121/>

[207] Van der Meer IM, Middelkoop BJC, Boeke AJP, Lips P. Prevalence of vitamin D deficiency among Turkish, Moroccan, Indian and sub-Sahara African populations in Europe and their countries of origin: an overview. *Osteoporosis International*. 2011;22(4):1009-1021. doi:10.1007/s00198-010-1279-1. <https://www.ncbi.nlm.nih.gov/pmc/articles/PMC3046351/>

[208] Daanen HAM, Van Marken Lichtenbelt WD. Human whole body cold adaptation. *Temperature: Multidisciplinary Biomedical Journal*. 2016;3(1): 104-118. doi:10.1080/23328940.2015.1135688. <https://www.ncbi.nlm.nih.gov/pmc/articles/PMC4861193/>

[209] Dympna Gallagher, Jeanine Albu, Qing He, Stanley Heshka, Lawrence Boxt, Norman Krasnow, Marinos Elia; Small organs with a high metabolic rate explain lower resting energy expenditure in African American than in white adults, *The American Journal of Clinical Nutrition*, Volume 83, Issue 5, 1 May 2006, Pages 1062–1067, https://doi.org/10.1093/ajcn/83.5.1062

game animals having a higher body fat percentage (i.e. temperate and subarctic Europe).

Thus, each race is biologically distinct and adapted to a specific habitat. Europeans are by Nature fit for living in the colder, darker, wetter Northern regions, and unfit for living in the hotter, brighter, drier southern regions of the Earth. Africans are by Nature fit for living most happily in African or similar habitats. Each race will enjoy best health when living in its homeland or similar habitat.

Nevertheless, all human ancestors in their native habitats were carnivores, whether African, European or Asian. Although humans have figured out ways to process plant foods to make them edible and more digestible by our carnivore-type gut, this has not changed the basic structure or function of the human gut or metabolism. Despite trying to adapt to plant-based diets for more than 10, 000 years, we still do not have plantivore guts, we still do not produce enzymes for digestion of fiber, and we still require animal protein, unique animal fats, and vitamin B12, regardless of race/subspecies.

Hence, we must conclude that no humans are natural plantivores. In fact, we are natural meso- or hyper- carnivores, adapted to a diet consisting largely or primarily of animal protein and fat and not well adapted to eating any significant quantity of plant matter other than low-sugar, low fiber fruits and some vegetables.

Due to genetic variation, individuals vary in their ability to tolerate plant-based diets. Those who best tolerate plant-based foods experience the least adverse effects from a plant-based diet and may mistakenly believe that everyone has a similar tolerance.

People who have a high tolerance for plant foods make up the ranks of long-term adherents to plant-based diets; apparently about 0.9 percent or less of the general population falls into this category. Many of these people believe that their own tolerance of a plant-based diet proves that all people can tolerate and should adopt a plant-based diet.

They do not understand that a plant-based diet is a selective factor, much like a professional sport. Basketball selects for tall people, and only people who have genetics favorable to the sport end up on professional basketball teams. Just so, a plant-based diet selects for people who have a high tolerance for plant foods and lower requirements for animal-derived nutrients, so only people who have genetics favorable to plant-based diets stick to those diets long-term; others simply drop out.

Because of ancestry, some people – particularly Europeans, all of whom are descendants of stone age people who were more carnivorous than the arctic fox – have very low to no tolerance for plant foods. These people develop various diseases of civilization when eating amounts of plant matter exceeding their tolerance. Often they do not realize they have exceeded their tolerance levels because the body finds ways to adapt to adverse circumstances, and it can be difficult to identify plant foods as the cause of one's conditions if one is always eating them.

Some people may have guts and metabolisms more or less damaged by chronic consumption of plant-based diets. Long-term consumption of low-fat plant-based diets can result in gall bladder disease, stones, and consequent gall bladder removal. Chronic consumption of high-fiber diets can result in inflammation and distention that deforms the colon, leading to irritable bowel and more or less difficulty adapting to THE HYPERCARNIVORE DIET. These people may have more or less difficulty regaining healthy gut function and metabolism when they first attempt to transition from a plant-based to an animal-based diet.

Nevertheless, with patience and persistence most people can recover healthy gut function and metabolism by eating a natural, whole foods animal-based diet.

5 POISONED BY PLANTS

Contrary to popular belief, the plants people choose to eat are not completely non-toxic. Plant foods can harm us through their provisions of fiber, sugars, fats, antioxidants, lectins, and other chemicals that are incompatible with our guts or may poison our cells.

Plants have occupied this planet longer than humans. Their roots, tubers, bulbs, stems, and leaves are as essential to their survival. Since they can't run and hide, they defend themselves from predators – microbes, insects, and animals – by producing chemicals that injure or even kill.

These chemicals generally have a bitter taste, and they kill microbes, fungi, insects, worms, and larvae. Since most function as neurotoxins, and our gut has a very high density of neurons, these phytochemicals can cause various levels of gut discomfort or damage.

Children almost universally reject vegetables because they can taste these bitter poisons (they have more bitter taste receptors than adults to protect them from these toxins) and have not yet been sufficiently programmed to erroneously believe that they need to eat vegetables.

In sufficient quantity, these bitter compounds can poison our digestive system, causing cramping, bloating, diarrhea (as the body attempts to rapidly expel the poison) or constipation (when the gut nerves are paralyzed by a sufficient quantity of the toxins).

Moreover, most vegetables primarily consist of the indigestible carbohydrates collectively called fiber, which has no nutritional benefit but reduces your absorption of essential nutrients causing them to be wasted in your defecation. Leaves, stems, bulbs, flowers, and other fibrous vegetables provide less energy than one expends in acquiring them.

No scientific evidence supports claims that people need to eat vegetables. Whole populations of humans – such as the Inuit, better known as Eskimos, the Masai, and many others already mentioned in Chapter 1 have lived for many generations without eating any nutritionally significant amount of plant foods. Simply put, we have no dietary requirement for fruits or vegetables.

We can reduce the toxicity and improve the nutrient availability of vegetables by cooking or saline fermentation (pickling). This processing can reduce or eliminate *some* (but never all) of the toxins in vegetables. Of interest, the word "salad" comes from the Latin root *sal* (salt) and originally referred to salted and fermented vegetables. In the original so-called Mediterranean diet almost all vegetables were cooked or pickled before consumption.

All that said, many of us have a natural taste for some plant products providing bitter tannins, and regular use of some individually determined small amount of these non-food plants or plant foods may provide some health benefits through *hormesis*.

Fatal Fiber

As discussed in Chapter 4, the human body does not produce enzymes for digestion of fiber, nor does it have any essential digestive organ devoted to microbial digestion of fiber.[1] Human infants live well on breast milk which contains no fiber, whereas foods containing fiber give many babies colic. Many native tribes have lived on diets containing little or no fiber. Gastroenterologists frequently prescribe low-residue diets to people who have gastrointestinal complaints caused by fiber. Humans never suffer any fiber deficiency disease, so, by definition, *fiber is not a nutrient*.

Contrary to propaganda and common belief, you don't need to eat fiber to have bowel movements. As explained in the previous chapter, the release of bile from the gall bladder in response to a meal containing adequate fat will stimulate peristalsis and consequent evacuation of bowel contents.

Given the current popular worship of fiber, you may find it hard to believe that dietary fiber is harmful, but in fact it is one of the most dangerous things we can ingest from plants. One of the most respected basic nutrition textbooks[2] clearly states that eating high fiber foods can have several adverse effects including:

- Making food so bulky it becomes difficult to ingest adequate nutrition: "The malnourished, the elderly, and young children adhering to all-plant (vegan) diets are especially vulnerable to this problem."

---

[1] "Dietary Fiber consists of nondigestible food plant carbohydrates and lignin in which the plant matrix is largely intact…Nondigestible means that the material is not digested and absorbed in the human small intestine." Institute of Medicine. Dietary Reference Intakes for Energy, Carbohydrate, Fiber, Fat, Fatty Acids, Cholesterol, Protein, and Amino Acids. National Academies Press, 2005. 341. <https://www.nap.edu/read/10490/chapter/9#341>

[2] Whitney E, Rolfes SR. Understanding Nutrition. 10th Edition. Thomson Wadsworth, 2005. Pages 125-26.

- Causing abdominal discomfort, gas, diarrhea, and intestinal obstruction.
- Limiting absorption of nutrients, particularly minerals.

I have suffered several digestive diseases and disorders – including tooth decay, acid reflux, painful abdominal bloating, hernia, hemorrhoids, and anal pruritis – as consequence of eating a high fiber whole foods plant based diet for many years, so much of what follows comes from my own experience and also medical literature research. However, I am extremely grateful to Konstantin Monstyrsky, author of *Fiber Menace*, for providing in that book and on his website a systematic review of the damage fiber does to the gut from top to bottom, which greatly helped me to write my similar review below.[3]

Oral Disorders

Like other carbohydrates, fiber feeds the growth of fermentative bacteria in all regions of the digestive tract. This fermentation starts in the mouth.

Fiber has a tendency to stick to the teeth and lodge between the teeth and gums at the gum line. Oral bacteria ferment fiber, producing acids that eat away at the tooth structure, producing tooth decay.

When fiber lodges in the gingival sulcus – the pocket between the teeth and the gums (gingiva) – bacteria there will ferment it, causing inflammation of the gums, the periodontal ligament, and the alveolar bone. This initially causes the gums to recede or bleed, and eventually produces periodontal disease and loss of teeth.

---

[3] Monastyrsky K. Fiber Menace. Ageless Press, 2nd edition, 2008. The full text is online: **<https://www.gutsense.org/fiber-menace/why-dietary-fiber-causes-harm.html>**

Our ancestors who ate animal-based diets had virtually no tooth decay, but once they started eating starchy roots or high fiber cereal grains and legumes, tooth decay became a common ailment.[4, 5]

If the pulverized fiber lodges in the small tubules of the salivary glands, it causes salivary gland obstruction. This produces a dry mouth, making mastication of food more difficult, and deprives the teeth of the protection provided by mineral-rich saliva.

Mechanical Damage

From the moment you swallow a high-fiber food, it starts to damage your digestive tract. High-fiber foods bang up against and tear open the cells lining the gut, causing them to rupture, and in response to this mechanical damage, the cells lose some of their contents and secrete much more mucus than they would in the absence of damage by fiber.[6, 7]

[4] Humphrey LT, De Groote I, Morales J, et al. Earliest evidence for caries and exploitation of starchy plant foods in Pleistocene hunter-gatherers from Morocco. *Proceedings of the National Academy of Sciences of the United States of America.* 2014;111(3):954-959. doi:10.1073/pnas.1318176111. <https://www.ncbi.nlm.nih.gov/pmc/articles/PMC3903197/>

[5] Adler CJ, Dobney K, Weyrich LS, et al.. Sequencing ancient calcified dental plaque shows changes in oral microbiota with dietary shifts of the Neolithic and Industrial revolutions. Nature Genetics 2013 April;45(4):450-55.

[6] Medical College of Georgia. "Scientists Learn More About How Roughage Keeps You 'Regular'." ScienceDaily. ScienceDaily, 23 August 2006. <www.sciencedaily.com/releases/2006/08/060823093156.htm>.

[7] Miyake K, Tanaka T, McNeil PL. Disruption-Induced Mucus Secretion: Repair and Protection. PLOS Biology 2006 Aug 22; Accessed Dec 14, 2017 from: <http://journals.plos.org/plosbiology/article?id=10.1371/journal.pbio.0040276>

Throat and Stomach Disorders

Fiber is hydrophilic (water-loving), so as it passes through the gut, it starts pulling water from the gut tissues and forming into large and expanding, pasty mass. In this process, fiber can expand to 4 or 5 times its original size.

When such a fibrous food mass reaches the stomach, it can stimulate nerves that trigger the regurgitation or vomiting reflex. As a result, you will burp or have acid reflux. The acid reaches up into and damages the lining of the esophagus, which is not designed for exposure to stomach acid. Over time this leads to Barrett's esophagus, ulceration, bleeding, and esophageal cancer.

The stomach has the function of churning food with acid to kill any pathogenic microbes, and dissolve the food mass into tiny particles. Most people have noticed that some whole plant foods, like sweet corn kernels, pass through the gut intact and show up practically unaltered in feces. This occurs because fiber, unlike animal protein, is resistant to dissolution by stomach acid.

This resistance to digestion means high fiber meals can delay stomach emptying after meals. Whereas a meal of meat will leave the stomach as a liquid within 6 hours, high fiber foods may remain in the stomach for 10 or more hours without dissolving at all.

Since the stomach is not designed for exposure to its own acid for this length of time, and fiber is indigestible, this causes the burning abdominal pain commonly and appropriately called "acid indigestion." Eventually this leads to chronic stomach inflammation and ulceration.

If the fibrous mass expands greatly in size during its prolonged time in the stomach, it can push upward against the upper region of the stomach and the diaphragm. In combination with 1) the muscular action of the stomach attempting to push the mass downward into the intestine and 2) packing of the abdomen with visceral fat, as in obesity, this can cause the upper portion of the stomach to push up through the esophageal hiatus of the diaphragm, a condition called *hiatal hernia* that affects more than 40% of the U.S. population.

If the fibrous mass obstructs the small passageway from the stomach to the duodenum (the first part of the small intestine), you can experience nausea and more acid regurgitation.

Small Intestine Disorders

The small intestine is about 7 meters (23 ft) of coiled muscular tubing that's only 3.5 to 4 cm (1.4 to 1.6 inches) in diameter. It has three sections: the upper duodenum (directly connected to the stomach), the middle jejunum, and the lower ileum (connected to the colon).

We call the acid-soaked stuff that the stomach delivers to the small intestine *chyme*. If you eat fiber-free food such as meat or fat, chyme is a liquid, but if chyme contains inherently indigestible fiber, it is a sticky mass – imagine oatmeal soaked in hydrochloric acid for several hours.

The common bile duct delivers bile from the gallbladder and liver, and pancreatic juice from the pancreas, into the small intestine. Bile is required for emulsification of fats for digestion, and pancreatic juice contains not only the enzymes required for digestion of protein, fat, and any carbohydrate consumed, but also bicarbonate needed to neutralize the acidity of the chyme so that it does not damage the duodenum.

When chyme is a sticky fiber mass it can block the common bile duct, preventing bile and pancreatic juice from flowing into the duodenum.

Hence high fiber chyme can have two bad effects. First, it reduces or blocks the entry of alkaline pancreatic juice into the duodenum, which means the duodenum is exposed to the acidic chyme instead of a neutral liquid. This will cause inflammation and eventually ulceration of the duodenum.

Second, blockage of the duct will cause the pancreatic juices and bile to back up into the pancreas and gallbladder. This can result in pancreatitis (inflammation of the pancreas) or cholecystitis (inflammation of the gallbladder).

Children have smaller diameter intestines hence a higher risk of bile duct blockage and pancreatitis from high fiber foods. Pancreatitis can result in the pancreas losing its ability to produce insulin, causing acute high blood sugar and diabetes.[8]

More women than men avoid meat and fat in favor of high fiber fruits, vegetables and grains,[9] especially when they have too much body fat and want to lose it, and women have a 2-to-3 times greater risk of cholecystitis than men.[10, 11]

When fibrous chyme blocks the common bile duct, digestive enzymes can't reach the intestine. Consequently, you are unable to extract adequate essential amino acids, fatty acids, or even carbohydrate from the food consumed.

Fiber itself binds proteins, fats, carbohydrates, vitamins and minerals, blocking their absorption, and the inflammation caused by fiber's mechanical assault on the intestinal tissue reduces your

---

[8] Raman VS, Loar RW, Renukuntla VS, Hassan KV, Fishman DS, Gilger MA, Heptulla RA. Hyperglycemia and diabetes mellitus in children with pancreatitis. J Pediatr. 2011 Apr;158(4):612-616.e1. doi: 10.1016/j.jpeds.2010.09.066. Epub 2010 Nov 20. PubMed PMID: 21093873.

[9] American Society for Microbiology. The difference in eating habits between men and women. Eurekalert 2008 Mar 19. Accessed Dec 15, 2017 from: <https://www.eurekalert.org/pub_releases/2008-03/asfm-tdi031408.php>

[10] Fialkowski E, Halpin V, Whinney RR. Acute cholecystitis. *BMJ Clinical Evidence*. 2008;2008:0411. <https://www.ncbi.nlm.nih.gov/pmc/articles/PMC2907986/>

[11] Novacek G. Gender and gallstone disease. Wien Med Wochenschr. 2006 Oct; 156(19-20):527-33. Review. PubMed PMID: 17103289.

assimilation of nutrients even further. Consequently you may not feel satisfied by your bulky meals, even though your abdomen aches from bloating and indigestion.

Ultimately this leads to chronically poor assimilation, multiple nutrient deficiencies and consequent degeneration of the cells, tissues and organs dependent on those nutrients. It is well known that people eating typical diets suffer from progressive loss of bone (osteopenia and osteoporosis), muscle (sarcopenia), organ mass, and brain tissue as they age. The body can't maintain itself when it can't extract nutrients from foods because of intestinal inflammation and blockage due to ingestion of high fiber, high carbohydrate diets.

Once the chyme manages to pass the duodenum it proceeds first to the jejunum and then the ileum. These latter two sections of the small diameter intestine primarily function as sponges for absorption of any nutrients liberated from the chyme by pancreatic enzymes.

As acid-soaked fiber-rich masses travel through these segments of the small intestine, the acidic fiber continues to tear open the cells, increase mucus production, and produce inflammation. The inflammation of intestinal mucosa reduces its ability to absorb nutrients and gases formed during digestion. Consequently the intestine frequently blows up like a balloon, causing bloating, cramping and pain.

When the gases inflate the intestines, the intestines become too large for their limited abdominal space, and firm enough to push through weaker seams between muscles of the abdominal wall. When an individual who has bloated intestines coughs, bears down to evacuate the bowels, or holds his/her breath to stabilize the spine when lifting a heavy weight, intra-abdominal pressure increases and can force the bloated intestine to penetrate the abdominal wall, producing a herniation. In the absence of fiber-induced gas and inflammation, the intestine would not be large or firm enough to do this damage.

If the inflammation progresses, the intestine closes in on itself as the inner lining grows in thickness from congestion of blood and fluids. This can evolve into a partial or complete intestinal obstruction. This most commonly occurs at the end of the ileum, where a mass of fiber can block the flow of small intestinal contents through the ileocecal valve into the colon. The fibrous mass can damage the valve, resulting in incomplete closure. A healthy small intestine is sterile, but this fiber-induced inflammation and blockage can allow bacteria from the colon to invade the small intestine.

Intestines chronically exposed to this stress will develop the inflammatory bowel disease iliitis or iliocolitis, more commonly known as Crohn's disease. This disease causes episodic diarrhea and abdominal pain; complications include abdominal abscesses and evolution of a fistula between the intestines and the skin. It occurs most commonly among people of Northern European and Anglo-Saxon (Germanic) origin eating a modern plant-based diet. These populations did not have this issue when they ate their traditional animal-based diet. Crohn's disease has been successfully treated with a strictly carnivorous diet (elimination of all plant-based foods).[12]

Colon Disorders

When the high-fiber mash finally gets into the colon (also called the large intestine), it continues to do further mechanical damage, tearing open cells and causing them to spill their vital fluids and secrete mucus to try to protect themselves from the fiber.

Since we *never* digest fiber, when it reaches the colon, it simply feeds the growth of fermentative bacteria, which produce acids and gases that wreak all manner of havoc.

---

[12] Tóth C, Dabóczi A, Howard M, Miller NJ, Clemens Z. Crohn's disease successfully treated with the paleolithic ketogenic diet. Int J Case Rep Images 2016;7(9):570-78.

The appendix attaches to the colon just past the ileocecal valve. When fiber accumulates in the appendix, bacteria therein start fermenting it, producing gas and acids that irritate and inflame the appendix. As this proceeds, the appendix swells, causing extreme pain, and if not surgically removed, the appendix can burst and release bacteria and fecal matter into the normally sterile peritoneal cavity, a life-threatening situation.

The acids produced by microbial fermentation of fiber further irritate the colon. This can initially or episodically cause frequent stools or diarrhea, which is the colon's proper reaction to exposure to a toxin: evacuate it as quickly as possible.

However, the colon is a muscle, and all muscles lose the ability to contract when exposed to high concentrations of acid. Consequently, the acids produced by microbial fermentation of fiber in the colon eventually poison the colon, making it weak so it has difficulty pushing out the stool.

In addition, dietary fiber makes stools larger, and larger stools are more difficult to pass through the rectum and anus.

Hence fiber can initially increase evacuation frequency in healthy individuals not previously loaded with fiber, but have no effect or decrease stool frequency in individuals who've been eating a high fiber diet for a long time.[13] It can therefore also cause or contribute to alternating constipation and diarrhea, sometimes called "irritable bowel." Research has failed to support claims that increasing dietary fiber helps this condition.[14]

Microbial fermentation of fiber in the colon produces large amounts of gases, and these gases rapidly expand in the warm environment,

---

[13] Tan K-Y, Seow-Choen F. Fiber and colorectal diseases: Separating fact from fiction. *World Journal of Gastroenterology: WJG*. 2007;13(31):4161-4167. doi: 10.3748/wjg.v13.i31.4161. <**https://www.ncbi.nlm.nih.gov/pmc/articles/PMC4250613/**>

[14] Ibid.

causing the colon to bloat. This is usually accompanied by cramping pain, because stretching of the intestines triggers pain receptors in the intestines. When people stop consuming fiber, they no longer suffer from abdominal bloating and pain.[15]

Authorities often claim that high fiber foods accelerate the passage of materials through the colon, keeping it "clean." In reality so long as you eat regularly, the colon is never "clean" as new material reaches the colon after every meal stimulating mass transit. There exists no evidence to support the claim that a long but normal residence of stools in the colon promotes any disease process.[15] Moreover, research has demonstrated that a high fiber diet retards propulsion of fecal matter and gases toward the rectum.[16] As already noted, as fiber accumulates in the colon, the stool becomes larger. Constipation is defined as difficulty passing a stool, regardless of frequency of evacuation. The larger the stool becomes, the harder it is to pass it through the colon, rectum and especially the anus. Removing fiber from the diet relieves constipation, anal bleeding, bloating, straining and abdominal pain in 100% of subjects (Figure 5.1).[15]

[15] Ho K-S, Tan CYM, Mohd Daud MA, Seow-Choen F. Stopping or reducing dietary fiber intake reduces constipation and its associated symptoms. *World Journal of Gastroenterology: WJG*. 2012;18(33):4593-4596. doi:10.3748/wjg.v18.i33.4593. <**https://www.ncbi.nlm.nih.gov/pmc/articles/PMC3435786/**>

[16] Gonlachanvit S, Coleski R, Owyang C, Hasler W. Inhibitory actions of a high fibre diet on intestinal gas transit in healthy volunteers. *Gut*. 2004;53(11): 1577-1582. doi:10.1136/gut.2004.041632. <**https://www.ncbi.nlm.nih.gov/pmc/articles/PMC1774297/**>

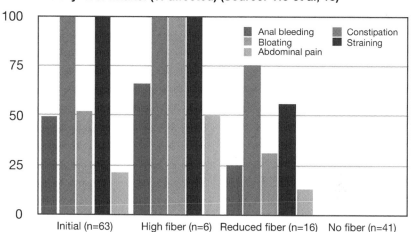

Figure 5.1: Initial symptoms and at 6 months following change in dietary fiber intake. (% affected) (Source: Ho et al, 15)

Large stools cause more than constipation. Combined with gases produced by microbial fermentation of fiber, they also produce deformations of the colon wall, known as diverticula, and when these get inflamed by the persistent accumulation of fiber and its fermentation to acids by flora, we call the condition diverticulitis.[17]

Peery and associates studied 2104 subjects aged 30-80 years old with colonoscopy.[18] They found that those who ate the most fiber (plants) had the highest prevalence of diverticulosis; and those who had more than 15 bowel evacuations per week had a 70% greater risk for diverticulosis than those with fewer than 7 bowel evacuations per

[17] Tan K-Y, Seow-Choen F. Fiber and colorectal diseases: Separating fact from fiction. *World Journal of Gastroenterology: WJG.* 2007;13(31):4161-4167. doi: 10.3748/wjg.v13.i31.4161. <**https://www.ncbi.nlm.nih.gov/pmc/articles/PMC4250613/**>

[18] Peery AF, Barrett PR, Park D, et al. A high fiber diet does not protect against asymptomatic diverticulosis. Gastroenterology 2012;142:266-72, <https://www.gastrojournal.org/article/S0016-5085(11)01509-5/pdf>

week. Neither red meat nor fat intake was associated with diverticulosis.

In another study Peery and colleagues reported that subjects who had bowel movements less than 7 times weekly had about half the risk of diverticulosis compared to those who had a bowel movement 7 times weekly.[19] People who reported hard stools also had a reduced risk of diverticulosis. High fiber intake did not reduce the risk of diverticulosis in this population.

The large stools produced by high fiber diets overstretch the colon, causing it to lose its contractibility, a condition called *megacolon*.[18] This can lead to accumulations of compressed stools which the poisoned, overstretched, weakened colon can't move, also known as fecal impactions.

Large stools overstretch the rectum and anus, resulting in nerve damage, which reduces the defecation reflex, making stool evacuation even more difficult. Regular passing of large stools over many years can also damage the anal sphincter, making one incapable of controlling evacuation, giving you bowel incontinence. Over-stretching by large plant-based stools eventually damages the rectal and anal muscles, resulting in prolapse. Straining to eliminate large stools containing undigested plant matter – fiber – through the anus results in hemorrhoids and tearing (fissure) of the anus.

A large body of research has failed to produce evidence to support the claim that high fiber foods help prevent colon cancer.[20]

---

[19] Peery AF, Sandler RS, Ahnen DJ, et al. Constipation and a Low-Fiber Diet are Not Associated with Diverticulosis. Clinical gastroenterology and hepatology: the official clinical practice journal of the American Gastroenterological Association. 2013;11(12):10.1016/j.cgh.2013.06.033. doi:10.1016/j.cgh.2013.06.033.

[20] Tan K-Y, Seow-Choen F. Fiber and colorectal diseases: Separating fact from fiction. *World Journal of Gastroenterology: WJG*. 2007;13(31):4161-4167. doi: 10.3748/wjg.v13.i31.4161. <**https://www.ncbi.nlm.nih.gov/pmc/articles/ PMC4250613/**>

High fiber intake promotes inflammation in the colon by the same mechanisms it causes inflammation in the small intestine. It is likely that fiber-induced cell damage, acidity and inflammation promotes or causes ulcerative colitis, intestinal obstruction, anal fistulas, intestinal or anal abscess, and creates the conditions that cause cells to malfunction, producing precancerous polyps and colorectal cancer.

Acids produced by microbial fermentation of fiber irritate the skin around the anus, producing anal itching (pruritis).

When you reduce fiber intake, you reduce the amount of indigestible material your gut will have to eliminate. Simply, less garbage in, less garbage out. Unfortunately, too many people have become convinced that one "must" drop a stool at least once a day.

Breast-feeding infants consume only milk – *an animal product* – containing no fiber and may go for long periods of time without any bowel evacuation. This is because breast milk is digested and absorbed with practically no residue. The same applies to meat, fat, eggs, and dairy products.

Therefore, if a person eats a fiber-free animal-based diet – as infants do – and consequently has infrequent bowel evacuations simply because he/she consumes less garbage – or *carbage* – this does not constitute disease or disorder. So long as one can evacuate the waste easily, one should have no concern about how often it happens.

When one first transitions from a plant-based diet to a diet with little or no fiber, one might initially have some difficulty with bowel evacuation. In *Life Without Bread*, Wolfgang Lutz M.D. explains that this occurs because a long-term high fiber diet can poison and damage the colon, making it too weak to move stools.[21]

As previously mentioned, this happened to me. When I first transitioned from a high fiber plant-based diet to a very low intake of

---

[21] Allan CB, Lutz W. Life Without Bread. Keats, 2000. 115-116, 204-205.

plants (and fiber), my bowel movement frequency dropped from daily to once every 3 to 7 days. For years previous to this, I mostly had loose, acidic, gaseous and sometimes somewhat explosive stools due to the prodigious amount of fermentation produced by my high fiber diet, so I was not accustomed to bearing down to move the stool. Consequently, when I finally got the urge, I found it difficult to get the stool started, and, since the stool had been in the colon for a while, the leading end of it was a bit dry and compact. However, once I got it moving out, the rest came out very smoothly.

To help my colon recover healthy function, I took 300-600 mg of magnesium daily. Magnesium improves bile flow, which stimulates healthy bowel movements, and it also draws water into the intestines, making the stool softer.

Since I was on a low-fat diet for many years, my bile production and flow was compromised. Also, I kept my fat intake no less than 60-65 percent of my energy (kcalorie) intake, and took digestive bitters and artichoke extract to establish a healthy bile flow. Coffee, digestive bitters and an adequately high fat intake stimulate strong post-meal bile flow, which stimulates intestinal movement and stool evacuation.

Over the course of about 6 months, my bowel function steadily improved. Eventually I had bowel movements at least 4 times weekly, and I regained the natural ability to bear down to move the stool out. At time of writing, I still take coffee, bitters and artichoke extract occasionally to keep bile production adequate.

Killer Carbohydrates

Dietary sugars and starches (grains, roots and tubers) promote tooth decay by feeding growth of oral bacteria that produce acids that eat away tooth enamel. It doesn't matter whether the plant is wild or modern, root, fruit or grain.

Ancient hunter-gatherers in North Africa who relied on wild plants rich in starch about 15 thousand years ago had dental decay rates

(51.2% of teeth in adults) comparable to modern industrialized populations consuming refined sugars and processed cereals.[22] Our hunting and gathering ancestors had virtually no dental decay, but when people adopted grain-based agricultural diets, tooth decay became a common ailment, and consumption of modern refined carbohydrates has made the problem worse.[23, 24, 25]

In 1974, British Royal Navy Surgeon-Captain T.L. Cleave published *The Saccharine Disease: Conditions caused by the Taking of Refined Carbohydrates, such as Sugar and White Flour,* in which he provided evidence that modern diseases of civilization did not occur among uncivilized populations, and all stem from the consumption of man-made refined carbohydrate foods such as sugar, white flour, and white rice.

Cleave's observation has received support from research suggesting that these dense acellular carbohydrates such as grains, beans, bread

---

[22] Humphrey LT, De Groote I, Morales J, et al. Earliest evidence for caries and exploitation of starchy plant foods in Pleistocene hunter-gatherers from Morocco. *Proceedings of the National Academy of Sciences of the United States of America.* 2014;111(3):954-959. doi:10.1073/pnas.1318176111. <https://www.ncbi.nlm.nih.gov/pmc/articles/PMC3903197/>

[23] Adler CJ, Dobney K, Weyrich LS, et al.. Sequencing ancient calcified dental plaque shows changes in oral microbiota with dietary shifts of the Neolithic and Industrial revolutions. Nature Genetics 2013 April;45(4):450-55.

[24] Sheiham A, James WPT. A reappraisal of the quantitative relationship between sugar intake and dental caries: the need for new criteria for developing goals for sugar intake. *BMC Public Health.* 2014;14:863. doi:10.1186/1471-2458-14-863. <https://www.ncbi.nlm.nih.gov/pmc/articles/PMC4168053/>

[25] Moynihan P. Sugars and Dental Caries: Evidence for Setting a Recommended Threshold for Intake. *Advances in Nutrition.* 2016;7(1):149-156. doi:10.3945/an.115.009365. <https://www.ncbi.nlm.nih.gov/pmc/articles/PMC4717883/>

and pasta promote inflammatory gut microbiota, and may be the primary causes of leptin resistance and obesity.[26]

High consumption of carbohydrates may accelerate aging. Every meal rich in sugars or starches increases the level of sugars in the blood. Insulin escorts glucose and fructose into cells where they react with proteins to produce advanced glycation end products (AGEs). These AGEs evidently promote diabetes, atherosclerosis, chronic kidney disease, cataracts, aging of muscle tissue, and Alzheimer's disease.[27]

Fructose sugar is the most potent of plant compounds to produce AGEs, up to 10 times more potent than glucose. Fructose consumption elevates triglycerides, cholesterol, uric acid and urea nitrogen in the blood, decreases glucose tolerance, increases insulin resistance, and raises VLDL levels. Animals fed a fructose (sugar) rich diet develop elevated blood levels of fructose and glycated hemoglobin, and excrete significantly more lipid peroxide products in urine compared to animals fed other sugars or low sugar diets. They also show accelerated skin and connective tissue aging.[28]

Dietary fructose has been found to have similar effects in humans. Fructose consumption appears to be an initiating factor in the

[26] Spreadbury I. Comparison with ancestral diets suggests dense acellular carbohydrates promote an inflammatory microbiota, and may be the primary dietary cause of leptin resistance and obesity. Diabetes, Metabolic Syndrome and Obesity: Targets and Therapy. 2012;5:175-189. doi:10.2147/DMSO.S33473. <https://www.ncbi.nlm.nih.gov/pmc/articles/PMC3402009/>

[27] Hous JM, Carrithers JA, Trappe SW, Trappe TA. Collagen, cross-linking, and advanced glycation end products in aging human skeletal muscle. J Appl Physiology 2007 Dec 1;103(6):2068-2076. <https://www.physiology.org/doi/10.1152/japplphysiol.00670.2007>

[28] Boaz Levi, Moshe J. Werman; Long-Term Fructose Consumption Accelerates Glycation and Several Age-Related Variables in Male Rats, *The Journal of Nutrition*, Volume 128, Issue 9, 1 September 1998, Pages 1442–1449, https://doi.org/10.1093/jn/128.9.1442

development of fatty liver, liver insulin resistance, metabolic syndrome, and diabetes along with ocular, renal, neural, musculoskeletal, and epidermal complications of diabetes such as cataracts, kidney failure, neuropathy, arthritis, asthma, and poor wound healing.[29]

Plants store fructose as fructans, also known as fructo-oligosaccharides or FOS. Mammals have no ability to digest fructans, but some gram-negative bacteria present in the gut can convert fructans to fructose. We have evidence that diets high in fructose or fructans increase intestinal bacteria overgrowth, leading to intestinal acidosis and permeability, resulting in endotoxemia and consequent disease.[30, 31]

By Nature we have a limited ability to absorb fructose and even more limited ability to absorb fructans (5-15%). Unabsorbed fructose or fructan rapidly draws water into the intestines, which causes rapid bowel movement of contents into the colon. There bacteria ferment the carbohydrates, resulting in abdominal pain, gas and bloating. In addition to fructose and fructans, plants contain

---

[29] Gugliucci A. Formation of Fructose-Mediated Advanced Glycation End Products and Their Roles in Metabolic and Inflammatory Diseases. *Advances in Nutrition*. 2017;8(1):54-62. doi:10.3945/an.116.013912. <https://www.ncbi.nlm.nih.gov/pmc/articles/PMC5227984/>

[30] Bergheim I, Weber S, Vos M, Krämer S, Volynets V, Kaserouni S, McClain CJ, Bischoff SC. Antibiotics protect against fructose-induced hepatic lipid accumulation in mice: role of endotoxin. J Hepatol. 2008 Jun;48(6):983-92. doi: 10.1016/j.jhep.2008.01.035. Epub 2008 Mar 14. PubMed PMID: 18395289.

[31] Johnson RJ, Rivard C, Lanaspa MA, et al. Fructokinase, Fructans, Intestinal Permeability, and Metabolic Syndrome: An Equine Connection? *Journal of equine veterinary science*. 2013;33(2):120-126. doi:10.1016/j.jevs.2012.05.004. <https://www.ncbi.nlm.nih.gov/pmc/articles/PMC3576823/>

galactans and polyols which have the same harmful effects (Table 5.1).[32]

Table 5.1 Foods high in fructans, galactans and polyols

	Food sources
Fructans	Wheat and wheat products (bread, pasta, etc), onions, shallots, scallions, garlic, barley, Brussels sprouts, cabbage, broccoli, pistachio, artichoke, inulin, chicory root
Galactans	Soy milk, soy protein isolate, miso, veggie-burgers, dried beans and peas, lentils, butter/lima beans, humus, coffee (more than 1 cup/d)
Polyols	Apples, plums, cherries, pear, cauliflower, sweet corn, snow peas, mushrooms, sugar-alcohol sweeteners (xylitol, sorbitol, etc.)

Glucose is among the least reactive of sugars, so the glucose the liver produces from amino acids or glycerol backbones of triglycerides is far less harmful than fructose. Diabetics produce some fructose, but there exists scant evidence that such endogenously produced fructose causes tissue damage; it is more likely that fructose ingested in plant-based foods drives the AGEing process.[33] People ingest fructose via fruits, honey, sugar, agave, maple syrup, corn syrup and some sweet tasting vegetables (e.g. sweet potatoes). Vegetarians evidently have higher AGE levels due to consuming more fructose-rich foods than non-vegetarians.[34]

---

[32] Fedewa A, Rao SSC. Dietary fructose intolerance, fructan intolerance and FODMAPs. *Current gastroenterology reports*. 2014;16(1):370. doi:10.1007/s11894-013-0370-0.

[33] Gugliucci A, op cit.

[34] Krajcovicova-Kulackova M, Sebekova K, Schinzel R, Klvanova J. Advanced Glycation End Products and Nutrition. Physiol Res 2002;51:313-316. <http://www.biomed.cas.cz/physiolres/2002/issue3/pdf/krajcovic.pdf>

Meat contains carnosine, a dipeptide that protects against glucose and fructose toxicity and suppresses glycation reactions, so a hypercarnivore diet may have strong anti-aging properties.[35, 36, 37] Carnosine has antioxidant, neuroprotective, antitoxic, anti-cataract, anti-glaucoma, anti-diabetic, anti-cancer and ergogenic properties.[38] Vegetarians have 26% lower carnosine levels than typical meat-eaters.[39] Typical meat-eaters eat a plant-based diet with meat providing only 10-20% of calories. Very likely a person eating a hypercarnivore diet with meat providing more than 70% of calories has an even higher carnosine level, therefore high protection against glycation reactions and premature aging.

Fatal Fats

Plants are rich in omega-6 polyunsaturated fatty acids and very poor sources of omega-3 fatty acids. In general, omega-6 fatty acids are proinflammatory while omega-3 fats are anti-inflammatory. People

[35] Hipkiss AR. Would carnosine or a carnivorous diet help suppress aging and associated pathologies? Ann N Y Acad Sci. 2006 May;1067:369-74. Review. PubMedPMID: 16804013.

[36] Pepper ED, Farrell MJ, Nord G, Finkel SE. Antiglycation Effects of Carnosine and Other Compounds on the Long-Term Survival of *Escherichia coli* . *Applied and Environmental Microbiology*. 2010;76(24):7925-7930. doi:10.1128/AEM. 01369-10. <https://www.ncbi.nlm.nih.gov/pmc/articles/PMC3008226/>

[37] Rashid I, van Reyk DM, Davies MJ. Carnosine and its constituents inhibit glycastion of low-density lipoproteins that promotes foam cell formation in vitro. FEBS Letters 2007; 581:1067-1070.

[38] Budzen S, Rymaszewska J. The Biological Role of Carnosine and Its Possible Applications in Medicine. Adv Clin Exp Med 2013;22(5):739-44. <http://www.advances.umed.wroc.pl/pdf/2013/22/5/739.pdf>

[39] Everaert I, Mooyaart A, Baguet A, Zutinic A, Baelde H, Achten E, Taes Y, De Heer E, Derave W. Vegetarianism, female gender and increasing age, but not CNDP1 genotype, are associated with reduced muscle carnosine levels in humans. Amino Acids. 2011 Apr;40(4):1221-9. doi: 10.1007/s00726-010-0749-2. Epub 2010 Sep 24. PubMed PMID: 20865290.

eating plant-based diets typically ingest 15 times more omega-6 fats than omega-3. As people have increased their intake of plant-based fats since the turn of the 20th century, we have experienced spectacular increases in chronic inflammatory diseases including nonalcoholic fatty liver disease (NAFLD), cardiovascular disease, obesity, inflammatory bowel disease (IBD), rheumatoid arthritis, and Alzheimer's disease. A high dietary intake of omega-6 fatty acids, characteristic of plant-based diets, promotes these conditions.[40] I discuss these fats further in Chapter 7.

Oxalates

Many vegetables contain oxalates. Plant-based foods rich in oxalates include:

- Spinach
- Rhubarb
- Almonds
- Cashews
- Miso soup
- Grits
- Baked potatoes with skin
- Beets
- Cocoa powder
- Okra
- Bran and shredded wheat cereals
- Raspberries
- Sweet potatoes
- Stevia

Also, high intakes of vitamin C, possible only with supplements or some plant foods very rich in vitamin C, raise oxalate levels.

---

[40] Patterson E, Wall R, Fitzgerald GF, Ross RP, Stanton C. Health Implications of High Dietary Omega-6 Polyunsaturated Fatty Acids. *Journal of Nutrition and Metabolism*. 2012;2012:539426. doi:10.1155/2012/539426. <**https://www.ncbi.nlm.nih.gov/pmc/articles/PMC3335257/**>

When your body excretes this useless oxalate, it combines with calcium and forms calcium oxalate stones. People with pre-existing kidney disease have suffered acute kidney failure from consuming oxalate-rich fruit and vegetable juices.[41] A 65-year-old woman who had no pre-existing kidney disease developed acute kidney injury that progressed to end-stage renal disease after consuming an oxalate-rich green smoothie juice "cleanse" prepared by juicing green leafy vegetables and fruits.[42]

Almond milk is a particularly rich source of dietary oxalate. Children have developed bloody urine, urinary pain, kidney stones and high blood oxalate by consuming almond milk regularly.[43]

Men who consume supplemental vitamin C (more than 1000 mg/d) have up to twofold increased risk of kidney stones.[44, 45]

---

[41] Getting JE, Gregoire JR, Phul A, Kasten MJ. Oxalate nephropathy due to 'juicing': case report and review. Am J Med. 2013 Sep;126(9):768-72. doi: 10.1016/j.amjmed.2013.03.019. Epub 2013 Jul 3. Review. PubMed PMID: 23830537.

[42] Makkapati S, D'Agati VD, Balsam L. "Green Smoothie Cleanse" Causing Acute Oxalate Nephropathy. Am J Kidney Dis. 2018 Feb;71(2):281-286. doi: 10.1053/j.ajkd.2017.08.002. Epub 2017 Dec 6. PubMed PMID: 29203127.

[43] Ellis D, Lieb J. Hyperoxaluria and Genitourinary Disorders in Children Ingesting Almond Milk Products. J Pediatr. 2015 Nov;167(5):1155-8. doi: 10.1016/j.jpeds.2015.08.029. Epub 2015 Sep 15. PubMed PMID: 26382627.

[44] Ferraro PM, Curhan GC, Gambaro G, Taylor EN. Total, Dietary, and Supplemental Vitamin C Intake and Risk of Incident Kidney Stones. *American journal of kidney diseases: the official journal of the National Kidney Foundation.* 2016;67(3):400-407. doi:10.1053/j.ajkd.2015.09.005.

[45] Thomas LDK, Elinder C, Tiselius H, Wolk A, Åkesson A. Ascorbic Acid Supplements and Kidney Stone Incidence Among Men: A Prospective Study. *JAMA Intern Med.* 2013;173(5):386–388. doi:10.1001/jamainternmed.2013.2296

Psychoactive Phytochemicals

Plants notoriously provide many psychoactive chemicals, some of which are very addictive, such as heroin, morphine and cocaine.

Some research indicates that plain table sugar is more addictive than cocaine. Ninety-four percent of animals given free choice of either sugar-sweetened water or intravenous cocaine choose the sugar water, even if already addicted to cocaine.[46] The authors of this study explain:

> "In most mammals, including rats and humans, sweet receptors evolved in ancestral environments poor in sugars and are thus not adapted to high concentrations of sweet tastants. The supranormal stimulation of these receptors by sugar-rich diets, such as those now widely available in modern societies, would generate a supranormal reward signal in the brain, with the potential to override self-control mechanisms and thus lead to addiction."

It appears probable that use of and/or addiction to psychoactive phytochemicals played an important or decisive role in the invention of agriculture and rise of civilization, since "a significant portion of the effort of early cultivators globally" was devoted to cultivation of mind-altering plants, including cereals, poppies, coca, sugar cane, tobacco, and cannibis.[47, 48]

---

[46] Lenoir M, Serre F, Cantin L, Ahmed S. Intense Sweetness Surpasses Cocaine Reward. PLoS ONE 2(8): e698. **https://doi.org/10.1371/journal.pone.0000698**

[47] Wadley G, Martin A. The origins of agriculture: a biological perspective and a new hypothesis. Australian Biologist 1993 June;6:96-105.

[48] Wadley G, Hayden B. Pharmacological Influences on the Neolithic Transition. Journal of Ethnobiology 2015;35(3):566-584.

Cereals contain exorphins, which at normal dietary doses have a potency comparable to morphine and enkephalin and have analgesic and anxiolytic effects.[49]

Schizophrenia and other psychoses appear linked to the amount and type of cereals in the diet. Individuals who have celiac disease (intolerance of gluten in wheat) have an unusually high risk of schizophrenia and other psychoses. Populations that transition to agricultural diets experience an emergence of previously absent psychoses including schizophrenia. Schizophrenia is most common in populations with high wheat consumption, less common in rice-based populations, and least common where grains are not staple foods. Patients suffering from schizophrenia have obtained relief by restricting cereal grains, especially wheat, or by limiting all plant foods.[50, 51, 52]

Research into food allergy and intolerance has shown that normal quantities of some plant foods – including most commonly wheat, corn, potato, coffee, rice, chocolate, tea, citrus, oats, and sugar cane – can have pharmacological, including psychoactive, effects. Some intolerance symptoms include anxiety, depression, epilepsy, hyperactivity, and schizophrenic episodes. People often have

---

[49] Wadley G, Martin A. The origins of agriculture: a biological perspective and a new hypothesis. Australian Biologist 1993 June;6:96-105.

[50] Dohan FC. Cereals and Schizophrenia: Data and Hypothesis. Acta Psychiatrica Scandinavica 1966 Jun 1;42(2):125-152.

[51] Kraft BD, Westman EC. Schizophrenia, gluten, and low-carbohydrate, ketogenic diets: a case report and review of the literature. *Nutrition & Metabolism*. 2009;6:10. doi:10.1186/1743-7075-6-10. <**https://www.ncbi.nlm.nih.gov/pmc/articles/PMC2652467/**>

[52] Palmer CM. Ketogenic diet in the treatment of schizoaffective disorder: Two case studies. Schizophrenia Research 2017 Nov;189:208-209.

cravings, withdrawal and addiction symptoms when attempting to remove these foods from their diets.[53]

The carbohydrate-restricted ketogenic diet "is now a proven therapy for drug-resistant epilepsy" and "there is mounting experimental evidence for its broad neuroprotective properties and in turn, emerging data supporting its use in multiple neurological disease states."[54] Ketogenic diets show promise for prevention of age-related neurodegeneration and treatment of Alzheimer's dementia, Parkinson's disease, amyotrophic lateral sclerosis, post-stroke brain damage, brain trauma, depression, autism, and migraine.

So far, no one knows exactly why a ketogenic diet has positive effects on neurological function. It is generally assumed that its benefits have something to do with reduction of blood glucose levels, increase of fatty acid metabolism and elevation of ketone bodies. Although the brain evidently readily utilizes and may even prefer ketones to glucose,[55, 56] no one has provided conclusive evidence that elevated ketones play the only or even key role.

Although it has been assumed that the proven anti-seizure properties of a very low carbohydrate ketogenic diet are due to elevation of

[53] Wadley G, Martin A. The origins of agriculture: a biological perspective and a new hypothesis. Australian Biologist 1993 June;6:96-105.

[54] Stafstrom CE, Rho JM. The ketogenic diet as a treatment paradigm for diverse neurological disorders. Front Pharmacol 2012 April 09; <**https://doi.org/10.3389/fphar.2012.00059**>

[55] Zhang Y, Kuang Y, Xu K, et al. Ketosis proportionately spares glucose utilization in brain. *Journal of Cerebral Blood Flow & Metabolism*. 2013;33(8): 1307-1311. doi:10.1038/jcbfm.2013.87. <https://www.ncbi.nlm.nih.gov/pmc/articles/PMC3734783/>

[56] LaManna JC, Salem N, Puchowicz M, et al. KETONES SUPPRESS BRAIN GLUCOSE CONSUMPTION. *Advances in experimental medicine and biology*. 2009;645:301-306. doi:10.1007/978-0-387-85998-9_45. <https://www.ncbi.nlm.nih.gov/pmc/articles/PMC2874681/>

ketone levels, several studies have provided evidence that non-ketogenic low carbohydrate diets have comparable anti-seizure activity, casting doubt on this assumption.[57, 58, 59] These studies found a lack of association between increased ketone levels and seizure control, and suggest that the benefits of the ketogenic diet for epilepsy may be largely due to reduction of total carbohydrate (i.e. plant food) intake, stabilization of blood sugar and insulin levels (e.g. removal of post-meal glucose and insulin spikes) and reduction of cellular glucose metabolism (less glycolysis). I discuss this in greater detail in Chapter 10.

It is common for the mind to focus on what is present, rather than what is absent, as an explanation for phenomena. This results in focus on the presence of ketones, rather than the absence of phytochemicals, including highly psychoactive sucrose, as the explanation for improved neurological health associated with ketogenic diets.

A ketogenic diet limits total carbohydrate intake, generally to less than 40 g per day, so it is per force an animal-based diet. Given the fact that plant foods contain many phytochemicals that have marked effects on the nervous system, it is reasonable to hypothesize that some of the positive effects of a ketogenic diet are produced not by the presence of ketones, but by the absence of psychoactive phytochemicals.

---

[57] Neal EG, et al. A randomized trial of classical and medium-chain triglyceride ketogenic diets in the treatment of childhood epilepsy. Epilepsia. 2009;50:1109–17. doi: 10.1111/j.1528-1167.2008.01870.x.

[58] Muzykewicz DA, et al. Efficacy, safety, and tolerability of the low glycemic index treatment in pediatric epilepsy. Epilepsia. 2009;50:1118–26. doi: 10.1111/j.1528-1167.2008.01959.x.

[59] Dallérac G, Moulard J, Benoist J-F, et al. Non-ketogenic combination of nutritional strategies provides robust protection against seizures. *Scientific Reports*. 2017;7:5496. doi:10.1038/s41598-017-05542-3. <https://www.ncbi.nlm.nih.gov/pmc/articles/PMC5511156/#CR28>

100% Natural Pesticides and Carcinogens

Compared to dangerous animals like wolves and lions, many plants appear defenseless and harmless, but they are not. Like all other organisms, they have to survive. They can't make noise, run or fight, so they have evolved sophisticated chemical weapons to protect themselves from predators, including worms, grubs, insects, animals and humans.

Non-food plants are among the most commonly ingested poisons for children under 5 years of age. However, most people do not know that food plants also contain poisonous compounds. Unfortunately, not many of these have been properly tested for health effects in humans.

Plants produce more of these poisons when under stresses such as high UV light, low temperatures, insect attack, pathogen infection, and nutrient deficiency.[60] Organic food production systems increase the pest and pathogen stress on plants, resulting in increased levels of these toxins in plants.[61] Whole grains provide more of these toxins than refined grains, typical whole grain intakes providing at least several hundred milligrams daily.

When tested in test tubes, many of these chemicals interfere with oxidation reactions, so they can also be called antioxidants. However, the fact that these chemicals behave as antioxidants in test tubes does not prove that they function likewise in the body. In fact it appears that some test-tube phytochemical antioxidants – including

---

[60] Young JE, Zhao X, Carey EE, et al.. Phytochemical phenolics in organically grown vegetables. Mol Nutr Food Res 2005;49:1136-1142.

[61] Baranski M, Srednicka-Tober D, Volakakis N, et al.. Higher antioxidant and low cadmium concentrations and lower incidence of pesticide residues in organically grown crops: a systematic literature review and meta-analysis. Br J Nutr 2014;112:794-811.

vitamin C – are pro-oxidative when in the body.[62] Consequently, it becomes difficult to support claims that the supposed benefits of these phytochemicals stem from their antioxidant effects.

Evidently, these "antioxidants" function as pesticides and antibiotics. They repel and kill pests and pathogens by poisoning cells, especially nerve cells.

Life depends on oxidation reactions. Oxidation reactions are essential to cellular metabolism. Our cells derive energy from fats through a series of reactions called beta-oxidation. We take in oxygen from the atmosphere to support oxidation of fats and other chemicals, without which we would die. Oxidation reactions can produce loose reactive oxygen species – commonly known as *free radicals* – that could cause collateral damage if not controlled.

Nature has not left us dependent on inconsistently available fruits and vegetables for protection from free radicals. We produce our own antioxidant compounds to prevent random undesirable oxidation in our bodies, including glutathione, alpha-lipoic acid, coenzyme Q10, uric acid, bilirubin, metallothioneine, melatonin, l-carnitine and l-carnosine. Meat is a rich source of the last two of these antioxidants.

People who assume that we benefit from eating plants have tried to "explain" the assumed (but never proven) benefits of eating plants as benefits of eating phytochemical antioxidants. However, direct studies have shown that eating antioxidant-rich plants (fruits and vegetables) probably provides no antioxidant benefit, and eliminating fruits and vegetables from the diet may even improve antioxidant status, indicating that our endogenous antioxidant

---

[62] Yin J-J, Fu PP, Lutterodt H, Zhou Y-T, Antholine WE, Wamer W. Dual Role of Selected Antioxidants Found in Dietary Supplements: Crossover between Anti- and Pro-oxidant Activities in the Presence of Copper. *Journal of agricultural and food chemistry*. 2012;60(10):2554-2561. doi:10.1021/jf204724w. <https://www.ncbi.nlm.nih.gov/pmc/articles/PMC3971523/>

mechanisms provide sufficient protection without any need for phytochemicals claimed to have antioxidant effects.[63, 64]

As mentioned, all of our life processes depend on oxidation reactions generating energy. A phytochemical that suppresses oxidation could in high enough concentration suppress energy metabolism in cells. This is one way the chemical can act as a poison. When cells can't produce enough energy from nutrients, they can't repair themselves and can die as a result.

This is why some of these natural antioxidants/pesticides have been shown to have anti-tumor cell properties. Simply, just like man-made chemotherapy, these chemicals interfere with cell metabolism, slowing the growth and repair systems of tumor cells. It is well known that synthetic chemotherapy for cancer is just as toxic to healthy cells as to tumor cells. We have no reason to believe that natural anti-cancer drugs taken from plants are any different.

In fact, more than 25% of anti-cancer drugs used in conventional medicine between 1989 and 2009 were derived from plants.[65] Anti-cancer chemotherapy drugs have so many undesirable side-effects –

---

[63] Møller P, Vogel U, Pedersen A, Dragsted LO, Sandström B, Loft S. No effect of 600 grams fruit and vegetables per day on oxidative DNA damage and repair in healthy nonsmokers. Cancer Epidemiol Biomarkers Prev. 2003 Oct;12(10): 1016-22. PubMed PMID: 14578137. <**http://cebp.aacrjournals.org/content/ 12/10/1016.long**>

[64] "The overall effect of the 10-week period without dietary fruits and vegetables was a decrease in oxidative damage to DNA, blood proteins, and plasma lipids, concomitantly with marked changes in antioxidative defense." Young JF, Dragsted LO, Haraldsdóttir J, et al.. Green tea extract only affects markers of oxidative stress postprandiallly: Lasting antioxidant effect of flavonoid-free diet. Br J Nutr 2002;87:343-355.

[65] Amin A, Gali-Muhtasib H, Ocker M, Schneider-Stock R. Overview of Major Classes of Plant-Derived Anticancer Drugs. *International Journal of Biomedical Science: IJBS*. 2009;5(1):1-11. <**https://www.ncbi.nlm.nih.gov/pmc/articles/ PMC3614754/**>

including promoting cancer[66] – because their modes of action, such as interfering with DNA replication, inhibiting energy metabolism (i.e. antioxidation), or triggering cell death, harm both tumor cells and normal cells.

The allegedly anti-cancer chemicals naturally occurring in plants are no different. A review[60] of these chemicals gives some interesting information such as:

- Phenols from tea have "cell-killing activity" and inhibit new blood vessel formation.
- High doses of sulforophane from cruciferous vegetables have been shown to induce oxidative stress and cause cell death.

About 99.99% of the pesticides in the typical American diet are phytochemicals that plants use to defend themselves.[67] Americans eat an estimated 1.5 g of natural pesticides daily, which is about 10,000 times more than they eat of synthetic pesticide residues. This includes 5,000 to 10,000 different natural pesticides and their breakdown products.

For example, cabbage contains at least 49 different natural pesticides and metabolites (Table 5.2).

---

[66] "For decades, clinicians and epidemiologists have recognized that radiotherapy and certain chemotherapies may increase risk for developing a second cancer." National Cancer Institute. Division of Cancer Epidemiology & Genetics. Discovering the causes of cancer and the means of prevention. Our Research > Second Primary Cancers. Accessed Dec 18, 2017 from: **<https://dceg.cancer.gov/ research/what-we-study/second-cancers>**

[67] Ames BN, Profet M, Gold LS. Dietary pesticides (99.99% all natural). Proc Natl Acad Sci USA 1990 Oct;87:7777-7781.

Table 5.2 Forty-nine natural pesticides and metabolites found in cabbage

Glucosinolates	2-propenyl glucoinolate (sinagrin), 2-methylthiopropyl glucosinolate, 33-methylsulfinylpropyl glucosinolate, 2-butenyl glucosinolate, 2-hydroxy-3-butenyl glucosinolate, 4-methylthiobutyl glucosinolate, 4-methysuflinylbutyl glucosinolate, 4-methylsulfonylbutyl glucosinolate, beyzyl glucosinolate, 2-phenylethyl glucosinolate, propyl glucosinolate, butyl glucosinolate
Indole glucosinolates and related indoles	3-indolylmethyl glucosinolate (glucobrassicin), 1-methoxy-3-indolylmethyl glocosinolate (neoglucobrassicin), indole-3-carbinol, indole-3-acetonitrile, bis(3-indolyl)methane
Isothiocyanates and goitrin	allyl isothiocyanate, 3-methylthiopropyl isothiocyanate, 3-methylsulfinylpropyl isothiocyanate, 3-butenyl isothiocyanate, 5-vinyloxazolidine-2-thione (goitrin), 4-methylthiobutyl isothiocyanate, 4-methylsulfinylbutyl isothiocyanate, 4-methylsulfonylbutyle isothiocyanate, 4-pentenyl isothiocyanate, benzyl isotyocyanate, phenylethyl isothyocyanate
Cyanides	1-cyano-2,3-epithiopropane, 1-cyano-3,4-epithiobutane, 1-cyano-3,4-epithiopentane, *threo*-1-cyano-2-hydroxy-3,4-epithiobutane, *erythro*-1-cyano-2-hydroxy-3,4-epithiobutane, 2-phenylpropionitrile, allyl cyanide, 1-cyano-2-hydroxy-3-butene, 1-cyano-3-methylsulfinylpropane, 1-cyano-4-methylsuflinylbutane
Terpenes	menthol, neomenthol, isomenthol, carvone
Phenols	2-methoxyphenol, 3-caffoylquinic acid (chlorogenic acid), 4-caffoylquinic acid, 5-caffoylqunic acid (neochlorogenic acid), 4-(*p*-coumaroyl)quniic acid, 5-(p-coumaroyl)quinic acid, 5-feruloylquinic acid

Source: Ames BN, Profet M, Gold LS. Dietary pesticides (99.99% all natural). Proc Natl Acad Sci USA 1990 Oct;87:7777-7781.

Some of the phytochemicals which have been touted as anti-cancer anti-oxidants have also been proven to be mutagenic and carcinogenic in the same type of animal studies used to test safety of man-made pesticides. Researchers have only tested 53 naturally occurring plant pesticides for carcinogenicity, but 27 have tested positive. These rodent carcinogens naturally occur in: anise, apple, apricot, banana, basil, broccoli, Brussels sprouts, cabbage, cantaloupe, caraway, carrot, cauliflower, celery, cherries, cinnamon, cloves, cocoa, coffee, collard greens, comfrey herb tea, currants, dill, eggplant, endive, fennel, grapefruit juice, grapes, guava, honey, honeydew melon, horseradish, kale, lentils, lettuce, mango, mushrooms, mustard, nutmeg, orange juice, parsley, parsnip, peach, pear, peas, black pepper, pineapple, plum, potato, radish, raspberries, rosemary, sesame seeds, tarragon, tea, tomato, and turnip. Probably every fruit and vegetable in the supermarket contains natural plant pesticides that are rodent carcinogens, at concentrations that are thousands of times higher than the levels of synthetic pesticides allowed on foods.[68]

At least 72 of these natural plant pesticides have been shown to be clastogenic – capable of breaking chromosomes – in at least one test, at doses far less than they naturally occur in foods. For example, allyl isothiocyanate exhibited clastogenicity at 0.0005 ppm, which is about 200,000 times less than the concentration of sinigrin, its glucosinolate, in cabbage. Caffeic acid proved clastogenic at a concentration of 260 and 500 ppm, which is less than its concentration in roasted coffee beans and close to its concentration in apples, lettuce, endive, and potato skin. Chlorogenic acid, a precursor of caffeic acid, proved clastogenic at a concentration of 150 ppm, which is 100 times less than its concentration in roasted coffee beans and similar to its concentration in apples, pears, plums, peaches, cherries, and apricots.[69] Chlorogenic acid and caffeic acid are also mutagens.

In plants, these compounds occur in measures of parts per thousand or million, whereas synthetic pesticide residues generally occur in parts per billion. Whereas you may be able to wash man-made pesticides off of foods, you can't wash naturally occurring pesticides out of foods.

---

[68] Ames BN, Profet M, Gold LS. Dietary pesticides (99.99% all natural). Proc Natl Acad Sci USA 1990 Oct;87:7777-7781.

[69] Ibid.

Many parts of plants taste quite bitter from high concentrations of these chemicals. Just the bitter flavor will repel many predators, but if it doesn't, the bitter stuff may injure or even kill healthy cells or tissues.

Remember, mutations and cancer are only the extreme effects of exposure to large amounts these chemicals. Any chemical that in high doses alters cell function enough to cause mutations or initiate tumors very likely will in smaller doses cause less severe disorders of cell function.

For example the goitrins in plants interfere with iodine metabolism, and about 8 million people world-wide have goiter and hypothyroidism because they consume plant-based, goitrin-rich diets.[70] Read more about this in Chapter 7, where I provide a list of goitrin-rich plant foods.

Compared to omnivores and carnivores, vegetarians and others who emphasize eating whole plant foods will consume greater amounts of these toxins. Some research indicates a higher incidence of cancer, allergies, and mental health disorders, a higher need and use of health care services, and a poorer quality of life for vegetarians, despite their mean lower body mass index, higher mean socioeconomic status, and better health behavior including greater physical activity and less use of alcohol and tobacco.[71]

Probably chronic consumption of these compounds causes or contributes to many maladies in humans, but no one conducts research on this topic because we all assume that eating fruits and vegetables promotes health, because some authorities have said so.

---

[70] Whitney EN and Rolfes SR. Understanding Nutrition 10th Edition. Thomson Wadsworth, 2005:451.

[71] Burkert NT, Muckenhuber J, Grobschadl F, et al.. Nutrition and Health – The Association between Eating Behavior and Various Health Parameters: A Matched Sample Study. PLoS One 9(2):e88278. doi:10.1371/journal.pone.0088278

Lectins

Lectins are carbohydrate-binding proteins that naturally occur in most plants (Table 5.3). They "are highly antinutritional and/or toxic substances being detrimental to various plant-eating organisms."[72] Seeds and tubers like cereals, beans, and potatoes have the highest lectin concentrations. In the service of plants, lectins appear to function primarily as insecticides.[73] Research has demonstrated that lectins are (a) present in most plant foods, (b) resistant to cooking and digestive enzymes, and (c) either toxic, inflammatory, or both.

Table 5.3 Partial list of foods containing lectins

Tomato, potato, beans, peas, carrots, soybeans, cherries, blackberries, wheat germ, rice, corn, garlic, peanuts, nuts, mushrooms, avocado, beetroot, leek, cabbage, tea, parsley, oregano, spices

These compounds cause acute gut poisoning, sometimes called "food poisoning." An article in the British Medical Journal recounts:

> "In 1988 a hospital launched a 'healthy eating day' in its staff canteen at lunchtime. One dish contained red kidney beans, and 31 portions were served. At 3 pm one of the customers, a surgical registrar, vomited in theatre. Over the next four hours 10 more customers suffered profuse vomiting, some with diarrhea. All had recovered by next day. No pathogens were isolated from the food, but the beans contained an abnormally high concentration of the lectin phytohaemaggluttin."[74]

---

[72] Vasconcelos IM, Oliveira JTA. Antinutritional properties of plant lectins. Toxicon 2004;44:385-403.

[73] Ibid.

[74] Freed DLJ. Do dietary lectins cause disease?: The evidence is suggestive — and raises interesting possibilities for treatment . *BMJ: British Medical Journal.* 1999;318(7190):1023-1024. <**https://www.ncbi.nlm.nih.gov/pmc/articles/ PMC1115436/**>

This story illustrates how ignoring Nature's warning not to eat a certain type of food (beans) and thinking you can make a non-food into a food by cooking it (cleverness, artifice) can lead to acute disaster. We think we can outsmart Nature. Our ancestors called this hubris.

Since that event we have learned that some food lectins make their way into our blood and deposit themselves into vital organs. Lectins also have been shown to strip away the healthy mucous coat from the small intestine, cause discharge of histamine and increase acid secretion from stomach cells, all three mechanisms promoting stomach infection with H. pylori and consequent ulcer. Finally, many lectins are powerful allergens.[71]

Researchers have linked lectins in wheat, soy, potato, peanuts, and tomatoes to metabolic and immune system diseases including obesity, nephropathy, diabetes, cancer, and autoimmune diseases such as rheumatoid arthritis.[75, 76, 77]

Lectins also have anti-nutritive effects.[78] They increase gut cell turnover, stimulate small intestine tissue hyperplasia, promote overgrowth of coliform bacteria (particularly E. coli), and interfere with protein digesting enzymes, resulting in pancreas hypertrophy (a potential prelude to pancreatic cancer) and nutrient malabsorption and facilitating passage of antigens into the blood circulation.

75 Jönsson, Tommy et al. "Agrarian Diet and Diseases of Affluence – Do Evolutionary Novel Dietary Lectins Cause Leptin Resistance?" BMC Endocrine Disorders 5 (2005): 10. PMC. Web. 1 Mar. 2017. **<https://www.ncbi.nlm.nih.gov/ pmc/articles/PMC1326203/>**

76 Lindeberg S, Food and Western Disease: Health and nutrition from an evolutionary perspective (Wiley, 2010): Sections 4.3, 4.6, 4.11, and 4.15.

77 Cordain, L., Toohey, L., Smith, M.J. and Hickey, M.S. (2000) 'Modulation of immune function by dietary lectins in rheumatoid arthritis', British Journal of Nutrition, 83(3), pp. 207–217. doi: 10.1017/S0007114500000271.

78 Vasconcelos IM, Oliveira JTA. Antinutritional properties of plant lectins. Toxicon 2004;44:385-403.

Lectins also interfere with insulin action and possibly insulin production.

Some other documented effects of dietary lectins include: liver enlargement, suppression of muscle protein synthesis leading to loss of muscle weight, lung enlargement, atherogenesis, and growth stunting.[79]

Clearly lectins can do a lot of damage. As carnivores we are not adapted to plant-based, lectin-laced diets. Reducing lectin intake – by reducing plant-food intake – will likely improve your health.

Alkylresorcinols

These chemicals occur primarily in cereals such as wheat, rye and barley. They "damage DNA and prevent its repair, a property that may be useful in cancer therapy."[80] However, as noted, while one may think it desirable to consume chemicals that "may be useful in cancer therapy," in reality, as already noted, a chemical that can damage and prevent the repair of DNA in cancer cells will also have the ability to damage and prevent the repair of DNA in healthy cells.

Alkylresorcinols also inhibit respiration (use of oxygen) and synthesis of nucleic acids and proteins in isolated thymocytes.[81] Thymocytes are progenitors for lymphocytes commonly known as T-cells, which play a key role in immune function. Cancer cells have inhibited respiration and active fermentation, which is known as the Warburg effect, named after Otto Warburg, the scientist who in 1924 first reported the phenomenon. Warburg produced evidence that he believed established that the Warburg effect is the root cause of cancers. In his words:

---

[79] Ibid.

[80] Ross AB, Kamal-Eldin A, Aman P. Dietary Alkylresorcinols: Absorption, Bioactivities, and Possible Use as Biomarkers of Whole-grain Wheat- and Rye-rich foods. Nutrition Reviews 2004 Mar 1;62(3):81-95.

[81] Ibid.

"Cancer, above all other diseases, has countless secondary causes. But, even for cancer, there is only one prime cause. Summarized in a few words, the prime cause of cancer is the replacement of the respiration of oxygen in normal body cells by a fermentation of sugar. All normal body cells meet their energy needs by respiration of oxygen, whereas cancer cells meet their energy needs in great part by fermentation. All normal body cells are thus obligate aerobes, whereas all cancer cells are partial anaerobes. From the standpoint of the physics and chemistry of life this difference between normal and cancer cells is so great that one can scarcely picture a greater difference. Oxygen gas, the donor of energy in plants and animals is dethroned in the cancer cells and replaced by an energy yielding reaction of the lowest living forms, namely, a fermentation of glucose"[82]

To reiterate, according to Warburg, "the prime cause of cancer is the replacement of the respiration of oxygen in normal body cells by a fermentation of sugar."[83] Inhibition of respiration shuts down the mitochondria (organelles of respiration) in cells, and the when mitochondria stop functioning, this disables the cells' programming for self-destruction (apoptosis). Hence inhibition of respiration may make a cell malignant. If thymocyte DNA gets damaged – perhaps by something that interferes with respiration and synthesis of nucleic acids, such as alkylresorcinols? – this can produce thymic lymphoma (cancer of lymphocytes). Do you really want to consume large or even "moderate" amounts of foods containing a substance that can damage your lymphocytes?

---

[82] Brand RA. Biographical Sketch: Otto Heinrich Warburg, PhD, MD. *Clinical Orthopaedics and Related Research.* 2010;468(11):2831-2832. doi:10.1007/s11999-010-1533-z. <**https://www.ncbi.nlm.nih.gov/pmc/articles/PMC2947689/**>

[83] Ibid.

Tannins and Salivary Proline-Rich Proteins

Plants contain large amounts of bitter-tasting polyphenols and flavonoids that are known collectively as tannins. Tannins are anti-nutrients because they bind and reduce the digestibility and bioavailability of dietary proteins.

Children reject many vegetables and fruits because they do not like the taste of tannins. This makes sense because children have a high need for protein and tannins would reduce their ability to acquire adequate dietary protein.

However, many (but not all) adults seek out and enjoy foods with a certain level of tannins – such as tea, red wine, beer, chocolate, smoked foods, herbs, and spices – leading some authors to suggest that adult humans have a natural taste for or attraction to tannins.[84]

In fact, we appear to have an evolved adaptation to inclusion of some tannins in our diets. About 70% of the proteins in adult human saliva consist of salivary proline-rich proteins (PRPs), which bind with dietary tannins.[85] Studies of mice and rats have shown that PRPs neutralize the detrimental effects of tannins.[86]

The hypothesis that we are naturally adapted to inclusion of some tannins in our diet is supported by the fact that some and perhaps all native uncivilized tribes – including some that are highly carnivorous – use tannin-rich herbs, gums and resins regularly in seasoning food, making beverages and as medicine.

For example, the African Maasai eat almost no plant matter as food, but they regularly use 28 herbs in meat-based soups and add a dozen

---

[84] Ibid., 424.

[85] Mehanso H, Butler LG, Carlson DM. **Dietary Tannins and Salivary Proline-Rich Proteins: Interactions, Induction, and Defense Mechanisms.** Annual Review of Nutrition 1987 Jul 1;7(1):423-40.

[86] Mehanso H, et al., op. cit., 424.

herbs to milk to prepare a tea-like beverage they call *orkiowa*. In interviews, the Maasai state that they believe that they must regularly consume these herbs to maintain health in their habitat. These herbs and gums contain phytochemicals that in small doses may improve digestion and metabolism of fats, so they complement the Maasai high fat diet.[87] The southern Inuit eat a nearly 100% animal food diet for at least half of every year, but they also seasonally may use spruce needle tea to prevent and treat scurvy.[88] Inuit also consumed kelp, sorrel grass, and blossoms of flowers, some of which they preserved in seal oil for winter use.[89]

Because of the universality of human consumption of non-food plants or plant extracts, it has been proposed that the use of herbs and spices evolved as a part of adapting to highly carnivorous diets.[90] We have evidence that in small doses tannins may act as important chemopreventers of infectious and chronic diseases in humans, and have antioxidant, anti-inflammatory, vasoprotective, vasodilatory, antibacterial, antiallergic, hepatoprotective, antithrombotic, antiviral, neuroprotective, and anticarcinogenic effects.[91, 92]

---

[87] Johns T. The Chemical Ecology of Human Ingestive Behaviors. Annu Rev Anthropol 1999;28:27-50.

[88] Brett HB. A Synopsis of Northern Medical History. Canad Med Ass J 1969 Mr 15;100:521-25.

[89] Price W. Nutrition and Physical Degeneration. Price-Pottenger Nutrition Foundation, 1970. 70-71.

[90] Johns T. The Chemical Ecology of Human Ingestive Behaviors. Annu Rev Anthropol 1999;28:27-50.

[91] Habauzit V, Morand C. **Evidence for a protective effect of polyphenols-containing foods on cardiovascular health: an update for clinicians**. Ther Adv Chronic Dis 2012 Mar;3(2):87-106. PMC3513903.

[92] Soobrattee MA, Bahorun T, Aruoma OI. **Chemopreventive actions of polyphenolic compounds in cancer.** Biofactors 2006 Jan 1:27(1):19-35. 21.

Although in large amounts the bitter, sour and spicy phytochemicals can be toxic to the digestive tract or other tissues, in small amounts the small stress they place on our physiology can have a hormetic effect, stimulating a beneficial response or adaptation.[93] Thus non-food phytochemicals such as tannins can have both direct and indirect chemopreventive and medicinal effects.

Normal metabolism includes anabolic and catabolic processes. Disease can occur if either anabolic or catabolic processes are excessive. For example, obesity is a disorder resulting from a predominance of anabolic over catabolic processes; while sarcopenia (loss of muscle mass) and osteoporosis result from a predominance of catabolic over anabolic processes.

From a nutritional perspective alone, while salty and sweet flavors represent minerals, protein and fats which provide nourishment and build the body up, small doses of herbs or spices having bitter, sour and spicy flavors stimulate flow of digestive juices and peristalsis, facilitating appetite, digestion and elimination.

Chinese medical theory maintains that everyone needs a balance between anabolic and catabolic influences depending on their present condition. For example an obese person needs to have fat catabolism dominate over fat anabolism, while a person with sarcopenia or an emaciated individual recovering from a fruitarian vegan diet needs to have some anabolic processes dominate over catabolic. Therefore some people who have diseases that resulted from excessive stimulation of anabolic processes (excess diseases) may benefit from strategic inclusion of bitter, sour and spicy foods or herbs to stimulate necessary increases in catabolic processes. On the other hand a person suffering from deficiency diseases will need to have a predominance of sweet and salty flavors is his/her diet and lesser amounts of bitter, sour and spicy flavors.

----

[93] Mattson MP. Hormesis Defined. Ageing research reviews. 2008;7(1):1-7. doi: 10.1016/j.arr.2007.08.007. <https://www.ncbi.nlm.nih.gov/pmc/articles/PMC2248601/>

When a person properly trained in Chinese herbal therapy formulates an herbal prescription containing rich, sweet and salty herbs to rectify a deficient condition, the formula almost always also includes some bitter, bland, sour or spicy herbs to prevent the rich herbs from causing congestion. Similarly, in not only Chinese but also European culinary arts, herbs and spices are added to rich foods to make them more enjoyable and facilitate digestion. A simple example is barbecued fatty meat, prepared with a marinade or sauce containing bitter, sour, and spicy seasonings.

Traditional herbal medicine theories of Europe, China and India agree with the Maasai, maintaining that in addition to the salty and sweet flavors dominant in meat and fat we need some bitter, sour and spicy flavors to maintain health via a balance of anabolic and catabolic processes.

Thus, the use of non-food plants as flavorings and medicines may have evolved into a universal Human practice (part of Human Nature) because it improves digestion and assimilation, and increases fitness and disease resistance. Similar evolutionary reasoning probably explains the felines' habit of regularly consuming grass and catnip.

Summary

Many authorities teach that we need to eat a plant-based diet to get starches, sugars, fiber, unsaturated fats and phytochemicals, but there exists no evidence that we have absolute dietary requirements for any of these. On the contrary, there exists much evidence that fiber, carbohydrates and phytochemicals have harmful effects on our guts, cells and tissues, and we have good reason to believe that plants we eat can have adverse effects on our brain function and health.

On the other hand, we have a specific physiological adaptation to consumption of tannin-rich plants (salivary proline-rich proteins); humans universally use non-food plants – herbs and spices – to make beverages, season staple foods, and as medicines; these non-food plants provide both direct and indirect (hormetic) effects when consumed in small amounts; and it seems likely that our use of non-food plant extracts co-evolved with our adaptation to highly carnivorous diets.

On this basis I believe that although we are not by Nature designed to subsist on plant-based diets providing large amounts of fiber, macronutrients or phytochemicals, we may be by Nature designed or adapted to regularly consume some small amounts of non-food plants and plant extracts as part of a meat-based diet, much as cats are evidently by Nature adapted to eating some grass (herbs) as part of their hypercarnivorous diets.

6 NATURE'S PREFERRED FUEL

Many people believe that human body cells "prefer" to use carbohydrates as their primary fuel source, and that they do not utilize fats as efficiently as carbohydrates. This has no basis in fact. Nature designed us to run primarily on fat and protein, without any need for dietary carbohydrate.

Evolution of Energy Usage

The first single-celled organisms to populate the earth had only the most primitive energy metabolism and relied on glucose (carbohydrate) as a fuel. They extracted energy from sugar through the anaerobic (oxygen-free) process of fermentation. Primitive micro-organisms that rely on sugar for fuel remain with us today. Bacteria, fungi, yeasts and cancer cells all rely primarily on fermentation of sugar for energy. These organisms can't use fat as a fuel because they either do not have mitochondria at all, or, in the case of cancer cells, do not have functional mitochondria.

About 2 billion years ago, eukaryotic cells – which contain internal 'organs' known as organelles – emerged on Earth. Biologists believe that eukaryotes evolved when one single cell organism engulfed another, and the two established a symbiotic relationship. The engulfed bacteria eventually became the organelle we call mitochondria.

During that same period, the first primitive plant cells containing another organelle called a chloroplast emerged. These organisms had the ability to take carbon dioxide out of the atmosphere, combine its carbon with water to produce sugar, and release its oxygen into the atmosphere. As a result, oxygen gradually accumulated in the atmosphere, making possible the emergence of organisms capable of the oxidation of fat, a great leap forward from fermentation because oxidation extracts more energy from organic fuels than fermentation.

All birds and mammals rely primarily on fats for fuel, for two main reasons. First, birds and mammals have very high energy requirements for maintaining stable body temperature in the face of climatic changes, and fats provide more than twice as much energy per gram than sugar or starch. Second, fats are a more highly concentrated fuel making them more portable. A gram of fat actually stores more than six times as much energy as a gram of glycogen, making carbohydrate an impractical fuel to carry around.[1]

To illustrate the superiority of fat as a fuel, consider the feats of migratory birds, such as the golden plover and ruby-throated hummingbird.[2] The plover flies from Alaska to the southern tip of South America, for 2400 miles of this trip traversing the skies over open ocean, with no opportunity of feeding. The hummingbirds can fly nonstop across the Gulf of Mexico. Fats provide the fuel for these fantastic feats. Carbohydrate stores having equivalent energy value would weigh the birds down with 6 times more mass than fat stores, making the trips impossible.

Ruminants such as cattle, sheep, and bison apparently eat only low-fat, high-fiber grass. However, this grass primarily consists of fiber and contains practically no starch or sugar. Microbes inhabiting the guts of these animals convert the fiber into short-chain saturated fatty acids. Consequently, ruminants depend on these saturated fats for at least 70% of their ongoing energy needs.[3]

Wild gorillas eat a nearly exclusively plant-based diet rich in fiber; about 74% of the dry matter in a gorilla's diet consists of fiber. Microbes in their hindgut (cecum and colon) convert this fiber into short-chain saturated fats. Consequently, a wild gorilla obtains

---

[1] Berg JM, Tymoczko JL, Stryer L. Biochemistry. 5th Edition. (WH Freeman, 2002). Section 22.1. <**https://www.ncbi.nlm.nih.gov/books/NBK22369/**>

[2] Ibid.

[3] Bergman EN. Energy Contributions of Volatile Fatty Acids From the Gastrointestinal Tract in Various Species. Physiological Reviews 1990 April;70(2): 567-590.

60-75 percent of its dietary energy from saturated fats and less than 15% from dietary starch or sugar.[4]

In comparison to these plantivores, wild carnivores may get a smaller portion of their dietary energy from fat. Wild (feral) cats obtain 52 percent of their dietary energy from protein, and 46 percent from fat.[5] Wild wolves may obtain 54 percent of their dietary energy from protein, 45 percent from fat, and a mere 1 percent from carbohydrate.[6]

Domestic dogs evolved from wild wolves that followed early human hunters, likely attracted to carcasses of large herbivores left over after people butchered them, or animals injured by men that escaped capture. These very large animals (aurochs, bison, rhinos, mastodons, elephants) would have had a higher fat content than the smaller animals habitually hunted by wild wolves (deer, moose, boar, hare, beaver).

Hence it is interesting to note that domestic dogs spontaneously choose a diet higher in fat than the wild wolf – 63 percent of energy from fat, 30 percent from protein – apparently as a result of evolutionary adaptation to human dietary habits.[7]

---

[4] Popovich DG, Jenkins DJA, Kendall CWC, et al. The Western Lowland Gorilla Diet Has Implications for the Health of Humans and other Hominoids. J Nutr 1997 Oct 1;127(10):2000-2005. <**http://jn.nutrition.org/content/127/10/2000.full**>

[5] Plantinga EA, Bosch G, Hendriks WH. Estimation of the dietary nutrient profile of free-roaming feral cats: possible implications for nutrition of domestic cats. Br J Nutr 2011 Oct 12;106(51):535-548. <**https://www.cambridge.org/core/journals/ british-journal-of-nutrition/article/estimation-of-the-dietary-nutrient-profile- of-freeroaming-feral-cats-possible-implications-for-nutrition-of-domestic- cats/2E0E827469FFC1AF51387E045C06759A/core-reader**>

[6] Bosch G, Hagen-Plantinga EA, Hendriks WH. Dietary nutrient profiles of wild wolves: insights for optimal dog nutrition? Br J Nutr 2015;113:S40-S54.

[7] Bosch G, Hagen-Plantinga EA, Hendriks WH. Dietary nutrient profiles of wild wolves: insights for optimal dog nutrition? Br J Nutr 2015;113:S40-S54.

The Fat-Fueled Human

Fat is clearly the dominant fuel in human metabolism.

In people eating "normal" mixed diets containing more than 150 g of carbohydrate daily, fats provide at least 60 percent of ongoing energy needs. Moreover, this increases to at least 70 percent when people engage in low- to moderate-intensity aerobic activity.[8] That's right, during aerobic exercise Nature increases the dominance of fat in the fuel mix, contrary to claims that carbohydrate is the preferred fuel in endurance activity.

Standard biochemistry textbooks all agree that, except for the brain and red blood cells, the major organs and tissues of the body derive the vast majority of their energy from fats and proteins[9]:

- Resting skeletal muscle obtains 85 percent of its energy needs from fat.[9]
- The heart has virtually no glycogen (carbohydrate) reserves, and generally derives its fuel from saturated fats, although it can use ketones as well, and prefers these to glucose.[9]
- The liver meets its own energy needs primarily via the catabolism of amino acids from protein, while exporting glucose (derived from amino acids and glycerol) to the brain and red blood cells and fats to the other vital organs.[9]

---

[8] Whitney EN, Rolfes SR. Understanding Nutrition. 6th Edition. West Publishing, 1993. 153

[9] Berg JM, Tymoczko JL, Stryer L. Biochemistry. 5th Edition. (WH Freeman, 2002). Section 30.2. <https://www.ncbi.nlm.nih.gov/books/NBK22436/>

- The brain readily uses ketones for up most of its energy needs when glucose supplies are restricted.[10, 11, 12, 13]

Owen et al. studied brain metabolism during fasting, a zero carbohydrate diet, and found that the brain adapted very thoroughly to use of ketones as its main fuel. They remarked:

"Finally, a few general comments seem in order. Man's capability to survive marked extremes in caloric intake depends, at least in part, on his ability to store fuel in an economical form. This means that the depot should have the highest calorie:weight ratio, should be capable of meeting substrate requirements for all tissues, and should be expendable without adverse effects. Survival during prolonged fasting, particularly in a primitive setting, obviously necessitates maximal sparing of nitrogen depots, of which the major portion is muscle. Fat has the greatest caloric potential per unit weight and is readily expendable. ß-Hydroxybutyrate and acetoacetate

[10] LaManna JC, Salem N, Puchowicz M, et al. KETONES SUPPRESS BRAIN GLUCOSE CONSUMPTION. *Advances in experimental medicine and biology*. 2009;645:301-306. doi:10.1007/978-0-387-85998-9_45. <https://www.ncbi.nlm.nih.gov/pmc/articles/PMC2874681/>

[11] Zhang Y, Kuang Y, Xu K, et al. Ketosis proportionately spares glucose utilization in brain. *Journal of Cerebral Blood Flow & Metabolism*. 2013;33(8): 1307-1311. doi:10.1038/jcbfm.2013.87. <https://www.ncbi.nlm.nih.gov/pmc/articles/PMC3734783/>

[12] Courchesne-Loyer A, Croteau E, Castellano CA, et al. Inverse relationship between brain glucose and ketone metabolism in adults during short-term moderate dietary ketosis: A dual tracer quantitative positron emission tomography study. J Cereb Blood Flow Metab. 2017 Jul;37(7):2485-2493. doi: 10.1177/0271678X16669366. Epub 2016 Jan 1. PubMed PMID: 27629100; PubMed Central PMCID: PMC5531346.

[13] Owen OE, Morgan AP, Kemp HG, Sullivan JM, Herrera MG, Cahill GF. Brain Metabolism during Fasting. *Journal of Clinical Investigation*. 1967;46(10): 1589-1595. <https://www.ncbi.nlm.nih.gov/pmc/articles/PMC292907/? page=6>

[ketone] utilization by the brain shows that fat products may even satisfy the central nervous system's substrate requirement, and therefore circumvent the need for gluconeogenesis and concomitant nitrogen depletion. Finally, our subjects failed to show any deficit on psychometric testing, and electroencephalographic tracings remained unchanged, which suggests that the keto acids did fulfill the predominant energy requirement in a satisfactory fashion."[15]

Although the brain and red blood cells require some glucose, the liver can produce enough glucose to meet these needs (via gluconeogenesis) if given enough dietary amino acids (from protein) and glycerol (from fats).

Some high intensity physical activities are partially fueled by glucose through glycolysis. However, skeletal muscle does not even have the enzymes required to completely oxidize glucose.[14] When muscle utilizes glucose it is only partially oxidized to pyruvic acid or, in anaerobic activity, lactic acid. These then travel to the liver which reconverts them to glucose which is then exported back to the muscles. In other words, glycogen is recycled so we may have no requirement for dietary carbohydrate to replenish it.

Thanks to our liver having the ability to produce all the glucose we need on demand from protein and fat via gluconeogenesis (see Chapter 10 for more details), we can go without any food – and thus without any dietary carbohydrate – for weeks and maintain all body functions. Consequently The Food and Nutrition Board of the U.S. National Academy of Sciences recognizes that *we have no dietary requirement for carbohydrate*.

"The lower limit of dietary carbohydrate compatible with life apparently is zero, provided that adequate amounts of protein and fat are consumed....There are traditional populations that ingested a high fat, high protein diet containing only a minimal amount of carbohydrate for extended periods of time (Masai),

---

[14] Marieb EN. Human Anatomy & Physiology. Benjamin Cummings, 2001: 980

and in some cases for a lifetime after infancy (Alaska and Greenland Natives, Inuits and Pampas indigenous people)… There was no apparent effect on health or longevity….

"The ability of humans to starve for weeks after endogenous glycogen supplies are essentially exhausted is also indicative of the ability of humans to survive without an exogenous supply of glucose or mono saccharides convertible to glucose in the liver (fructose and galactose)."[15]

Nature shows us the relative importance of fats, protein and carbohydrate as human fuels in the way we store these in reserves. A typical 70-kg man with 15% body fat carries fuel reserves of 95,000 kcal in fats, 70,000 kcal in protein, 800 kcal in glycogen,[16] and only 40 kcal in circulating glucose, a stored fuel ratio of 57 percent fats, 42 percent protein and only 1 percent carbohydrate.

Human fuel use was selected by Nature during the Ice Ages when carbohydrate-rich plant foods were quite scarce much of the time, especially for Europeans and Asians. To succeed at tracking, chasing and capturing prey and escaping predators, our ancestors had to perform both long duration low intensity and short duration high intensity exertions on an empty stomach, fueled only by on-board reserves. Evidently Nature identified this high fat, low carbohydrate stored fuel mix as the most efficient for supporting intense physical activity in a fasted state. If stone age humans had needed dietary carbohydrate to prepare for, perform or recover from hunting mammoths and other large animals, they would have gone extinct and we would not be here today.

---

[15] Food and Nutrition Board, National Academy of Sciences. Dietary Reference Intakes for Energy, Carbohydrate, Fiber, Fat, Fatty Acids, Cholesterol, Protein, and Amino Acids. National Academies Press, 2005. Pages 275-6. **<https://www.nap.edu/read/10490/chapter/8?term=carbohydrate+requirement#275>**

[16] 100 g in the liver and 100 g in muscle: Marieb EN. Human Anatomy & Physiology. Benjamin Cummings, 2001: 980

Summary

Nature has designed all mammals, including humans, to rely primarily on fat and secondarily on protein for fuel. We need comparatively little carbohydrate for basic metabolic functions and what we do need our liver can obtain from protein and fat via gluconeogenesis. We have no dietary requirement for carbohydrate when we consume adequate animal protein and fat. For humans and all other higher animals, fat is Nature's preferred fuel.

7 A SHORT FAT PRIMER

There is no nutrition topic more clouded by misunderstanding and prejudice than fat. Thanks to a relentless campaign of incomplete information, most Americans believe that saturated fats and cholesterol are akin to poisons, and unsaturated vegetable oils and artificial fats made from them (margarine, shortening) are practically panaceas.

However, saturated fat is natural to the human body, and people have eaten saturated animal fats for many centuries. Animal fats have been highly valued in all traditional cultures.[1] Since hunter-gatherers and herdsmen who got most of their calories from partially saturated animal fats had very high resistance to all the degenerative diseases blamed on those nutrients, modern conceptions are clearly amiss.

Let me dispel some big fat myths and replace them with some fat facts.

Saturated Facts

As animals, we produce saturated animal fats. On a fat-free diet, or whenever the body synthesizes fats from excess carbohydrate or protein, it produces saturated and monounsaturated, but not polyunsaturated, fatty acids. According to Dr. Germain J. Brisson, Ph.D., former professor of nutrition at Laval University (Quebec, Canada) and author of *Lipids in Human Nutrition*, when we eat large amounts of polyunsaturated fatty acids, enzymatic processes in the intestines will, as much as possible, convert them into saturated fatty acids before absorption.[2]

---

[1] Abrams HL. The Preference for Animal Protein and Fat: A Cross-Cultural Survey. In: Harris M and Ross EB, eds. *Food and Evolution*. Philadelphia, PA: Temple University Press, 1987: 207.

[2] Brisson GJ. *Lipids In Human Nutrition*. Englewood: Jack K. Burgess, Inc., 1981:107.

The body makes saturated fats because they are essential to health. They are used to make cell walls resistant to penetration by parasites, viruses, and bacteria. The fat pads that protect bony surfaces (palms, soles, sitting bones) and fat deposits that cushion the internal organs are made up largely of saturated fat.

Saturated fats are also very important in the nervous system and brain. The gray matter of the nervous system is made up largely of sphingomyelin, a compound that incorporates 1 fatty acid, most commonly saturated stearic acid or palmitic acid – both richly supplied by animal fats.[3, 4] The white matter of the brain is composed largely of phospholipids incorporating palmitic or stearic acids.[5] All told, about a third of the brain's fat is saturated.

How does human body fat stack up against common dietary animal and vegetable fats? Look at Table 7.1

Surprise! Forty-three percent of the fat produced and stored by our bodies is saturated! Beef tallow, butter, lard, and human fat are all quite similar. Lard is most like human fat. Palm oil also is very similar to human fat; but most vegetable oils are a world apart. Fats much like our own are loudly denounced; fats most unlike our own are most loudly praised. What's up?

3 Bettelheim FA, Brown WH, March J. Introduction to General, Organic, & Biochemistry, sixth edition. Brooks/Cole, 2001:482.

4 Enig M. Know Your Fats. Silver Spring, MD: Bethesda Press, 2000:270.

5 Ibid., p. 60.

Table 7.1 Average Fatty Acid Profiles of Some Common Fats and Oils

	Saturated (%)	Monounsaturated (%)	Polyunsaturated (%)
Animal			
Human	42.9	46.9	10.2
Beef tallow	47.8	49.6	2.6
Butter	62.6	28.6	3.4
Lard	40.0	50.0	10.0
Chicken fat	29.6	44.5	21.0
Vegetable			
Almond	8.2	69.9	17.4
Avocado	11.6	70.6	13.5
Canola	7.4	63.3	28.1
Coconut	82.5	6.3	1.7
Corn	8.0	24.2	58.8
Flax	9.6	17.0	68.8
Olive	14.3	77.1	9.3
Palm	49.3	36.8	9.6
Sesame	14.0	39.7	41.2
Sunflower	10.3	19.5	65.7
Sunflower, high oleic	9.9	83.7	3.8

Sources: Human fat: Bettelheim FA, Brown WH, March J, *Introduction to General, Organic, & Biochemistry*, sixth edition (Brooks/Cole, 2001), p. 474. All others: USDA via **cronometer.com**

In Nature, tissues of temperate or northern plants, fish, and other cold-blooded animals typically produce highly unsaturated fats, whereas warm-blooded animals (including people) and tropical plants (palm, coconut) typically produce more saturated fats. Why?

This distribution is due not to nutritional properties but to the melting points of the fats. Creatures inhabiting cold climates or having low body temperatures (northern plants, reptiles, ocean fish) have more unsaturated fats (oils) because they are sufficiently fluid at low temperatures. Saturated fats are too stiff at those temperatures. If an Alaskan salmon contained much saturated fat, it would freeze solid in the cold Pacific waters; saturated fats would be immovable in a flax plant on the Canadian plains.

In contrast, at tropical temperatures – including human core body temperature (98.6° F, 37° C) –unsaturated fats alone are too fluid for making fat pads, storage depots, or strong cell membranes. Also, unsaturated fats are prone to produce dangerous, carcinogenic peroxides in warm oxygen-rich environments – such as our innards – so Nature combines them with saturated fats which act as antioxidants and protect the essential unsaturates.

For those readers who are more technically inclined, consider this. Some experts claim that saturates with different carbon chain lengths have different health effects. They say myristic acid (14 carbons) and palmitic acid (16 carbons) are the major factors raising total and LDL cholesterol and risk of cardiovascular disease, but stearic acid (18 carbons) is supposed to have little or no harmful effect.

Putting aside the fact that the body can convert the myristic or palmitic acids into stearic acid—or vice versa—consider Table 7.2 showing the average percentage of these fatty acids in human fat, tallow, and lard.

Table 7.2 Average percentage of major saturated fatty acids in common animal fats

	Myristic	Palmitic	Stearic
Fat			
Human	2.7	24.0	8.4
Beef tallow	6.3	27.4	14.1
Lard	1.3	28.3	11.9

Sources: Human fat: Bettelheim FA, Brown WH, March J, *Introduction to General, Organic, & Biochemistry*, sixth edition (Brooks/Cole, 2001), p. 474.

Beef tallow has more "bad" myristic and palmitic acids than human fat, but also more neutral or "good" stearic acid. Lard actually has less "bad" myristic acid than human fat, as well as more "good" stearic. But the differences are so small it is unlikely that tallow or lard has properties significantly different from our own body fat.

Here's why I bring this up: Although this seems forgotten by critics of saturated fats, animals store fat mainly as a reservoir of energy for use between meals or when food is scarce. As discussed in Chapter 6, the heart, liver, and resting muscles together consume most of the energy used by the body, and these tissues prefer fat for fuel.[6] The fat they burn – your own body fat – is about 43% saturated (Table 7.1).

Clearly, Nature has selected saturated fatty acids as safe for use as fuel, fuel storage and structural applications. Since not only humans but all mammals use saturated fats for all these purposes, and the heart prefers using saturated fats for fuel, it is extremely unlikely that saturated fats cause cardiovascular disease.

---

[6] Marieb EN. Human Anatomy and Physiology, fifth edition. New York: Benjamin Cummings, 2001:983.

In the 1990's, experts stopped heavily promoting polyunsaturated oils and switched to promoting monounsaturates such as oleic acid. Human tissues can convert saturated palmitic and stearic acids into monounsaturated oleic acid – just like in olive oil.[7] Hence, 95 percent of tallow and 90 percent of lard is either monounsaturated or readily convertible to monounsaturated. Olive oil is only 77 percent monounsaturated.

If now you're confused, you're not alone. The experts themselves are confused. While hypnotically fixed on the real and imagined effects of degrees of saturation, they apparently have forgotten many basic fat chemistry facts.

Dr. Michael I. Gurr, Ph.D., a professor of biochemistry at the school of Biological and Molecular Sciences at Oxford Brookes University, UK, and former editor-in-chief of Nutrition Research Reviews, says that the preponderance of research on the topic does not support the idea that saturated fats promote cardiovascular diseases.[8] Brisson shares this view.[9]

Since 1990, Dr. Uffe Ravsnkov, M.D., Ph.D. has published more than 30 critical articles and letters addressing the alleged link between saturated fats and cholesterol and cardiovascular disease in peer-reviewed Scandinavian and international medical journals. In *The Cholesterol Myths* Dr. Ravsnkov shows that despite millions of dollars spent on research, scientists have repeatedly failed to produce good evidence that diets rich in saturated fats or cholesterol promote heart disease or cancer.[10]

---

[7] Enig, op cit:31.

[8] Gurr MI. Role of Fats in Food and Nutrition. London: Elsevier Applied Science, 1992.

[9] Brisson, op cit, Chapters 4 and 5.

10 Ravsnkov U. The Cholesterol Myths: Exposing the Fallacy that Saturated Fat and Cholesterol Cause Heart Disease. Washington D.C.: New Trends Publishing, 2000.

216

History fails to support the idea that saturated fats are responsible for soaring rates of cardiovascular disease in western nations. In 1909, cardiovascular disease was rare in America, but by 2000, it affected 60 million people and was the leading cause of deaths. Table 7.3 (next page) shows that while total daily per capita fat consumption increased by about 33 percent between 1909 and 1999, saturated fat consumption remained nearly constant. A marked (67 percent) rise in intake of polyunsaturated fats (from vegetable oils) accounted for almost all (97 percent) of the increased dietary fat during this time.

Table 7.3 Changes in U.S. dietary fats during the twentieth century

Time period	Total Fat	Saturated Fat	Unsaturated Fat
1909-19	120	50	60
1990-99	159	51	100

Adapted from Cordain L, Eades MR, Eades MD, "Hyperinsulinemic diseases of civilization: more than just Syndrome X," *Comparative Biochemistry and Physiology*, Part A, 136 (2003): 95-112, p. 100.

Essential Fat Facts

The body does not make polyunsaturated fatty acids. Two kinds are essential for health, the omega-3s (ω-3) and the omega-6s (ω-6). These must be obtained from foods.

The ω-3 family includes alpha-linolenic acid, eicosapentaenoic acid (EPA), and docosahexaenoic acid (DHA). Alpha-linolenic acid (LNA) is available from both vegetable and animal sources. Some blue-green algae and sea plankton contain traces of DHA, but only animal fats –especially sea animal fats – contain enough EPA or DHA to be significant sources for humans.

The ω-6 family includes linoleic acid, available from both vegetable and animal sources, and arachidonic acid, found only in animal sources. None of these can be synthesized in laboratories, and because they are very sensitive to heat and light, improper processing of foods (i.e. over-exposure to heat and light) destroys them.

Alpha-linolenic acid and linoleic acid are considered the parent fatty acids of their respective families because they have the shortest chains (18 carbons), which can be elongated to form the longer family members, which are essential for numerous body functions and structures.

DHA is particularly important in the nervous tissue, brain, and eyes of higher mammals. Herbivorous animals can convert alpha-linolenic acid first to EPA (20 carbons) and then to DHA (22 carbons), and linoleic acid to AA (20 carbons). Carnivorous animals have more sophisticated nervous systems than herbivores and consequently have a higher DHA requirement. Yet according to biochemist Dr. Michael Crawford, Ph.D., a leading expert on essential fatty acids, the meat-eating animals are less efficient at converting the alpha-linolenic acid into EPA and especially DHA. Although cats have a high need for DHA, they are completely incapable of producing it from alpha-linolenic acid.[11]

We have the most sophisticated central nervous system of all animals. Do we produce enough EPA and DHA to meet our needs? According to Dr. Eleanor N. Whitney, Ph.D., R.D. and Sharon R. Rolfes, M.S., R.D., authors of the textbook *Understanding Nutrition*, although we can make the conversion, the process is so inefficient, "the most effective way to sustain body stores of arachidonic acid, EPA, and DHA is to obtain them directly from foods."[12] DHA is the

11 Crawford M, Marsh D. Nutrition and Evolution. New Canaan, CT: Keats, 1995:127-128.

12 Whitney EN, Rolfes SR. Understanding Nutrition. Minneapolis/St. Paul, MN: West Pub. Co., 1993:141.

218

most difficult to produce, yet the most important for health of the brain and nervous system.

In 1999, scientists from the Departments of Food Science and Medical Laboratory Science, RMIT University, Melbourne reported that vegetarians produce little DHA even if fed diets rich in vegetable source omega-3 alpha-linolenic acid.[13, 14] Studies performed in the 1990s supported this finding and reported that the milk of vegetarian women contains only one-third the DHA of omnivores, indicating that dietary DHA is the main source of DHA in the blood.[15] The children of vegetarian women who have no dietary EPA or DHA have a smaller head circumference,[16] indicating lesser brain development. DHA is necessary for growth and development of the brain and eyes.

The omega-3s are also very important for cardiovascular health. In 1996 Italian scientists compared free-living vegetarians and fish-eaters in Tanzania and found that the vegetarians had lower blood levels of omega-3s, higher blood pressure, and blood profiles suggesting increased risk of cardiovascular diseases.[17] Thus animal

[13] Li D, Sinclair A, Wilson A, Nakkote S, Kelly F, Abedin L, Mann N, Turner A. Effect of dietary alpha-linolenic acid on thrombotic risk factors in vegetarian men. Am J Clin Nutr 1999;69:872-82.

[14] Ågren, Jyrki, Marja-Leena Törmälä, Mikko Nenonen, and Osmo Hänninen. "Fatty acid composition of erythrocyte, platelet, and serum lipids in strict vegans." Lipids 30.4 (1995): 365-369.

[15] Sanders TA, Reddy S. The influence of a vegetarian diet on the fatty acid composition of human milk and the essential fatty acid status of the infant. J Pediatr. 1992 Apr;120(4 Pt 2):S71-7. PubMed PMID: 1560329.

[16] Reddy S, Sanders TA, Obeid O. The influence of maternal vegetarian diet on essential fatty acid status of the newborn. Eur J Clin Nutr. 1994 May;48(5):358-68. PubMed PMID: 8055852.

17 Pauletto P, et al. Blood Pressure and Atherogenic Lipoprotein Profiles of Fish-Diet and Vegetarian Villagers in Tanzania: The Lugalawa Study. The Lancet 1996 Sept. 21;348:784-88.

fats rich in omega-3s may be essential for prevention of heart disease. An animal-based diet easily provides adequate omega-3 fats, including EPA and DHA. More about this in Chapter 8.

Unfriendly Fats

For years doctors and dietitians have been blaming animal fats for heart disease and cancer, and recommending people eat vegetable oils instead. However, history and research suggest vegetable oils are more likely the culprits.

For more than 2 million years before the industrial revolution, these oils were very rare and fake fats made from those oils, such as margarine and shortening, were unknown. Each tablespoon of vegetable oil provides about 15 grams of fat and 130 to 150 calories – 3 times as much fat, twice the calories, and none of the protein or micronutrients found in an egg!

Table 7.4 Changes in U.S. dietary fats 1909-1988 (grams/capita/day)

Time period	Animal fat	Vegetable fat/oil
1909-13	100	20
1957-59	100	40
1988	90	80

Source: Enig M, *Know Your Fats* (Bethesda Press, 2000), p. 94

As shown in Table 7.4, in America during the past 100 years animal fat intake has declined slightly, while consumption of processed unsaturated vegetable oil products has increased four-fold, parallel with rates of major degenerative diseases – obesity, heart disease, cancer, and diabetes.[18]

Polyunsaturated oils are highly susceptible to rancidity from exposure to heat, light, and oxygen. They must be extracted without being heated, then refrigerated in dark bottles to prevent formation of highly toxic, sticky lipid peroxides, which are a lot like plastic.[19] This is why boiled linseed (flaxseed) oil is still used as a varnish. After the boiled oil is applied to wood it reacts with oxygen in the air to produce a thick plastic coat.

In the industrial processes used to extract vegetable oils for sale in supermarkets, oils are exposed to enough heat, light, and oxygen to produce peroxides. These give the oils a bad taste and smell so they are bleached and deodorized before being put on the market or used to make synthetic fats (margarine and shortening).

Even if the oils were to survive industrial processing undamaged, they are typically packaged in clear bottles and stored in brightly lit groceries at room temperature. They are more or less rancid by the time someone takes them home. Then people at home usually store them at room temperature (why not, that's what they do in the stores), and often use them for cooking. (If you want to witness oil turning to plastic, brush a baking pan with safflower oil, then bake it at 350° F – you'll have trouble getting the glue off the pan with any solvent).

Even if you get cold-pressed oils packaged in dark bottles and keep them refrigerated, as soon as you eat them conditions are correct for converting them to the pesky peroxides. Remember, your innards are always hot (98.6° F), and loaded with oxygen. What happens

---

18 Rizek RL, Welsh SO, Marston RM, Jackson EM. Levels and Sources of Fat in the U.S. Food Supply and in Diets of Individuals. In: Dietary Fats and Health. Champaign, IL: American Oil Chemists' Society, 1983:13-43 .

19 Bettleheim, et al, op cit:273.

when peroxides get loose in your blood? Damage to arterial tissue and plaque.

That's right – unsaturated oils are a large part of the plaque that blocks coronary arteries. Lipid expert Dr. Mary Enig, Ph.D., president of the Maryland Nutritionists Association says "The major fatty acids in the cholesterol esters in the atheroma blockages are unsaturated (74 percent of total fatty acids). Proportionally, there are, by far, many more polyunsaturates (41 percent) than saturates (26 percent) in these lesions."[20]

Since polyunsaturates are so unstable and easily damaged by oxygen, they increase the body's need for antioxidants, especially vitamin E. Whole foods rich in unsaturated fat typically are also rich in vitamin E. But when oils are industrially refined, virtually all the natural vitamin E that was in the source is destroyed. Synthetic vitamin E is about half as effective as natural E and lacks the full E complex of multiple tocopherols and tocotrienols. Consequently, unless people who eat a lot of vegetable oils also take a full-spectrum natural vitamin E supplement, they may suffer from vitamin E deficiency.

The brain may incorporate more polyunsaturated fats when they are a significant portion of the diet.[21] If so, the brain may become more vulnerable to dangerous peroxidation reactions.[22] The brain has low levels of vitamin E required to prevent these reactions. One study reports chickens fed polyunsaturated oil developed brain damage very quickly.[23]

---

20 Enig, op cit:187.

21 Brisson, op cit:62.

22 Samhan-Arias AK, Ji J, Demidova OM, Sparvero LJ, et al.: Oxidized phospholipids as markers of tissue and cell damage with a focus on cardiolipin. Biochim Biophys Acta - Biomembranes 2012 Oct;1818(10):2413-2423. <https://www.sciencedirect.com/science/article/pii/S0005273612000946#s0060>

23 Ransnkov, op cit: 224.

When food fabricators hydrogenate those oils to produce synthetic fats marketed as shortening and margarine, they produce trans fats unknown to Nature. When trans fats are taken up into heart muscle cells, the rate of energy production drops dramatically – by about 200 percent. When under stress, the heart's need for energy rises rapidly; if trans fats are major part of its fuel supply, it may not be able to generate adequate energy.[24]

The National Academy of Sciences Institute of Medicine states that artificial trans fats increase the risk for cardiovascular disease and there is no safe level of these fake fats in the diet.[25] Trans fats have also been linked to infertility, depressed sperm counts and testosterone levels, abnormal sperm formation, lactation insufficiency, low birth weight, and reduced visual acuity in developing infants. They also impair the enzyme system that detoxifies carcinogens and drugs.[26]

Omega-6 Overload

We need no more than 12 grams of omega-6 fat daily; we can get more than enough from meat, eggs, dairy products and animal fats. But these days people are eating about 80 grams of vegetable oils daily (Table 7.4). These oils supply lots of omega-6s and little or no omega-3s. Consequently, the typical American consumes about 8 times as much omega-6s as needed. Vegetarians typically consume far more of these fats than omnivores.

Medical detectives have found that excess omega-6s increase inflammation, cell proliferation, blood clotting, vasospasm,

---

24 Brisson, op cit:54-55.

25 CDC. Trans Fats: The Facts.<**https://www.cdc.gov/nutrition/downloads/ trans_fat_final.pdf**>

26 Enig, op cit:85-86.

vasoconstriction, and cardiac arrhythmia.[27] Omega-6 overload suppresses immune functions and promotes atherosclerosis, cancer (including skin cancer), inflammatory diseases, insulin resistance, and some neurological disorders.[28, 29, 30, 31, 32]

In 2001 scientists at the University of Minnesota Hormel Institute, Austin, published a study in the Proceedings of the National Academy of Sciences showing how the omega-6 fat arachidonic acid promotes while the omega-3s EPA and especially DHA inhibit nonmelanoma skin cancer cell development. The authors concluded "the dietary ratio of omega-6 to omega-3 fatty acids may be a significant factor in mediating tumor development."[31] This research partly explains why skin cancer is more common in 2003 than in 1903, although people in 2003 spend less time in the sun.

Summary

If we follow Nature, the safest fats are those most like our own, i.e. the animal fats. If monounsaturated fats are preferable, then lard, tallow, butter and other ruminant fats are preferable to almost all plant fats, including olive oil. The safest vegetable fats are those

---

27 Simopoulos AP. Essential fatty acids in health and chronic disease. Am J Clin Nutr 1999 Sept.;70(3 Suppl):560S-569S.

28 Enig, op cit.

29 Ravnskov, op cit.

30 Braden LM, Carroll KK. Dietary polyunsaturated fat in relation to mammary carcinogenesis in rats. Lipids 1986; 21:285-88.

31 Liu G, Bibus DM, Bode AM, Ma WY, Holman RT, Dong Z. Omega 3 but not omega 6 fatty acids inhibit AP-1 activity and cell transformation in JB6 cells. PNAS 2001 June 19;98(13): 7510-7515.

32 Toborek M, Lee YW, Garrido R, Kaiser S, Hennig B. Unsaturated fatty acids selectively induce an inflammatory environment in human endothelial cells. Am J Clin Nutr 2002; 75:119-125.

most similar to our own, namely those that are mostly saturated or monounsaturated, about 10% polyunsaturated fats or less.

In Table 7.1, the plant fats with less than 10% polyunsaturates are coconut (1.7%), high oleic sunflower (3.8%), olive (9.3%) and palm (9.6%). Of those, high oleic sunflower and olive have the most monounsaturates (84% and 77% respectively), palm has the profile most similar to animal fats, and coconut has the most saturated fats. Avocado oil is 14% polyunsaturated fat and 71% monounsaturated fat, fairly close to animal fats

The bottom line: Plant-based omega-6-rich refined oils and man-made vegetable fats are dangerous. Your body will thank you for dumping them out and substituting time-tested, delicious, safe and healing animal fats.

8 NUTRIENTS AND ANTINUTRIENTS

An animal-based diet including little plant food is nutritionally superior to a plant-based diet. Eating large amounts of plants increases our nutrient requirements because plants contain anti-nutrients that block nutrient absorption, and their carbohydrate content causes hormonal and metabolic imbalances that increase demands for some vitamins and minerals.

Animal-Based Diets: Natural and Artificial Experiments

Both natural and controlled experiments have shown that humans eating whole foods animal-based diets including very little or no plant matter for long periods of time will develop no nutrient deficiencies.

Several hunting and pastoralist tribes have lived for many generations without nutrient deficiencies eating whole foods animal-based diets containing little or no plants. These include the Inuit (Eskimos), Siberian tribes, Mongols, Masai, Samburu, North American plains hunting tribes, Gauchos, Saami and Lapps.

In addition, as already recounted, a team of medical professionals studied the effects of an exclusive meat diet on health on two individuals – arctic explorers Vilhjalmur Stefansson and Karsten Anderson – for more than a year.[1] They reported finding no evidence of vitamin or mineral deficiencies in either individual.

Animals require all the same nutrients we require. These nutrients are present in the organs, muscles and fats of the animals we eat. Hence, we should not be surprised that when we eat only animal products, we can obtain all of the nutrients we require.

---

[1] McClellan WS, DuBois EF. Clinical Calorimetry XLV. Prolonged meat diets with a study of kidney function and ketosis. J Bio Chem 1930 July 1;87:651-668. <http://www.jbc.org/content/87/3/651.full.pdf+html>

Indigestibility of Plants

Plants are composed primarily of cellulose, commonly known as fiber. All the nutrients (vitamins, minerals) in plants are locked inside the cells ("cell" is the root of "cellulose").

Most people have at one time or another noticed that corn kernels and other plant matter will pass through our digestive tract intact, unaltered by our stomach acid or pancreatic enzymes. This occurs because we do not produce any cellulase, the enzyme required for the digestion of cellulose.

Consequently, unlike Natural plantivores, no human can effectively digest raw plant cells in order to gain access to the vitamins and minerals locked inside those cells. Cooking plants markedly increases nutrient availability by bursting the cell walls, allowing the gut access to the nutrient-rich intracellular juices.

However, many nutrients in plants are not in the forms that we require. Consequently, those who rely on plants for nutrients are prone to nutrient deficiencies that are best remedied by eating animal products.

Vitamins

Vitamin A

Contrary to suggestions made by advocates of plant-based diets, plants do not provide vitamin A. They only provide so-called pro-vitamin A carotenoids, such as beta-carotene. Carotenoids are poorly absorbed and inefficiently converted to vitamin A. Preformed vitamin A – also known as retinol – is found only in animal products.

Vitamin A deficiency affects more than 100 million children in developing nations, where plant foods are abundant but animal foods scarce, making them vulnerable to infectious disease and blindness.[2] Scientists have done a lot of research on carotenoid and retinol (true vitamin A) metabolism, trying to find a way to prevent this vitamin deficiency disease without animal foods.

Studies have shown that giving these children two large doses of retinol (animal-source vitamin A) twice a year can reduce infectious disease death rates by 26 to 54 percent.[3] Unfortunately, plant foods rich in carotenoids do not seem as effective for this purpose.

We only absorb 9 to 22 percent of doses of B-carotene ranging from 45 mcg to 39 mg, and the absorption efficiency decreases as the amount of dietary carotenoids increases. Many factors affect the bioavailability and bioconversion of carotenoids. Carotene bioavailability varies with different processing methods of the same

---

[2] "A clinical sign of vitamin A deficiency, night blindness, is prevalent in developing countries where animal and vitamin A-fortified products are not commonly available." Institute of Medicine (US) Panel on Micronutrients. Dietary Reference Intakes for Vitamin A, Vitamin K, Arsenic, Boron, Chromium, Copper, Iodine, Iron, Manganese, Molybdenum, Nickel, Silicon, Vanadium, and Zinc. National Academies Press (US), 2001. <**https://www.ncbi.nlm.nih.gov/books/NBK222318/#ddd00139**>

[3] Whitney EN, Rolfes SR. Understanding Nutrition. 6th Edition. West Publishing, 1993. 342.

foods, and among different foods containing similar levels of carotenoids.[4]

In contrast, according to the Institute of Medicine Food and Nutrition Board, "The absorption of preformed vitamin A is generally high, in the range of 70-90%."[5] This is largely because our intestinal cells produce a specific retinol transport protein to facilitate retinol uptake. The presence of this transporter protein provides evidence that we are naturally adapted or designed by Nature to ingest and assimilate retinol. Since retinol only occurs in animal tissues, this also provides evidence that we are naturally adapted or designed by Nature to ingest animal foods rich in retinol, such as liver.

If you think in evolutionary terms, this low and variable bioavailability of plant-based carotenoids suggests that human ancestors did not depend upon plant-based carotenoids for vitamin A. If our ancestors were dependent on plant-based carotenoids for vitamin A, people who could not efficiently absorb and convert plant-based carotenoids would have developed vitamin A deficiency, which would have eliminated them from the gene pool. In other words, natural selection would have favored individuals who were highly efficient at absorbing and converting plant-based carotenoids, and today we would find that humans have a high efficiency of absorption and conversion. Since this is *not* the case, and we do have a specific intestinal adaptation to retinol, the logical conclusion is that human ancestors depended on animal source retinol for vitamin A.

---

[4] Ibid.

[5] Food and Nutrition Board, Institute of Medicine. Dietary Reference Intakes for Vitamin A, Vitamin K, Arsenic, Boron, Chromium, Copper, Iodine, Iron, Manganese, Molybdenum, Nickel, Silicon, Vanadium, and Zinc. National Academies Press. <https://www.ncbi.nlm.nih.gov/books/NBK222318/#ddd00139>

Carotenoid absorption from whole plant foods is limited by fiber.[6, 7] We absorb only 4% of the carotenoids in green leafy vegetables, 18-26 percent of those in carrots, 11 to 12 percent of those in broccoli, and only 5% of those in spinach. We absorb *86% less* ß-carotene from a mixed vegetable diet than from isolated ß-carotene emulsified in oil i.e fat.[8, 9, 10, 11] Make a mental note of this: ß-carotene is most bioavailable when isolated from plants – that is, not in a fiber matrix – and dissolved in fat. I will come back to this fact later.

We appear to convert carotenoids from more fleshy fruits (presumably including pumpkins and squashes) more efficiently than carotenoids from vegetables, most likely due to fruits containing less fiber.[12]

------

[6] Riedl J, Linseisen J, Hoffmann J, Wolfram G. Some Dietary Fibers Reduce the Absorption of Carotenoids in Women. J Nutr 1999 Dec 1;129(12):2170-2176. <http://jn.nutrition.org/content/129/12/2170.full>

[7] van het Hof KH, West CE, Westrate JA, Hautvast JGAJ. Dietary Factors That Affect the Bioavailability of Carotenoids. J Nutr 2000 Mar 1:130(2):503-506. <http://jn.nutrition.org/content/130/3/503.full>

[8] Ibid.

[9] Rao CN, Rao BSN. Absorption of Dietary Carotenes in Human Subjects. Am J Clin Nutr 1970 Jan;23(1):105-109. <http://ajcn.nutrition.org/content/23/1/105.full.pdf+html>

[10] van het Hof KH, West CE, Westrate JA, Hautvast JGAJ. Dietary Factors That Affect the Bioavailability of Carotenoids. J Nutr 2000 Mar 1:130(2):503-506. <http://jn.nutrition.org/content/130/3/503.full>

[11] Haskell MJ. The challenge to reach nutritional adequacy for vitamin A: ß-carotene bioavailability and conversion–evidence in humans. Am J Clin Nutr 2012 Nov;96(5);1193S-1203S. <http://ajcn.nutrition.org/content/96/5/1193S.full>

[12] de Pee S, West CE, Permaesih D, et al.. **Orange fruit is more effective than are dark-green, leafy vegetables in increasing serum concentrations of retinol and ß-carotene in schoolchildren in Indonesia.** Am J Clin Nutr 1998 Nov;68(5): 1058-1067.

A lot of the variability found in research stems from degrees of processing and cooking applied to the plant foods before consumption. Absorption of carotenoids is lowest from raw plant foods because we have no enzymes for digesting fiber, and all the carotenoid in raw plants is locked inside cellulose walls. Cooking, homogenizing, slicing and juicing releases carotenoids from their cellulose cells, making them more bioavailable.[13] We can absorb only about 11 percent of the ß-carotene from raw carrots, but as much as 75 percent from stir-fried carrots.[14]

However, when researchers study blood levels of carotenoids after ingestion of cooked plant foods, they still often find low absorption rates. One study found that a large dose of cooked broccoli (600 g/1.3 lb) or tomato juice (180 g) produced no change in blood carotenoid levels, while a large dose of cooked carrots (270 g/0.6 lb) produced only a small change.[15] Another research team concluded

[13] van het Hof KH, West CE, Westrate JA, Hautvast JGAJ. Dietary Factors That Affect the Bioavailability of Carotenoids. J Nutr 2000 Mar 1:130(2):503-506. <http://jn.nutrition.org/content/130/3/503.full>

[14] Ghavami A, Coward A, Bluck LJC. The effect of food preparation on the bioavailability of carotenoids from carrots using intrinsic labelling. Br J Nutr 2012;107:1350-1366. <https://www.cambridge.org/core/services/aop-cambridge-core/content/view/C4E2B9F580B2F6D142A7E48DC52953D9/S000711451100451Xa.pdf/effect_of_food_preparation_on_the_bioavailability_of_carotenoids_from_carrots_using_intrinsic_labelling.pdf>

[15] Brown ED, Micozzi MS, Craft NE, et al.. Plasma carotenoids in normal men after a single ingestion of vegetables or purified beta-carotene. Am J Clin Nutr 1989 June;49(6):1258-1265. <http://citeseerx.ist.psu.edu/viewdoc/download?doi=10.1.1.976.4236&rep=rep1&type=pdf>

that the human intestine "possesses only an extremely limited ability to absorb unchanged dietary ß-carotene into the lymph."[16]

We poorly assimilate even crystalline ß-carotene completely removed from plant fiber. A study of 11 men found that they absorbed on average only about 2 percent of crystalline ß-carotene ingested with adequate dietary fat.[17] However, only 6 of the 11 men had detectible response to the ingestion of the carotenoid, and they only absorbed about 4 percent of what they ingested. Absorption of ß-carotene in the non-responder group was too low to be measured.

A study of 11 women found they absorbed on average only about 3 percent of crystalline ß-carotene ingested with adequate dietary fat.[18] However, 5 of the 11 subjects absorbed no more than 0.01 (one-one hundredth) percent of ingested purified ß-carotene, while the other 6 had a mean absorption of about 6 percent of the isolated carotenoid.

In both of these studies, 45-55 percent of subjects had no change in blood levels of either carotenoids or retinol vitamin A after ingesting the purified ß-carotene, which as already noted is far more bioavailable than carotenoids from whole plant foods. The remaining subjects had only a limited response. Carotenoids proved to have little effect on vitamin A levels.

In addition to being poor absorbers of carotenoids, we are poor converters of absorbed carotenoids into retinol. Evidently, to get just

---

[16] Goodman DS, Blomstrand R, Werner B, et al.. The Intestinal Absorption and Metabolism of Vitamin A and ß-Carotene in Man. J Clin Invest 1966(45(10): 1615-1623. <https://www.ncbi.nlm.nih.gov/pmc/articles/PMC292843/pdf/jcinvest00268-0107.pdf>

[17] Hickenbottom SJ, Follett JR, Lin Y, et al.. Variability in conversion of β-carotene to vitamin A in men as measured by using a double-tracer study design. Am J Clin Nutr 2002 May;75(5):900-907.

[18] Lin Y, Dueker SR, Burri BJ, et al.. Variability of the conversion of ß-carotene to vitamin A in women measured by using a double-tracer study design. Am J Clin Nutr 2000 June;71(6):1545-1554.

one mg of true vitamin A, we need to absorb 10 to 28 mg of ß-carotene from plants.[19]

One research team documented marginal vitamin A deficiency in pregnant Indonesian women who were consuming amounts of whole plant foods that would be expected to provide 3 times the recommended daily allowance for vitamin A using the generally accepted conversion factors.[20] This team found that adding carotene-rich vegetables to diets of deficient individuals in developing nations "did not improve vitamin A status," whereas doses of isolated ß-carotene dissolved in oil did. They report that intervention studies in developing nations attempting to prevent or reverse vitamin A deficiency with whole plant foods have found this strategy is not reliable – using the known carotenoid conversion rates, populations eating plant-based diets in developing nations could not achieve adequacy – and, while animal-source foods are reliable, they are often too expensive for poor people, so vitamin A fortified foods are becoming the preferred tool for this job.

Humans evidently have higher tissue levels of carotenoids than the great apes, probably due to lower activity of the enzyme that converts ß-carotene into retinol.[21] Logically natural selection could have preserved this mutation only if our ancestors were obtaining vitamin A directly from animal products.

---

[19] Tang G. Bioconversion of dietary provitamin A carotenoids to vitamin A in humans. *The American Journal of Clinical Nutrition*. 2010;91(5):1468S-1473S. doi:10.3945/ajcn.2010.28674G. **<https://www.ncbi.nlm.nih.gov/pmc/articles/ PMC2854912/#bib15>**

[20] West CE, Eilander A, van Lieshout M. Consequences of revised estimates of carotenoid bioefficacy for dietary control of vitamin A deficiency in developing countries. J Nutr 2002 Sept;132(9):2920S-2926S. <https://doi.org/10.1093/jn/ 132.9.2920S>

[21] Cutler RG. **Carotenoids and retinol: their possible importance in determining longevity of primate species.** PNAS, December 1, 1984; 81(23): 7627-7631.

In fact, meat, fat and eggs from wild or grass-fed animals are good sources of both retinol (true vitamin A) and ß-carotene. Meat from steers raised exclusively on pasture contains an average of 7 times (range: 4-16 times) as much carotenoids as meat from grain-finished steers. That's why the fat of wild game and pastured animals, and the yolks of eggs, are yellow. The color comes from carotenoids; the more yellow the fat or yolk, the more carotenoids present. Therefore ancestral humans who ate meat, milk and eggs from grass-feeding animals got both retinol and carotenoids from those foods.

However, meat and eggs from grain-finished animals also provide some dietary carotenoids. Egg yolks from grain-fed chickens, and butter from grain-fed cows, are yellow because they contain carotenoids. Thus, if you eat animal products, whether from wild, grass-fed or grain-fed animals, you will get carotenoids from those products.

Moreover, all ß-carotene provided by meat and eggs is isolated from fiber and dissolved in fat. In other words, the carotenoids in animal products, whether grass-fed or not, are in the form known to be most bioavailable for humans. As I noted above, the Food and Nutrition Board of the National Academies states that isolated ß-carotene dissolved in fat is on average more than 6 times more bioavailable than the carotenoids in whole plant foods. Therefore, the carotenoids in meat, milk and eggs are more than 6 times more bioavailable than those found in plants.

Since we evidently are best adapted to absorbing carotenoids that are dissolved in fats and not bound by fiber, and in Nature such carotenoids only occur in animal products, one can reasonably argue that we are best adapted to obtaining both carotenoids and retinol from animal products, and poorly adapted to obtaining carotenoids from whole plant foods. Plants provide no retinol, and only provide carotenoids in forms that have a low bioavailability in our gut.

Recall that, despite consuming far less dietary carotenoids from plants, we have much higher tissue carotenoids than the great apes, and this may have a role in supporting our much longer life expectancy than the apes.[21] Since meat-eating provides retinol directly, it has a carotenoid-sparing effect. That is, if we eat retinol-rich animal products, we don't have to use the carotenoids for vitamin A, so we can use them for other purposes.

Thus, an ancestral human eating a diet consisting largely or exclusively of wild game meat and eggs would get both highly bioavailable retinol and highly bioavailable carotenoids. His intake of retinol would make it unnecessary to convert carotenoids to retinol to meet vitamin A needs.

Consequently, a meat-based diet makes it possible to maintain both adequate retinol levels and high tissue carotenoid levels even in the face of low intake from plants. Since high tissue levels of carotenoids are positively related to maximum life span, it is reasonable to hypothesize that meat-eating makes it possible for a human to maintain the high tissue levels of carotenoids not found in other primates, and therefore played (plays) an important role in making it possible for us to have a maximum life span at least 40% greater than the longest lived great apes.

Individuals vary in their ability to convert carotenoids to retinol due to genetics. Multiple studies have found that many people have genetic variations called single nucleotide polymorphisms – SNPs – that dramatically reduce their ability to convert carotenoids to retinol. Carriers of both the 379V and 267S+379V BCMO1 variant alleles have limited ability to convert ß-carotene to retinol, and 44% of Europeans have the 379V haplotype, so a "a high percentage of the Western population may therefore not be able to achieve adequate vitamin A intake if dietary ß-carotene is a major source of their vitamin A intake."[22, 23]

SNPs in 12 genes affect an individual's ability to convert of ß-carotene into retinoids; some of these SNPs reduce ß-carotene conversion rates by 48 to 59%.[24, 25] More importantly, these SNPs that reduce the ability to convert carotenoids into vitamin A occurred in the study population at high allele frequencies ranging from 30 to 71%.[26] Homozygous rs11645428G allele carriers evidently have a 51% decreased conversion ability compared to homozygous A carriers. Homozygous A allele carriers of another SNP, rs6420424 show a reduced conversion efficiency by 59% compared to homozygous G allele carriers. Homozygous A allele of rs6420424

[22] Lietz G. Do genetic polymorphisms in a beta-carotene metabolizing key enzyme influence dietary Vitamin A requirements? UK Research and Innovation, 2011. <http://gtr.ukri.org/projects?ref=BB%2FG004056%2F1>

[23] Pizzorno L. Common Genetic Variants and Other Host-related Factors Greatly Increase Susceptibility to Vitamin A Deficiency. Longevity Medicine Review 2010. <http://www.lmreview.com/articles/print/common-genetic-variants-and-other-host-related-factors-greatly-increase-susceptibility-to-vitamin-a-deficiency/>

[24] Lietz G, Oxley A, Leung W, Hesketh J. Single nucleotide polymorphisms upstream from the β-carotene 15,15'-monoxygenase gene influence provitamin A conversion efficiency in female volunteers. J Nutr. 2012 Jan;142(1):161S-5S. doi: 10.3945/jn.111.140756. Epub 2011 Nov 23. PubMed PMID: 22113863.

[25] Borel P, Desmarchelier C, Nowicki M, Bott R. A Combination of Single-Nucleotide Polymorphisms Is Associated with Interindividual Variability in Dietary β-Carotene Bioavailability in Healthy Men. J Nutr. 2015 Aug;145(8): 1740-7. doi: 10.3945/jn.115.212837. Epub 2015 Jun 10. PubMed PMID: 26063065.

[26] Lietz G, Oxley A, Leung W, Hesketh J. Single nucleotide polymorphisms upstream from the β-carotene 15,15'-monoxygenase gene influence provitamin A conversion efficiency in female volunteers. J Nutr. 2012 Jan;142(1):161S-5S. doi: 10.3945/jn.111.140756. Epub 2011 Nov 23. PubMed PMID: 22113863.

occurs at a frequency of about 70% in Asian populations, ~30% in European populations and ~20% in African populations.

On the basis of this one allele, one would expect that Asians will be less efficient at converting ß-carotene to retinol than Europeans, and Europeans less efficient than Africans. However, remember that this is considering only one of the SNPs that affect the activity of the enzyme that converts carotene to retinol. In fact as noted here there are multiple SNPs that reduce this enzyme's activity. Evidently at least 25 SNPs can have an affect on an individual's ability to utilized ß-carotene or retinol.[27]

As a side note, this study showed that, contrary to propaganda, racial groups do indeed differ genetically and biochemically, no doubt due to specific adaptations to different native habitats (e.g. sunny tropical Africa versus temperate or subarctic Europe). Further, within each racial population, individuals vary markedly, so it is irresponsible to claim that all people will be able to derive adequate vitamin A from conversion of carotenoids obtained from plants.

When you consider that Europeans and Asians are adapted to northern bioregions that would have lacked plant foods during the Ice Ages, the widespread genetic mutations that limit carotenoid conversion to retinol make perfect sense. Microevolutionary theory would predict that mutations such as these that mute the activity of this enzyme would have been favored among our ancestors if they were eating meat-based diets rich in animal-source retinol vitamin A.

To review the reasoning: If our ancestors were eating meat-based diets rich in retinol, those individuals among them who had mutations that reduced the activity of the enzyme that converts B-carotene to vitamin A would have had less energy going to that task, and therefore more energy available for other actually necessary tasks. In short those who did not invest in the unnecessary task of

---

[27] Borel P, Desmarchelier C. Genetic Variations Associated with Vitamin A Status and Vitamin A Bioavailability. *Nutrients*. 2017;9(3):246. doi:10.3390/nu9030246. <https://www.ncbi.nlm.nih.gov/pmc/articles/PMC5372909/>

converting ß-carotene to retinol were more efficient users of the energy available in their environment, so they would have had more offspring than those who did the unnecessary conversion. Consequently, over many generations the population would become dominated by people who were less able or unable to convert ß-carotene to vitamin A.

For 2 million years the cold and dry Ice Age climate produced long winters and short summers, which favored the growth of abundant grasses, but not trees or succulent vegetation. The vast grasslands of Eurasia supported large herds of very large grazing animals, but produced very little if any plant food that humans can support human life. That Europeans hunted those animals is undeniable; they left us with cave paintings depicting their hunts. No cave paintings depicting harvesting of plants exist. During those millions of ice age years, Nature favored the reproduction of people who didn't need to eat plants and didn't waste energy trying to convert ß-carotene to vitamin A because they had guts that produced a specific transporter to uptake animal-source retinol, and plenty of retinol-rich meat, including liver, was available. Consequently, we, their descendants, have these SNPs that reduce the activity of the enzyme that would convert ß-carotene to retinol, along with the specific retinol transporter protein.

Given how poorly we absorb ß-carotene from raw plant foods, and how inefficiently we convert it to retinol, it appears that in Nature we – at least Europeans and Asians – could not obtain adequate vitamin A from plants alone. Nature appears to have made us dependent on animal products to meet our vitamin A needs. The richest sources of true vitamin A (retinol) are liver, fish liver oils, eggs, butter, and milk and milk products.

B-Group Vitamins

Vitamin B1

Vitamin B1 is also known as thiamin. Beriberi, the disease caused by deficiency of vitamin B1 does not occur in people eating sufficient animal products, because all animals require and have thiamin in their muscles and organs.

Thiamin plays an important role in carbohydrate, amino acid, and fat metabolism. Diabetics have been found to have blood thiamin concentrations 75 percent lower and renal clearance of thiamin 16 to 24 times greater than healthy subjects.[28] In diabetics high blood glucose appears to increase excretion of thiamin and induces thiamin deficiency.[29] In support of this, high dose thiamin supplementation has been shown to improve glucose tolerance in diabetics.[30] This suggests that increased exposure to blood glucose, which inevitably occurs with high carbohydrate plant-based diets as well as diabetes, may increase thiamin excretion and requirements.

---

[28] Thornalley PJ, Babaei-Jadidi R, Al Ali H, et al. High prevalence of low plasma thiamine concentration in diabetes linked to a marker of vascular disease. *Diabetologia*. 2007;50(10):2164-2170. doi:10.1007/s00125-007-0771-4. **<https://www.ncbi.nlm.nih.gov/pmc/articles/PMC1998885/>**

[29] Larkin JR, Zhang F, Godfrey L, et al. Glucose-Induced Down Regulation of Thiamine Transporters in the Kidney Proximal Tubular Epithelium Produces Thiamine Insufficiency in Diabetes. Das A, ed. *PLoS ONE*. 2012;7(12):e53175. doi:10.1371/journal.pone.0053175. **<https://www.ncbi.nlm.nih.gov/pmc/articles/PMC3532206/>**

[30] Alaei Shahmiri F, Soares MJ, Zhao Y, Sherriff J. High-dose thiamine supplementation improves glucose tolerance in hyperglycemic individuals: a randomized, double-blind cross-over trial. Eur J Nutr. 2013 Oct;52(7):1821-4. doi: 10.1007/s00394-013-0534-6. Epub 2013 May 29. PubMed PMID: 23715873. Abstract.

Some studies have shown that thiamin-deficient rats had impaired insulin synthesis and secretion.[31, 32] This provides more reason to believe that thiamin requirements may increase when one consumes a plant-based high carbohydrate diet, because high carbohydrate intake – unlike high fat intake – requires increased insulin secretion.

Of common dietary items, pork and pork products (ham, bacon) provide the highest concentrations of thiamin. Liver is also rich in thiamin.

Vitamin B2

Vitamin B2 is also known as riboflavin. Riboflavin deficiency does not occur in individuals who consume adequate fresh animal products. The richest dietary sources are whole milk products, meats, and green vegetables.

Some types of dietary fiber reduce riboflavin absorption.[33]

Vitamin B3

Vitamin B3 is also known as niacin. Pellagra, the niacin deficiency disease, does not occur in people who consume adequate fresh animal products. It is common in populations relying on corn-based diets.

[31] Rathanaswami P, Sundaresan R. Effects of thiamine deficiency on the biosynthesis of insulin in rats. Biochem Int. 1991 Aug;24(6):1057-62. PubMed PMID: 1781784. Abstract.

[32] Rathanaswami P, Pourany A, Sundaresan R. Effects of thiamine deficiency on the secretion of insulin and the metabolism of glucose in isolated rat pancreatic islets. Biochem Int. 1991 Oct;25(3):577-83. PubMed PMID: 1805801. Abstract.

[33] Roe DA, Kalkwarf H, Stevens J. Effect of fiber supplements on the apparent absorption of pharmacological doses of riboflavin. J Am Diet Ass 1988 Feb 01;88(2):211-213. Abstract.

Our liver can produce niacin from the amino acid tryptophan, which an animal-based diet supplies in abundance. Milk, eggs, meat, poultry, and fish all provide an abundance of niacin and tryptophan. Liver is the richest dietary source.

Vitamin B5

Vitamin B5 is also known as pantothenic acid, so-called because it is ubiquitous ("pantos" = everywhere). Deficiency of this vitamin never occurs in people eating adequate animal products. Organ and muscle meats provide plenty.

Vitamin B6

Vitamin B6 is also known as pyridoxine. Pyridoxine from animal-derived foods is highly bioavailable, up to 100 percent. Meat, poultry, fish and dairy products all provide pyridoxine.

Vitamin B6 bioavailability from plant-derived foods is limited. For instance, up to 80 percent of the vitamin B6 naturally occurring in grains is unavailable because it is bound by pyridoxine glucosides impervious to human digestion.[34]

Vitamin B6 deficiency is prevalent in type 2 diabetics,[35] suggesting that high blood sugar and metabolism of carbohydrates increases requirements for pyridoxine.

---

[34] Reynolds RD. Bioavailability of vitamin B-6 from plant foods. Am J Clin Nutr 1988 Sep;48(3 Suppl):863-7.

[35] Nix WA, Zirwes R, Bangert V, et al.. Vitamin B status in patients with type 2 diabetes mellitus with and without incipient nephropathy. Diabetes Research and Clinical Practice 2015;107(1):157-165. <**http://www.diabetesresearchclinicalpractice.com/article/S0168-8227(14)00458-6/fulltext**>

Folate

Folate is named after leaves (foliage). Among plant foods, the best sources are green leafy vegetables and legumes, but "entrapment of folates in the cellular structure of plant materials [i.e. fiber] partially inhibits their absorption."[36] Folate from animal products is more bioavailable. Meat, eggs and dairy products all provide folate, but the richest source is liver. Regular consumption of liver, egg yolks, or low carbohydrate leafy vegetables can easily satisfy requirements. Ten whole eggs (~ 800 kcal) provides 440 mcg, more than the RDA.

Table 8.1: Folate contents of selected foods (mcg/100 g)

Food	Folate
Chicken liver	578
Beef liver	253
Spinach, raw	194
Pork liver	163
Lamb liver	73
Egg, whole (folate is in the yolk only), cooked or raw	44
Cheese, cheddar	27
Yogurt, whole milk (1 cup)	17
Milk, whole (1 cup)	12
Beef, grass fed, ground	6

Source: USDA, cronometer.com

---

[36] Gregory III JF. Case Study: Folate Bioavailability. J Nutr 2001 April 1;131(4): 1376S-1382S. <http://jn.nutrition.org/content/131/4/1376S.full>

Vitamin B12

No plants provide vitamin B12, while meat provides it abundantly. People who choose to avoid or restrict animal products are "destined" for vitamin B12 deficiency.[37, 38]

Vitamin C

Contrary to popular belief, human vitamin C requirements are very low and we can meet our needs for this vitamin from fresh animal foods or very small amounts of plants.

Dietary deficiency of ascorbic acid produces a disease caused scurvy. One of the primary symptoms of scurvy is scorbutic gingivitis. According to the Institute of Medicine, adults require less than 10 mg vitamin C daily to prevent scurvy.[39]

The Institute recommends 75 mg per day to maintain near maximal concentrations of vitamin C in neutrophils (white blood cells), because "this should potentially protect intracellular proteins from oxidative injury when these cells are activated during infectious and inflammatory processes." However, it also states "There are no data

---

37 "The present study confirmed that an inverse relationship exists between plasma tHcy and serum B12, from which it can be concluded that the usual dietary source of vitamin B12 is animal products and those who choose to omit or restrict these products are destined to become vitamin B12 deficient. At present, the available supplement, which is usually used for fortification of food, is the unreliable cyanocobalamin." Obersby D, Chappell DC, Dunnett A and Tsiami AA, "Plasma total homocysteine status of vegetarians compared with omnivores: a systematic review and meta-analysis," Br J Nutr 2013;109:785-794.

38 Kelly G, "The coenzyme forms of vitamin B12: towards an understanding of their therapeutic potential," Alt Med Rev 1997;2:459–471.

39 Institute of Medicine (US) Panel on Dietary Antioxidants and Related Compounds. Dietary Reference Intakes for Vitamin C, Vitamin E, Selenium, and Carotenoids. National Academies Press, 2000. <**https://www.ncbi.nlm.nih.gov/books/NBK225480/**>

to quantify directly the dose-response relation between vitamin C intake and in vivo antioxidant protection" and:

"Although it is known that the classic disease of severe vitamin C deficiency, scurvy, is rare in the United States and Canada, other human experimental data that can be utilized to set a vitamin C requirement, based on a biomarker other than scurvy, are limited. Values recommended here are based on an amount of vitamin C that is thought to provide antioxidant protection as derived from the correlation of such protection with neutrophil ascorbate concentrations.

"It is recognized that there are no human data to quantify directly the dose-response relationship between vitamin C intake and in vivo antioxidant protection. In addition, only one study (Levine et al., 1996a) with seven apparently healthy males reported plasma, neutrophil, and urinary ascorbate concentrations during vitamin C depletion and repletion to steady state. Thus, there are wide uncertainties in the data utilized to estimate the vitamin C requirements. However, in the absence of other data, maximal neutrophil concentration with minimal urinary loss appears to be the best biomarker at the present time. It must be emphasized that research is urgently needed to explore the use of other biomarkers to assess vitamin C requirements."[40]

Thus, evidently there exists no evidence that failure to maximize concentrations of vitamin C in neutrophils results in any deficiency disease, nor any evidence for any deficiency disease associated with vitamin C other than scurvy. Therefore, the Institute makes its recommendation for an intake of 75 mg daily on purely hypothetical grounds (i.e. it might have antioxidant benefits).

---

[40] Institute of Medicine (US) Panel on Dietary Antioxidants and Related Compounds. Dietary Reference Intakes for Vitamin C, Vitamin E, Selenium, and Carotenoids. National Academies Press, 2000. <**https://www.ncbi.nlm.nih.gov/books/NBK225480/**>

The bottom line is that we know that we need 5-10 mg vitamin C daily to prevent scurvy, and have no strong evidence we require or benefit from larger amounts.

Since so many people hold firmly to the idea that a meat-based diet will cause scurvy, it bears repeating again that a team of medical professionals studied the effects of an exclusive meat diet on health on two individuals – arctic explorers Vilhjalmur Stefansson and Karsten Anderson – for more than a year, and neither individual developed scurvy.[41] In fact, Stefansson started the experiment with a mild case of gingivitis, one of the symptoms of vitamin C deficiency, which resolved on the exclusive meat diet.

Stefansson and other arctic explorers learned from the Inuit (Eskimos) that eating fresh meat prevents and cures scurvy. In a synopsis of Arctic medical history, Brett recounts:

> "In fact, instead of the European bringing medical attention to the Eskimo, the latter ministered to the explorer in matters of health by instructing him in the principles of Arctic survival and in preventing scurvy by the simple expedient of eating fresh raw meat or, in the more southerly latitudes, consuming a distillate of the bark of the spruce tree."[42]

Every mammal needs vitamin C to form collagen, and collagen is an integral part of muscle and organ tissue, so fresh meat from any animal contains some vitamin C. However, the USDA does not

---

[41] McClellan WS, DuBois EF. Clinical Calorimetry XLV. Prolonged meat diets with a study of kidney function and ketosis. J Bio Chem 1930 July 1;87:651-668. <http://www.jbc.org/content/87/3/651.full.pdf+html>

[42] Brett HB. A synopsis of northern medical history. *Canadian Medical Association Journal*. 1969;100(11):521-525. <https://www.ncbi.nlm.nih.gov/pmc/articles/PMC1945783/>

measure the vitamin C content of beef.[43] Despite admitting that it does not measure vitamin C in beef, the USDA declares in its food nutrient database that beef contains no vitamin C (it should instead say "not measured"). Consequently many experts and laypeople alike incorrectly believe that meat contains no vitamin C.

A 1953 textbook on the biochemistry and physiology of nutrition provides a table listing the vitamin C contents of various tissues of the ox, horse, dog, sheep, rat, guinea pig, and human.[44] I have listed those from ox, horse, and sheep in Table 8.2 (next page).

---

[43] See Roseland JM, Nguyen QV, Williams JR, Patterson KY. USDA Nutrient Data Set for Retail Beef Cuts from SR, Release 3.0. USDA Nutrient Data Laboratory, ARS, 2013 September. Accessed Dec 4, 2017 at: <**https://www.ars.usda.gov/ ARSUserFiles/80400525/Data/Meat/Retail_Beef_Cuts03.pdf**> When you read through the Nutrient Analysis section (starting on page 6) you will see that they report testing beef for every nutrient except vitamin C. Thanks to Amber O'Hearn for pointing me to this document in her blog post "C is for Carnivore" <http:// www.empiri.ca/2017/02/c-is-for-carnivore.html>.

[44] Lloyd BB, Sinclair HM. Vitamin C. Chapter 11 in: Biochemistry and Physiology of Nutrition, Vol 1, edited by GH Bourne and GW Kidder; Academic Press Inc, 1953: 381. <**https://ia801602.us.archive.org/13/items/in.ernet.dli. 2015.549607/2015.549607.Biochemistry-and.pdf**> Thanks to Amber O'Hearn for providing a lead to this book in her blog post "C is for Carnivore" <http:// www.empiri.ca/2017/02/c-is-for-carnivore.html>.

Table 8.2: Distribution of ascorbic acid in ox, horse and sheep (mg/100g).

	ox	horse	sheep
Brain	16.6	18.5	15.4
Hypophysis	126	136	139.6
Testicle	30	46	34
Thyroid	17	18	31.7
Stomach	6.3	8	6.5
Small intestine	18	17	20.2
Large intestine	7.3	6.8	10.4
Lymphatic ganglion	51	44	45.4
Lung	18.2	18	12.6
Skeletal muscle	1.6	1.3	2.55
Cardiac muscle	3.8	3.3	6.2
Smooth muscle	6.3	5.3	10.8
Liver	20-37	N.V.[a]	N.V.[a]
Spleen	27.5	29	34
Adrenal	97-160	N.V.[a]	N.V.[a]

[a] N.V. = no value given
Source: Lloyd BB, Sinclair HM. Vitamin C. Chapter 11 in: Biochemistry and Physiology of Nutrition, Vol 1, edited by GH Bourne and GW Kidder; Academic Press Inc, 1953: 381.

Thus beef muscle, heart, and liver provide 1.6, 3.8, and a median of 29 mg vitamin C per 100 g, respectively. Sheep muscle and heart provide 2.55 and 6.2 mg vitamin C per 100 g, respectively.

A recent analysis of game meats consumed by Inuit (Eskimos) shows similar vitamin C contents for muscle and organ meats.[45] Raw caribou muscle, heart, liver, and kidney contained 0.86, 2.60, 23.76, and 8.88 mg vitamin C per 100 g, respectively. Since all ruminants have similar biochemistry, probably the meat and organs of all ruminants have similar vitamin C contents.

Thus, just 50 g of fresh raw beef liver would likely supply 10-19 mg vitamin C, more than enough to meet the daily requirement. One kilogram (2.2 lb.) of fresh beef, raw or very rare, contains about 16.0 mg of vitamin C, also enough to meet the daily need, yet supplies only about 1980 kcal, about two-thirds the energy requirement of an active adult male. A man eating a whole foods meat-based diet has to eat at least a pound of fresh meat daily just to get adequate calories.

Since cooking reduces the vitamin C content of plants, one might think that cooking would reduce the vitamin C content of animal products. However, data from USDA tests suggest otherwise. According to the USDA, raw spinach contains 28 mg vitamin C in 100 g, but cooked spinach only 9.8 mg/100 g. In contrast, the USDA reports that raw and cooked pork liver contain comparable amounts of vitamin C, the former 25 mg/100 g and the latter 23.6 mg/100 g. Evidently, cooking has a large destructive effect on plant-based vitamin C but little effect on the vitamin C content of animal organs.[46]

Hunters consume the offal as well. One would need no more than 10 g of hypophysis or adrenal gland to obtain a day's requirement of vitamin C. Aboriginal hunters were well aware that eating adrenal gland could prevent and cure acute scurvy. Weston Price reported:

---

[45] Fediuk K. Vitamin C in the Inuit diet: past and present. Master's Thesis. School of Dietetics and Human Nutrition, McGill University, Montreal, Canada, July 2000.

[46] Clemens Z, Toth C. Vitamin C and Disease: Insights from the Evolutionary Perspective. Journal of Evolution and Health 2016:1(1):Article 13.

"When I asked an old Indian, through an interpreter, why the Indians did not get scurvy he replied promptly that that was a white man's disease. I asked whether it was possible for the Indians to get scurvy. He replied that it was, but said that the Indians know how to prevent it and the white man does not. When asked why he did not tell the white man how, his reply was that the white man knew too much to ask the Indian anything. I then asked him if he would tell me. He said he would if the chief said he might.

"He went to see the chief and returned in about an hour, saying that the chief said he could tell me because I was a friend of the Indians and had come to tell the Indians not tot eat the food in the white man's store. He took me by the hand and led me to a log where we both sat down. He then described how when the Indian kills a moose he opens it up and at the back of the moose just above the kidney there are what he described as two small balls in the fat. These he said the Indian would take and cut up into as many pieces as there were little and big Indians in the family and each one would eat his piece. They would eat also the walls of the second stomach. By eating these parts of the animal the Indians would keep free from scurvy, which is due to the lack of vitamin C. The Indians were getting vitamin C from the adrenal glands and organs. Modern science has very recently discovered that the adrenal glands are the riches sources of vitamin C in all anima or plant tissues."[47]

Traditionally Europeans and Asians have incorporated the intestines, spleen, lungs, and other offal into sausages.

Dairy products also provide small amounts of vitamin C. Human breast milk provides about 50 mg vitamin C per liter, and exclusively breast-fed infants consume about 36-42 mg vitamin C

---

[47] Price W. Nutrition and Physical Degeneration. Price-Pottenger Nutrition Foundation, 1974: 75.

per day.[48] This translates to about 13 mg vitamin C per cup; thus one cup would be enough to satisfy adult requirements. One would expect raw cow milk to have similar vitamin C contents. Indeed, one source reports it contains between 3 and 23 mg per kg (liter).[49] Mammals appear to produce milks containing similar amounts of vitamin C: another source reports camel, cow, buffalo, sheep, goat, human, ass, and mare milks contain 52, 27, 22, 29, 16, 35, 49 and 61 mg/L respectively.[50]

Yet the USDA food nutrient database declares that whole cow milk contains no vitamin C. One might guess that perhaps pasteurization destroys most of the vitamin C in commercial milk. However, a review and meta-analysis of research investigating the effects of pasteurization on vitamin contents of cow milk found some studies reporting losses ranging from -6.83 x 10^{-6} to -7.27 mg/L, others reporting gains ranging from +0.76 to +25.46 mg/L.[51]

You might wonder how pasteurization could increase ascorbic acid concentrations in milk, since heat destroys vitamin C. First, leaving aside the possibility of measurement error, as already noted the USDA data on cooked vs. raw liver suggests that vitamin C in animal products is less vulnerable to destruction by heat (cooking). Further, pasteurization evaporates some water from milk, thus condensing the nutrient contents.

[48] Institute of Medicine (US) Panel on Dietary Antioxidants and Related Compounds. Dietary Reference Intakes for Vitamin C, Vitamin E, Selenium, and Carotenoids. National Academies Press, 2000. <**https://www.ncbi.nlm.nih.gov/ books/NBK225480/**>

[49] Park YW, Haenlein GFW, Wendorff WL. Handbook of Milk of Non-Bovine Mammals. John Wiley & Sons, 2017: 1946. Table 6.10.

[50] Ibid..

[51] MacDonald LE, Brett J, Kelton D, et al. A Systematic Review and Meta-Analysis of the Effects of Pasteurization on Milk Vitamins, and Evidence for Raw Milk Consumption and Other Health-Related Outcomes. J Food Protect 2011;74(11):1814-1832. <**http://jfoodprotection.org/doi/pdf/ 10.4315/0362-028X.JFP-10-269?code=fopr-site**>

Nevertheless, the authors of this review state that pasteurization "significantly" reduces the vitamin C content of milk, "but milk also is not an important source" of this vitamin in the typical diet.

However, if we take the average ascorbic acid content of cow milk to be 27 mg/L as cited above, and subtract the maximum reported pasteurization-induced reduction of 7.27 mg/L (a significant 27% reduction), we would still have roughly 20 mg vitamin C in every liter of pasteurized cow milk. A half-liter (about 2 cups) would then supply 10 mg, satisfying the absolute adult daily vitamin C requirement.

We need vitamin C mainly for its function as a co-factor in the synthesis of collagen and carnitine.[52] Meat is a rich source of both collagen and carnitine. We absorb collagen peptides from meat, bones and skin we consume (especially if hydrolyzed, i.e. prepared

---

[52] [52] Institute of Medicine (US) Panel on Dietary Antioxidants and Related Compounds. Dietary Reference Intakes for Vitamin C, Vitamin E, Selenium, and Carotenoids. National Academies Press, 2000. <**https://www.ncbi.nlm.nih.gov/books/NBK225480/**>

as soup by long cooking in water)[53, 54, 55, 56] and these improve the health of collagenous tissues, including skin, joint cartilage and bones.[57, 58] Consuming preformed collagen and carnitine from meat very likely reduces the dietary requirement for ascorbic acid.

Clinicians using a paleolithic ketogenic animal-based diet restricting fruit and vegetable intake to less than 30% of diet (by weight) to

[53] Iwai K, Hasegawa T, Taguchi Y, Morimatsu F, Sato K, Nakamura Y, Higashi A, Kido Y, Nakabo Y, Ohtsuki K. Identification of food-derived collagen peptides in human blood after oral ingestion of gelatin hydrolysates. J Agric Food Chem. 2005 Aug 10;53(16):6531-6. PubMed PMID: 16076145. <https://www.ncbi.nlm.nih.gov/pubmed/16076145>

[54] Ichikawa S, Morifuji M, Ohara H, Matsumoto H, Takeuchi Y, Sato K. Hydroxyproline-containing dipeptides and tripeptides quantified at high concentration in human blood after oral administration of gelatin hydrolysate. Int J Food Sci Nutr. 2010 Feb;61(1):52-60. doi: 10.3109/09637480903257711. PubMed PMID: 19961355. <https://www.ncbi.nlm.nih.gov/pubmed/19961355>

[55] Sato K. The presence of food-derived collagen peptides in human body-structure and biological activity. Food Funct. 2017 Dec 13;8(12):4325-4330. doi: 10.1039/c7fo01275f. Review. PubMed PMID: 29114654.

[56] Shigemura Y, Kubomura D, Sato Y, Sato K. Dose-dependent changes in the levels of free and peptide forms of hydroxyproline in human plasma after collagen hydrolysate ingestion. Food Chem. 2014 Sep 15;159:328-32. doi: 10.1016/j.foodchem.2014.02.091. Epub 2014 Mar 12. PubMed PMID: 24767063.

[57] Figueres Juher T, Basés Pérez E. [An overview of the beneficial effects of hydrolysed collagen intake on joint and bone health and on skin ageing]. Nutr Hosp. 2015 Jul 18;32 Suppl 1:62-6. doi: 10.3305/nh.2015.32.sup1.9482. Review. Spanish. PubMed PMID: 26267777. <http://www.aulamedica.es/nh/pdf/9482.pdf>

[58] Bello AE, Oesser S. Collagen hydrolysate for the treatment of osteoarthritis and other joint disorders: a review of the literature. Curr Med Res Opin. 2006 Nov;22(11):2221-32. Review. PubMed PMID: 17076983. <https://www.ncbi.nlm.nih.gov/pubmed/17076983>

treat chronic diseases have not found scurvy in their patients despite prolonged adherence to the diet.[59] A trial comparing a high-protein low-carbohydrate diet to a high-protein moderate-carbohydrate diet in obese men found that plasma vitamin C concentrations increased in the low-carbohydrate diet group.[60]

On the other hand, eating a carbohydrate-rich diet probably increases vitamin C requirements. Plants, some animals and pharmaceutical companies that manufacture vitamins all use glucose to synthesize ascorbic acid, and it has the chemical structure resembling a monosaccharide.[61] Insulin promotes and elevated blood sugar inhibits cellular uptake of vitamin C,[62] so blood sugar and vitamin C compete for entry into cells; high carbohydrate intake and high blood sugar evidently reduce vitamin C status.[63]

Elevated blood sugar also inhibits kidney reabsorption of of vitamin C. Consequently, diabetics evidently have an increased ascorbic acid requirement and susceptibility to vitamin C deficiency resulting in susceptibility to slow wound healing, and microvascular and red

---

[59] Clemens Z, Toth C. Vitamin C and Disease: Insights from the Evolutionary Perspective. J Evol and Health 2016;1(1). Article 13.

[60] Johnstone, A., Lobley, G., Horgan, G., Bremner, D., Fyfe, C., Morrice, P., & Duthie, G. (2011). Effects of a high-protein, low-carbohydrate v. high-protein, moderate-carbohydrate weight-loss diet on antioxidant status, endothelial markers and plasma indices of the cardiometabolic profile. *British Journal of Nutrition, 106*(2), 282-291. doi:10.1017/S0007114511000092

[61] Bettelheim FA, Brown WH, March J. Introduction to General, Organic & Biochemistry. 6th Edition. Brooks/Cole, 2001: 449.

[62] Cunningham JJ. The glucose/insulin system and vitamin C: implications in insulin-dependent diabetes mellitus. J Am Coll Nutr. 1998 Apr;17(2):105-8. Review. PubMed PMID: 9550452. Abstract.

[63] Clemens Z, Toth C. Vitamin C and Disease: Insights from the Evolutionary Perspective. J Evol and Health 2016;1(1). Article 13.

blood cell fragility,[64, 65] probably due to defects in collagen synthesis.

These data provide evidence that eating copious carbohydrates may increase ascorbic acid requirements; conversely, an animal-based diet low in carbohydrates probably drastically reduces vitamin C requirements. Since 5-10 mg ascorbic acid daily prevents scurvy in people eating carbohydrate-rich diets, an individual eating an animal-based diet containing little dietary carbohydrate but plenty of collagen and carnitine may need no more than 5 mg daily. This would explain why Eskimos and many arctic explorers and seamen reported that a diet consisting exclusively or almost exclusively of fresh meat could reliably cure scurvy. The absence of high-carbohydrate plants ensured that the fresh meat was sufficient.

Aside from this, nothing prevents a natural carnivore from consuming some small amount of fruits and vegetables rich in vitamin C. As already noted, wild wolves, bears and even crocodiles eat some plant matter; wolves have been found to eat many species of berries.[66] Although cats are universally acknowledged to be

---

64 Wilson R, Willis J, Gearry R, et al. Inadequate Vitamin C Status in Prediabetes and Type 2 Diabetes Mellitus: Associations with Glycaemic Control, Obesity, and Smoking. *Nutrients*. 2017;9(9):997. doi:10.3390/nu9090997. <https://www.ncbi.nlm.nih.gov/pmc/articles/PMC5622757/>

65 Tu H, Li H, Wang Y, et al. Low Red Blood Cell Vitamin C Concentrations Induce Red Blood Cell Fragility: A Link to Diabetes Via Glucose, Glucose Transporters, and Dehydroascorbic Acid. *EBioMedicine*. 2015;2(11):1735-1750. doi:10.1016/j.ebiom.2015.09.049. <https://www.ncbi.nlm.nih.gov/pmc/articles/PMC4740302/>

66 Bosch G, Hagen-Plantinga EA, Hendriks WH. Dietary nutrient profiles of wild wolves: insights for optimal dog nutrition? Br J Nutr 2015;113:S40-S54.

obligate carnivores, they intentionally consume some grass and other plant matter on a regular basis.[67]

Although natural history and controlled trials show we can obtain all the vitamin C (or collagen and carnitine) that we need from fresh (raw) or lightly cooked meat and dairy products, we also can consume small amounts of fruits, berries and vegetables – or, like the Eskimos or North Amerindian tribes, spruce bark or pine needle tea – that provide some vitamin C.

[67] Plantinga EA, Bosch G, Hendriks WH. Estimation of the dietary nutrient profile of free-roaming feral cats: possible implications for nutrition of domestic cats. Br J Nutr 2011 Oct 12;106(51):535-548. <https://www.cambridge.org/core/journals/british-journal-of-nutrition/article/estimation-of-the-dietary-nutrient-profile-of-freeroaming-feral-cats-possible-implications-for-nutrition-of-domestic-cats/2E0E827469FFC1AF51387E045C06759A/core-reader>

Vitamin D

Fair skinned people (Europeans) evolved in a habitat with significant ongoing cloud cover, heavy forests and low sunlight exposure for 6 months or more every year. These people are by Nature sun-intolerant, prone to sun burn and sun cancer, so they tend to avoid direct sun exposure. In prehistory and historical times they would have gotten vitamin D from eggs, organ meats, and fatty fish. Contemporary fair-skinned Europeans tend to have low levels of vitamin D in the absence of a vitamin D-rich diet.[68, 69] European children raised on vegetarian diets lacking vitamin D-rich animal foods develop nutritional rickets, suggesting that sun exposure alone can't meet vitamin D requirements.[70, 71] Adults eating diets low in vitamin D have high rates of dental, skeletal, metabolic, immune, and psychiatric diseases linked to vitamin D deficiency.[72] Thus, Caucasians and perhaps other racial types may require dietary vitamin D *in addition to* sun exposure.

---

[68] Davies, J.R., Chang, YM., Snowden, H. et al. The determinants of serum vitamin D levels in participants in a melanoma case-control study living in a temperate climate. Cancer Causes Control (2011) 22: 1471. https://doi.org/10.1007/s10552-011-9827-3

[69] Hedlund L, Brembeck P, Olausson H. Determinants of Vitamin D Status in Fair-Skinned Women of Childbearing Age at Northern Latitudes. Anderson ML, ed. *PLoS ONE*. 2013;8(4):e60864. doi:10.1371/journal.pone.0060864.

[70] Dwyer JT, Dietz WH, Hass G, Suskind R. Risk of Nutritional Rickets Among Vegetarian Children. *Am J Dis Child*. 1979;133(2):134–140. doi:10.1001/archpedi.1979.02130020024004

[71] P C Dagnelie, F J Vergote, W A van Staveren, H van den Berg, P G Dingjan, J G Hautvast; High prevalence of rickets in infants on macrobiotic diets, *The American Journal of Clinical Nutrition*, Volume 51, Issue 2, 1 February 1990, Pages 202–208, https://doi.org/10.1093/ajcn/51.2.202

[72] Wang H, Chen W, Li D, et al. Vitamin D and Chronic Diseases. *Aging and Disease*. 2017;8(3):346-353. doi:10.14336/AD.2016.1021.**<https://www.ncbi.nlm.nih.gov/pmc/articles/PMC5440113/>**

Plants do not make cholesterol in any significant quantity, so no plants provide the form of vitamin D that we utilize. Only animal products provide vitamin D, including fatty fish (particularly fish liver), liver, egg yolks, and full fat dairy products (Table 8.3).

Table 8.3: Food Sources of Vitamin D

Food	Serving	IUs
Cod liver oil	1 tablespoon	1360
Swordfish, cooked	6 ounces	1132
Salmon (sockeye), cooked	6 ounces	894
Sardines	200 g	984
Halibut	200 g	462
Liver, beef	100 g	49
Egg, chicken, whole, raw	1 whole large	44
Butter	1 tablespoon	1.5

Source: USDA, cronometer.com

Vitamin E

Vitamin E deficiency rarely occurs in humans; it is usually associated with diseases that impair fat absorption, such as cystic fibrosis.[73] In addition, eating plant products rich in polyunsaturated fats increases vitamin E requirements. Avoidance of plant fats reduces vitamin E requirements.

Fatty fish, liver, egg yolks and animal fats provide all the vitamin E that a carnivorous human requires.

Vitamin K

There exist two forms of vitamin K: K1 and K2. Vitamin K1 is required for the process of blood clotting, and vitamin K2 is required for the formation of bone and tooth protein, the fixation of minerals in bones and teeth, regulation of the actions of vitamin A and D, and for normal function of the nervous system.

Evidently the human gut absorbs a higher percentage of dietary animal-derived vitamin K2 than of plant-derived K1. Unlike some other species, we evidently do not efficiently convert K1 to K2 in quantities sufficient to meet metabolic needs, so we require dietary sources of K2. Deficiency of K2 evidently contributes to tooth decay, osteopenia, osteoporosis, atherosclerosis, seizure disorders, and dementia.[74]

Green vegetables provide vitamin K1 only. Fermented plants and fresh animal products – liver, egg yolks, and milk products – provide both vitamin K1 and K2 (Table 8.4).

---

[73] Whitney EN, Rolfes SR. Understanding Nutrition 10th Ed. Thompson/Wadsworth 2005. 381.

[74] Masterjohn C. On the Trail of the Elusive X-Factor: A Sixty-Two-Year-Old Mystery Finally Solved. 2008 Feb 13.

Table 8.4 Vitamin K2 in Foods (mcg/100 g)

Food	Vitamin K2 (mcg/100 g)
Natto	1103.4
Goose liver paste	369
Hard cheeses	76.3
Soft cheeses	56.5
Egg yolk (Netherlands)	32.1
Goose leg	31.0
Curd cheeses	24.8
Egg yolk (United States)	15.5
Butter	15.0
Chicken liver	14.1
Salami	9.0
Chicken breast	8.9
Chicken leg	8.5
Ground beef (medium fat)	8.1
Bacon	5.6
Calf liver	5.0
Sauerkraut	4.8
Whole milk	1.0

Source: Masterjohn C. On the Trail of the Elusive X-Factor: A Sixty-Two-Year-Old Mystery Finally Solved. 2008 Feb 13.

Choline

We need dietary choline to maintain the health of our nervous system. Plant foods are poor sources of choline, and people who avoid animal products have difficulty obtaining an adequate intake.[75] Egg yolks and liver are the best dietary choline sources.

Minerals

Phosphorus

I have personal experience with attempting to obtain phosphorus from a plant based diet. In 2016, after 5 years eating a diet free of animal products, I had my blood chemistry tested, and the results showed that my phosphorus level was significantly below normal. This had never occurred on any previous blood test.

The only possible explanation for this was my diet. I knew that plants provide phosphorus in the form of phytate, a compound that we can't break down. This compound binds not only phosphorus, but also other minerals found in plant foods. In contrast, animal flesh provides highly bioavailable phosphorus.[76]

I decided to return to eating animal products, and had my blood chemistry tested again a few months later. My phosphorus level improved, but was still a little below the normal range. Apparently I had significantly depleted my phosphorus stores by eating a whole foods plant-based diet for 5 years, and only partially recovered by a few months of eating animal products.

---

75 "Strict vegetarians, who consume no meat, milk, or eggs, may be at risk for inadequate choline intake." Linus Pauling Institute Micronutrient Information Center, Oregon State University, "Choline," <http://lpi.oregonstate.edu/mic/other-nutrients/choline>

76 Whitney EN, Rolfes SR. Understanding Nutrition. 10th edition. Wadsworth/Thompson Learning 2005: 419.

Calcium

Plants contain fiber and other compounds – including phytate and oxalate – that bind calcium so that it is not available for absorption. Some green vegetables – mustard greens, kale, parsley, watercress, and broccoli – supply calcium in a form that is as bioavailable as the calcium in dairy products. However, "the quantity of vegetables required to reach sufficient calcium intake make an exclusively plant-based diet impractical for most individuals unless fortified foods or supplements are included."[77]

Bones are 50% protein by volume and 20% calcium by weight. Bone calcium is a reservoir for metabolic calcium. If dietary calcium is insufficient, bone calcium is released into circulation to serve ongoing needs. Some calcium is lost daily in urine and shedding of skin and intestinal cells. Dietary calcium deficiency therefore eventually results in bone mineral loss. Consequently, long-term maintenance of bone health requires a high intake of both protein and calcium, which was sustained by our ancestors.

Calcium plays very important metabolic roles. Calcium binds to many cellular proteins to activate them. Calcium activation of these proteins produces cell movement, muscle contraction, nerve transmission, glandular secretion, blood clotting, and cell division and differentiation. Dietary or tissue calcium deficiency can cause or contribute to muscle cramping, edema, and skin disorders

---

[77] Connie M Weaver, William R Proulx, Robert Heaney; Choices for achieving adequate dietary calcium with a vegetarian diet, *The American Journal of Clinical Nutrition*, Volume 70, Issue 3, 1 September 1999, Pages 543s–548s, https://doi.org/10.1093/ajcn/70.3.543s

(psoriasis, atopic dermatitis).[78, 79, 80] Calcium plays a critical role in the immune system and the killing of cancer cells is most likely calcium-dependent.[81] Calcium is required for maintaining intestinal integrity and prevention of leaky gut.[82]

Wild primates and humans may give us some idea how much calcium we require. An early study of calcium metabolism in rhesus macaques concluded that a growing 3-kg monkey requires 150 mg calcium daily for each kg bodyweight.[83] Later studies found that this was not sufficient to prevent osteoporosis in the monkeys.[84] If human calcium requirements are similar, a 150 pound (68 kg) man

---

[78] J M Belizán, J Villar; The relationship between calcium intake and edema-, proteinuria-, and hypertension-gestosis: an hypothesis, *The American Journal of Clinical Nutrition*, Volume 33, Issue 10, 1 October 1980, Pages 2202–2210, https://doi.org/10.1093/ajcn/33.10.2202

[79] Floriana Elsholz, Christian Harteneck, Walter Muller, Kristina Friedland. Calcium - a central regulator of keratinocyte differentiation in health and disease. European Journal of Dermatology. 2014;24(6):650-661. doi:10.1684/ejd. 2014.2452

[80] Hung AKD. Severe hypocalcaemia as a cause of seemingly idiopathic bilateral lower limb oedema. *BMJ Case Reports*. 2014;2014:bcr2013201387. doi:10.1136/ bcr-2013-201387. <https://www.ncbi.nlm.nih.gov/pmc/articles/ PMC3902373/>

[81] Schwarz, E., Qu, B., & Hoth, M. (2013). Calcium, cancer and killing: The role of calcium in killing cancer cells by cytotoxic T lymphocytes and natural killer cells. Biochimica et Biophysica Acta (BBA) - Molecular Cell Research, 1833(7), 1603-1611.

[82] Gomes JMG, Costa JA, Alfenas RC. Could the beneficial effects of dietary calcium on obesity and diabetes control be mediated by changes in intestinal microbiota and integrity? *British Journal of Nutrition*. 2015;114(11):1756-1765. doi:10.1017/S0007114515003608

[83] National Academies: Nutrient Requirements of Nonhuman Primates: Second Revised Edition. National Academies Press, 2003. Chapter 6 Minerals. Page 95.

[84] Ibid.

would require 10 grams of calcium daily, an amount more than 10 times the current recommended daily allowance.

Table 8.5: Estimated mineral intakes of wild howler monkeys compared to the human RDA.

Mineral	Total daily intake–7 kg adult monkey (mg)	RDA, 70 kg adult male (mg)
Calcium	4571	800
Phosphorus	728	800
Potassium	6419	2000
Sodium	182	500
Chloride	1778	750
Magnesium	1323	350
Iron	39	10
Manganese	18	5
Copper	3	3

Source: Milton K. **Nutritional Characteristics of Wild Primate Foods**. Nutrition 1995;15(6): 488-98. 493.

A 7 kg wild howler monkey consumes about 4600 mg of calcium daily (Table 8.5). Wild chimpanzees in their native habitat have diets that supply 80-100 mg calcium per 100 kcal, and both prehistoric and contemporary human hunter-gatherers have very high calcium intakes, in range of 70-80 mg per 100 kcal, or in excess of 2000 mg (50 mmol) per day.[85, 86] The latter obtained calcium from

---

[85] Heaney RP. The roles of calcium and vitamin D in skeletal health: an evolutionary perspective. <http://www.fao.org/docrep/W7336T/W7336T03.HTM>

[86] Eaton SB, Nelson DA: Calcium in evolutionary perspective. *Am. J. Clin. Nutr. 1991;* 54: 281S-287S.

bones, egg shells, mineral-rich ground water and ashes. It is important to realize that hunter-gatherers had dietary customs that may at first glance seem inconsequential but on further examination played a very important role in meeting their nutritional needs. For example, the Navajo tribe habitually used an ash prepared from branches and needles of the juniper tree as a dietary seasoning and supplement. Just one teaspoon of this ash provides about as much calcium as a cup of cow milk (i.e. 300 mg).[87]

In contrast to wild primate and hunter-gatherer calcium intakes, the median intake for women in modern North America and European nations is less than 600 mg (15 mmol) per day.

A high protein diet increases calcium absorption but also increases urinary calcium excretion, and a person on a high protein diet probably needs a calcium intake of 20 mg per gram of dietary protein to protect the skeleton from depletion.[88, 89] Given that high protein and calcium intakes appear synergistic in promoting bone health and characteristic of preagricultural diets, it appears likely that we are by nature adapted to a diet that is very high in protein and calcium.[83, 84, 86] Since a hypercarnivore diet will provide 100-200 grams of protein daily, this would translate to a requirement for 2000-4000 mg calcium daily, which remarkably corresponds to the estimated calcium intakes of wild chimpanzees and hunter-gatherers.

Some proponents of plant-based or paleolithic diets suggest that we don't need this much calcium. Advocates of plant-based diets claim that the idea that we may have a high calcium requirement is just

---

[87] Whitney EN, Rolfes SR. Understanding Nutrition. 10th edition. Wadsworth/ Thompson Learning 2005: 417.

[88] Gaffney-Stomberg E, Sun B, Cucchi CE, et al. The Effect of Dietary Protein on Intestinal Calcium Absorption in Rats. *Endocrinology*. 2010;151(3):1071-1078. doi:10.1210/en.2009-0744.

[89] Heaney RP: Excess Dietary Protein May Not Adversely Affect Bone, *The Journal of Nutrition*, Volume 128, Issue 6, 1 June 1998, Pages 1054–1057, https:// doi.org/10.1093/jn/128.6.1054

dairy industry propaganda. Advocates of paleolithic diets reason that since ancient hunter-gatherers didn't use dairy products, dietary dairy products are incompatible with our genes and we don't need the amount of calcium provided by a dairy-rich diet. Plant-based and psuedo-paleolithic diets are generally low in both amount and bioavailability of calcium because they tend to rely on plant sources of calcium (mostly green leafy vegetables), although paleolithic diet advocates may also use some bone broth.

I followed diets (plant-based or pseudo-paleo) providing only 500-1000 mg of calcium daily for more than 25 years during which I was unable to obtain a remission of psoriasis. However, after my hypercarnivore revelation, I started trusting my own experience, and I found that I need a high calcium intake to thrive. I have already cited evidence indicating it is unlikely that I am unique in this requirement.

When I first adopted a hypercarnivore diet I used dairy products liberally, along with bone broth and a tablet desiccated liver supplement that also provided some calcium. I initially included the dairy products because I like them, I find them easily digestible, and my Hungarian, French and German ancestors used them, not because I believed I needed more calcium. Nevertheless, as a result, I had a very high calcium intake. During my first 6 hypercarnivore months, I had a steady improvement in my psoriasis, at which point some of the rashes I had suffered with for 40 years had improved by an estimated 50-90% (less itching and flaking) depending on location.

At that point I thought the improvement was primarily due to restricting the plant foods and carbohydrates that had given me so much gut distress. Then, influenced by paleo-diet arguments suggesting that dairy products might contribute to leaky gut and conditions like psoriasis, I tried a dairy-free hypercarnivore diet for several months, to see if removing milk and yogurt would improve the results. (Since cream has been reported to not increase intestinal permeability[90] I did not eliminated cream or butter.) Since I was eating almost no plant foods, my carbohydrate intake dropped to below 20 g daily – often below 10 g daily – during this experiment.

I expected good results, but was surprised to find that the rashes that had improved during the first 6 months got noticeably worse again (more itching and flaking) the longer I avoided dairy. I wondered if removing the dairy products resulted in some nutrient deficiency that might influence psoriasis. Although I had continued to consume homemade bone broth, which was providing me some unknown amount of calcium, I knew I had been getting a lot more calcium when using milk and yogurt.

When I searched the medical literature, I discovered reports linking low calcium to proliferative skin disorders. Low serum calcium is a risk factor for psoriasis;[91] vitamin D improves psoriatic skin by increasing calcium levels in skin cells (which promotes differentiation);[92] calcium channel blocking drugs (which reduce intracellular calcium concentrations) frequently cause psoriasiform skin eruption as a side effect;[93] low tissue levels of calcium impair skin cell differentiation and maturation, characteristic of atopic

---

[90] Beate Ott, Thomas Skurk, Ilias Lagkouvardos, Sandra Fischer, Janine Büttner, Martina Lichtenegger, Thomas Clavel, Andreas Lechner, Michael Rychlik, Dirk Haller, Hans Hauner; Short-Term Overfeeding with Dairy Cream Does Not Modify Gut Permeability, the Fecal Microbiota, or Glucose Metabolism in Young Healthy Men, *The Journal of Nutrition*, Volume 148, Issue 1, 1 January 2018, Pages 77–85, https://doi.org/10.1093/jn/nxx020

[91] Qadim HH, Goforous F, Nejad SB, Goldust M: Studying the Calcium Serum Level in Patients Suffering from Psoriasis. Pakistan Journal of Biological Sciences 2013;16:291-94. <https://scialert.net/fulltext/?doi=pjbs. 2013.291.294#913896_ja>

[92] Shahriari M, Kerr P, Slade,K, & Grant-Kels J: Vitamin D and the skin. Clinics in Dermatology, 2010; 28(6), 663-668.

[93] Kitamura,K, Kanasashi M, Suga C, Saito S, et al.: Cutaneous Reactions Induced by Calcium Channel Blocker: High Frequency of Psoriasiform Eruptions. The Journal of Dermatology (1993;20(5), 279-286.

dermatitis and psoriasis;[94] and high calcium intakes (including from milk) may improve intestinal integrity and reduce permeability.[95] I hypothesized that by removing milk and yogurt from my diet, I had reduced my intestinal and skin cell levels of calcium, and this was responsible for the exacerbation of my psoriasis.

When I resumed liberally consuming milk, yogurt and cheese and if necessary taking a multi-mineral supplement to achieve a calcium intake of 2000-2500 mg most days, my psoriasis started improving again. (The Institute of Medicine recommends not habitually exceeding 2500 mg daily.) On average I consume 1-2 quarts of whole milk or whole milk yogurt daily, plus 1-2 ounces of aged cheese. A high dairy hypercarnivore diet has given *me* the best results *so far*, albeit not complete resolution of all lesions. I will continue to experiment to improve the results.

Based on this experience I strongly urge people who adopt a hypercarnivore diet to take steps to ensure adequate – that is, high – calcium intake. Recall that a high protein diet probably increases your dietary calcium requirement, and if you fail to consume enough calcium, your body will draw down your bone reserves to obtain calcium for other vital functions.

---

[94] Floriana Elsholz, Christian Harteneck, Walter Muller, Kristina Friedland. Calcium - a central regulator of keratinocyte differentiation in health and disease. European Journal of Dermatology. 2014;24(6):650-661. doi:10.1684/ejd. 2014.2452

[95] Gomes JMG, Costa JA, Alfenas RC. Could the beneficial effects of dietary calcium on obesity and diabetes control be mediated by changes in intestinal microbiota and integrity? *British Journal of Nutrition*. 2015;114(11):1756-1765. doi:10.1017/S0007114515003608

A hypercarnivore can consume any dairy products that one enjoys and tolerates. Most people can tolerate fermented dairy products.[96, 97, 98] Milk products are excellent food sources of calcium. Whole milk and yogurt provide about 275 mg of calcium per 8 ounce serving, and and aged cheeses provide about 200 mg calcium per 1 ounce serving. Four or more servings (serving = 8 oz milk or yogurt, 1 oz cheese) daily will satisfy requirements.

If you don't consume milk products, other rich sources of calcium include:[99]

- The soft bones of small animals, particularly fish (e.g. sardines and salmon) and birds (the ends of chicken bones are often edible).
- Bone broth made by boiling (or better yet, pressure cooking) bones in water and vinegar, which can provide more than 100 mg of calcium per tablespoon (1600 mg per cup).
- Mineral waters, some of which provide as much as 500 mg calcium per liter.[100]

---

[96] Brown-Riggs C. Nutrition and Health Disparities: The Role of Dairy in Improving Minority Health Outcomes. Edberg M, Hayes BE, Rice VM, Tchounwou PB, eds. *International Journal of Environmental Research and Public Health*. 2016;13(1):28. doi:10.3390/ijerph13010028. <https://www.ncbi.nlm.nih.gov/pmc/articles/PMC4730419/>

[97] Jarvis JK, Miller GD. Overcoming the barrier of lactose intolerance to reduce health disparities. *Journal of the National Medical Association*. 2002;94(2):55-66. <https://www.ncbi.nlm.nih.gov/pmc/articles/PMC2594135/>

[98] Gaskin DJ, Ilich JZ. Lactose maldigestion revisited: Diagnosis, Prevalence in Ethnic Minorities, and Dietary Recommendations to Overcome it. Am J Lifestyle Med 2009 May 1;3(3):7.

[99] Whitney EN, Rolfes SR. Understanding Nutrition. 10th edition. Wadsworth/Thompson Learning 2005: 417.

[100] Quattrini S, Pampaloni B, Brandi ML. Natural mineral waters: chemical characteristics and health effects. *Clinical Cases in Mineral and Bone Metabolism*. 2016;13(3):173-180. doi:10.11138/ccmbm/2016.13.3.173. <**https://www.ncbi.nlm.nih.gov/pmc/articles/PMC5318167/**>

- Egg shells (dried and powdered, 370-415 mg calcium/g powder).[101]

Of these I consider egg shells the most reliable, inexpensive way to get a specific amount of calcium. Many wild carnivores eat whole eggs including the shells. One teaspoon of eggshell powder provides 750-830 mg calcium (as calcium carbonate) along with magnesium, phosphorus and 11 trace minerals, of which only one, strontium, is in significant amounts. Egg shells contain less heavy metals than oyster shells or mineral calcium carbonate, far below acceptable intakes, even in amounts providing 1,200 mg calcium. Calcium absorption from eggshell powder has been reported to be greater than from mineral calcium carbonate. Eggshell powder has been shown to improve bone mass more effectively than calcium carbonate in both animal and human studies. It has also been shown to promote fracture healing and have an analgesic effect. In addition, eggshell powder has been reported to promote cartilage growth in *in vitro* experiments. Eggshell powder has been found to be well-tolerated by most people.[102] I explain how to make it in Chapter 8.

Non-human animals will eat whatever necessary – including rocks and soil – to obtain the nutrients they require. For example, deer require large amounts of calcium and phosphorus to support antler growth, and will chew on cast-off antlers, eat soil surrounding decayed bones, lick rocks, and drink brackish water to obtain the minerals, if the plants they normally consume do not provide enough.[103]

---

[101] Rovensky J, Stancikova M, Masaryk P, et al.: Eggshell calcium in the prevention and treatment of osteoporosis. Int J Clin Pharm Res 2003;XXIII(2/3): 83-92.

[102] Ibid.

[103] Engel C. Wild Health: Lessons in Natural Wellness from the Animal Kingdom. Houghton Mifflin Harcourt, 2003. 29.

Calcium is not the only important nutrient for maintaining bones. As noted, bone is by volume 50% protein, and it is this protein, not the calcium and other minerals deposited in the protein matrix of bone, that gives bone its resistance to shearing forces and breakage. A growing body of evidence indicates that people who eat higher amounts of animal protein and adequate calcium have a lower risk of bone fracture.[104] Also, vitamins A, D and K2, found only in animal fats, are essential for forming healthy bone protein. Magnesium, boron, and strontium are also important for bone health.

Potassium

Many people associate potassium with vegetables and fruits (especially bananas) and do not know that meat, milk and eggs all provide abundant potassium. Every animal needs potassium in its tissues and diet, so all animal foods provide potassium. Since we need to eat food to meet our energy needs, it is best to ask whether we would get enough potassium if we ate enough meat, eggs and milk to satisfy our energy requirements.

Official estimated requirements for potassium vary. Canadian authorities have stated that an average adult needs a minimum of 1170 mg daily, while U.S. authorities have set the "estimated minimum daily requirement" at 2000 mg. Clearly there exists disagreement.

As shown in Table 8.6, meats, eggs and dairy provide between 800 and 3385 mg potassium per 1000 kcal. Given that the typical individual needs no less than 2000 kcal daily, we can see that an energy-adequate diet consisting of whole meat, eggs and dairy would provide between 1600 and 6770 mg potassium daily. A 2000 kcal

---

[104] Mangano KM, Sahni S, Kerstetter JE. Dietary protein is beneficial to bone health under conditions of adequate calcium intake: an update on clinical research. *Current opinion in clinical nutrition and metabolic care*. 2014;17(1):69-74. doi: 10.1097/MCO.0000000000000013. <**https://www.ncbi.nlm.nih.gov/pmc/articles/PMC4180248/**>

diet consisting entirely of 80% lean ground beef would provide 2890 mg potassium.

Table 8.6: Potassium content of selected animal source foods

Food	Potassium (mg/1000 kcal)
Beef, ground 80% lean (500 g)	1445
Chicken, ground meat (500 g)	3385
Pork, ground (333 g)	1205
Lamb, ground (350 g)	879
Cod, Atlantic (1 kg)	2440
Eggs (13 large)	819
Milk, whole (7 cups)	2255

Source: USDA, cronometer.com

Clearly a strictly animal based diet can provide plenty of potassium. One would have trouble getting adequate potassium only if one chose to get too large a portion of one's energy from fats separated from the whole food, such as tallow, lard, cream, and butter. For this reason sedentary people who have limited energy expenditure should focus on whole animal foods and use separated fats sparingly.

Moreover, you can include low sugar fruits, berries and vegetables in your HYPERCARNIVORE DIET at your own discretion. Some of these provide significant amounts of potassium with little carbohydrate (Table 8.7).

Table 7.7: Potassium content of selected fruits and berries.

Food (100 g)	Carbohydrate (net g)	Potassium (mg)
Cucumber (peeled)	2	136
Zucchini (peeled, cooked)	2	264

Food (100 g)	Carbohydrate (net g)	Potassium (mg)
Tomato	2	237
Blackberry	4	162
Raspberry	5	151
Strawberry	6	153
Cantaloupe	7	267
Watermelon	8	112
Orange	9	181
Peach	8	190
Tangerine	11	166
Apple	11	107
Blueberry	12	77
Cherries, sweet	14	222

Source: USDA, cronometer.com

Insulin causes a dose-dependent decline in plasma potassium concentration so reliably that physicians use IV insulin as a treatment for hyperkalemia (too much potassium in the blood).[105] Since high carbohydrate diets increase post-meal insulin levels, and this would drive down plasma potassium levels, it seems possible that high carbohydrate plant-based diets increase potassium requirements. On the other had avoidance of plant foods and their carbohydrates will result in a very low serum insulin level, which probably reduces dietary potassium requirements.

[105] Stone MS, Martyn L, Weaver CM. Potassium Intake, Bioavailability, Hypertension, and Glucose Control. *Nutrients*. 2016;8(7):444. doi:10.3390/nu8070444. <https://www.ncbi.nlm.nih.gov/pmc/articles/PMC4963920/>

Since reducing dietary carbohydrate results in marked reductions in chronic serum insulin levels, and insulin stimulates the kidneys to retain sodium, reducing carbohydrate intake results in greatly reduced sodium and water retention. Consequently, when one first transitions to a carnivorous diet, one will lose water and minerals, including potassium. To prevent electrolyte imbalance you should maintain an adequate sodium intake and prepare your meat in ways that minimizes loss of its potassium.

In Nature, carnivores eat meat fresh (raw), therefore retaining all of its minerals. Cooking meat for long periods over an open fire or in any way in which you lose juices from the meat will lead to loss of some of its potassium and other minerals. If you want to succeed with minimal plant intake you should prepare meat with a method that preserves its juices. Aside from eating meat raw, you can achieve this by searing meats to seal in the juices, then cooking at high temperature only briefly (rare or medium rare), or by roasting slowly at low temperatures (≤200 °F), or making stews and soups, and by using the juices of oven-roasted meats as sauce for the meat.

Also, you can reduce urinary losses of potassium and prevent or reverse muscle cramping in the transition phase by consuming adequate sodium in the form of salt. Simply, use salt to taste in preparation of meat or at the table.

Magnesium

Magnesium plays a crucial role in glucose and insulin metabolism,[106] which suggests that high carbohydrate diets would increase magnesium requirements.

Authorities often claim that whole grains, legumes, seeds and nuts are good sources of magnesium. However, fibers, phytate and oxalate in these foods binds the magnesium and reduces absorption

---

[106] Gröber U, Schmidt J, Kisters K. Magnesium in Prevention and Therapy. *Nutrients*. 2015;7(9):8199-8226. doi:10.3390/nu7095388. <https://www.ncbi.nlm.nih.gov/pmc/articles/PMC4586582/>

by as much as 58 percent.[107, 108] Green leafy vegetables also contain magnesium because magnesium is part of the chlorophyll molecule, but oxalate in some types of greens reduces magnesium absorption.[109] However, the magnesium content of vegetables and grains has significantly decreased since 1900, and up to 90% of people eating conventional plant-based diets fall short of recommended magnesium intakes by up to 65%.[110] Since our preagricultural ancestors did not eat modern grains or vegetables, they obtained required magnesium from some other source.

All animals need magnesium, so all animal tissues contain some magnesium. Marine fish are particularly good sources. Moreover, animal protein and medium-chain-triglycerides found in animal fats enhance magnesium uptake.[83]

However, meat and eggs are not very good sources of magnesium. Since 1940 the magnesium content of animal products has declined by up to 70%: beef (–4 to –8%), bacon (–18%), chicken (–4%), cheddar cheese (–38%), parmesan cheese (–70%) and whole milk (–

---

[107] Bohn T, Davidsson L, Walczyk T, Hurrell RF. Phytic acid added to white-wheat bread inhibits fractional apparent magnesium absorption in humans. Am J Clin Nutr. 2004 Mar;79(3):418-23. PubMed PMID: 14985216.

[108] Schuchardt JP, Hahn A. Intestinal Absorption and Factors Influencing Bioavailability of Magnesium-An Update. Current Nutrition and Food Science. 2017;13(4):260-278. doi:10.2174/1573401313666170427162740. <https://www.ncbi.nlm.nih.gov/pmc/articles/PMC5652077/>

[109] Bohn T, Davidsson L, Walczyk T, Hurrell RF. Fractional magnesium absorption is significantly lower in human subjects from a meal served with an oxalate-rich vegetable, spinach, as compared with a meal served with kale, a vegetable with a low oxalate content. Br J Nutr 2004 Apr;91(4):601-6.

[110] Rosanoff A. The high heart health value of drinking-water magnesium. Medical Hypotheses 2013 Dec;81(6):1063-1065. https://doi.org/10.1016/j.mehy.2013.10.003

21%).[111] Five hundred grams of beef T-bone steak provides only 110 mg magnesium, only about 26% of the recommended intake; 1 kg will still get you only 52% of the recommendation. Dairy products are the best animal sources of magnesium, but still not adequate.

Many people focus on food as the primary source of magnesium, but for our ancestors and many rural people today drinking water was/is probably the major source. Hard water and mineral waters from wells and springs contain no magnesium binders and can provide more than 50 mg magnesium per liter.[112] In some areas drinking water easily provides 300-400 mg magnesium daily (the recommended intake) and water-borne magnesium occurs as hydrated ions which have a higher bioavailability than magnesium in food.[113] Modern urban populations generally use surface waters which supply far less magnesium than groundwaters.

Magnesium-rich water has a laxative effect, could potentially prevent 4.5 million heart disease and stroke deaths annually worldwide, probably protects against kidney stones and

---

[111] DiNicolantonio JJ, O'Keefe JH, Wilson W. Subclinical magnesium deficiency: a principal driver of cardiovascular disease and a public health crisis. *Open Heart*. 2018;5(1):e000668. doi:10.1136/openhrt-2017-000668. <https://www.ncbi.nlm.nih.gov/pmc/articles/PMC5786912/>

[112] Quattrini S, Pampaloni B, Brandi ML. Natural mineral waters: chemical characteristics and health effects. *Clinical Cases in Mineral and Bone Metabolism*. 2016;13(3):173-180. doi:10.11138/ccmbm/2016.13.3.173. **<https://www.ncbi.nlm.nih.gov/pmc/articles/PMC5318167/>**

[113] Sengupta P. Potential Health Impacts of Hard Water. *International Journal of Preventive Medicine*. 2013;4(8):866-875. <https://www.ncbi.nlm.nih.gov/pmc/articles/PMC3775162/>

osteoporosis, and is associated with reduced risk of diabetes, some birth defects, and various types of cancer.[114, 115, 116]

If you don't drink hard water rich in magnesium, I recommend using an inexpensive magnesium supplement daily. I personally take 300-600 mg per day.

Iron

Iron deficiency is the most common nutrient deficiency in the world, affecting more than 1.2 billion people. In developing nations, almost half of the pre-school children and pregnant women exhibit iron-deficiency anemia. It occurs most often among infants less than 2 years of age, teenage girls, pregnant women, and the elderly. In the U.S., 10 percent of toddlers, adolescent girls, and women of childbearing age have iron-deficiency.[117]

[114] Sengupta P. Potential Health Impacts of Hard Water. *International Journal of Preventive Medicine*. 2013;4(8):866-875. <https://www.ncbi.nlm.nih.gov/pmc/articles/PMC3775162/>

[115] Rosanoff A. The high heart health value of drinking-water magnesium. Medical Hypotheses 2013 Dec;81(6):1063-1065. https://doi.org/10.1016/j.mehy.2013.10.003

[116] Seelig MS. Magnesium Deficiency In The Pathogenesis of Disease: Early Roots of Cardiovascular, Skeletal and Renal Abnormalities. Goldwater Memorial Hospital, New York University Medical Center, 1980. <http://www.mgwater.com/Seelig/Magnesium-Deficiency-in-the-Pathogenesis-of-Disease/chapter1.shtml#toc1-6>

[117] Whitney EN, Rolfes SR. Understanding Nutrition. 10th edition. Wadsworth/Thompson Learning 2005: 442.

Iron deficiency commonly occurs in regions where the people consume a primarily plant-based diet.[118] Fiber and phytates in plant-based diets interfere with iron absorption.

Heme (animal-source) iron is at least 3 times more bioavailable than non-heme (plant) iron. Vegetarians need 1.8 times as much iron as meat-eaters to make up for the lower bioavailability of iron from plant foods.[119]

Some people claim that eating heme iron from animal products leads to a build up of excess iron in the body that promotes many diseases. However, "adults with normal intestinal function have very little risk of iron overload from dietary sources of iron."[120] In fact, the body has a system for removing excessive heme iron from circulation, and reutilizes the iron only as needed depending on the state of body iron stores.[121]

Zinc

Animal foods supply the highest concentrations of zinc in the most bioavailable forms. Oysters have the highest zinc concentration, but red meats (including dark meat of poultry) and fish provide plenty.

Plant foods have much lower concentrations of zinc, and the zinc in plant foods has a low bioavailability because phytic acid (phytate) in

---

118 Zimmermann MB, Chaouki N, Hurrell RF, "Iron deficiency due to consumption of a habitual diet low in bioavailable iron: a longitudinal cohort study in Moroccan children," Am J Clin Nutr 2005 Jan;81(1):115-121.

[119] Whitney EN, Rolfes SR. Understanding Nutrition. 10th edition. Wadsworth/ Thompson Learning 2005: 445.

[120] National Institutes of Health. Office of Dietary Supplements. Iron. Dietary Supplement Fact Sheet. <**https://ods.od.nih.gov/factsheets/Iron-HealthProfessional/**>

[121] Sears DA. Disposal of plasma heme in normal man and patients with intravascular hemolysis. *Journal of Clinical Investigation*. 1970;49(1):5-14. <**https://www.ncbi.nlm.nih.gov/pmc/articles/PMC322438/**>

plants binds zinc into a complex that we can't break down to access the zinc.

Zinc deficiency never occurs in people who consume adequate amounts of red meats, but was first identified in the 1960s among Middle Eastern children raised on plant-based diets containing little meat. The legumes and whole grains they were relying on as staple foods have high fiber and phytate contents which inhibit zinc absorption.[122]

Children eating plant-based diets have an increased risk of zinc deficiency.[123, 124, 125]

Iodine

Land plants are poor sources of iodine, and many plants contain goitrogens which interfere with iodine utilization and cause hypothyroidism in about 8 million people world-wide.[126] Examples of goitrogen-containing foods include:

- Vegetables: Arugula, asparagus, bok choy, broccoli, broccolini, Brussels sprouts, cabbage, cauliflower, Chinese broccoli, Chinese

---

[122] Whitney EN, Rolfes SR. Understanding Nutrition. 10th edition. Wadsworth/ Thompson Learning 2005: 449.

[123] Strict vegetarians have an increased risk for zinc deficiency. Linus Pauling Institute Micronutrient Information Center, Oregon State University, "Zinc," <http://lpi.oregonstate.edu/mic/minerals/zinc>

[124] "Supplements [of zinc and iron] may be necessary for vegetarian children following very restricted vegan diets." Gibson RS, Heath AL, Szymlek-Gay EA, "Is iron and zinc nutrition a concern for vegetarian infants and young children in industrialized countries?," Am J Clin Nutr 2014 Jul;100 Suppl 1:459S-68S.

[125] Hunt JR, "Bioavailability of iron, zinc, and other trace minerals form vegetarian diets," Am J Clin Nutr 2003 Sep:78(3 Suppl):633S-639S.

[126] Whitney EN and Rolfes SR. Understanding Nutrition 10th Edition. Thomson Wadsworth, 2005:451.

cabbage, choy sum, collard greens, kale, kohlrabi, mizuna, mustard greens, onions, parsley, radishes, rapini, rutabagas, spinach, turnips, wasabi, watercress
- Roots and tubers: Cassava, horseradish, sweet potato,
- Grains: Millet, corn
- Seeds: Flax, canola, mustard
- Legumes: Soybeans, soy products, peanuts, lima beans
- Fruits: Apples, apricots, blueberries, citrus fruits, cranberries, grapes, peaches, strawberries

Cooking the listed vegetables reduces their goitrogen contents; thus if you have health problems I suggest that you avoid eating the listed foods and thoroughly cook them if you eat them. In the U.S. most people get their iodine from iodized salt. However, all seafoods (animal and vegetable) are good sources of iodine.

People who avoid eating animal products have a much higher risk of iodine deficiency than people who eat animal products. One study reported that one-fourth of vegetarians and 80 percent of vegans suffer from iodine deficiency compared to only 9 percent of meat-eaters.[127]

Essential Fats

Linoleic and Arachidonic Acids

Omega-6 linoleic acid is conventionally considered one of the essential fatty acids. We can not make linoleic acid from scratch. In theory, we need it primarily as a precursor to gamma-linoleic, dihomo-gamma-linoleic, and arachidonic acids. We need dihomo-gamma-linoleic acid to produce some series-1 prostaglandins, and we need arachidonic acid to maintain cell membrane fluidity, ion channel function, heal injuries, fight infections, and control the cell cycle (programmed cell death).

---

[127] Kajcovincová-Kudláčková M, Bucková K, Klimes I, Seboková E. Iodine deficiency in vegetarians and vegans. Ann Nutr Metab 2003;47(5):183-5.

If we consume sufficient gamma-linoleic, dihomo-gamma-linoleic, and arachidonic acids directly from foods, we do not need any dietary linoleic acid. While plants typically only provide linoleic acid or gamma-linoleic acid, animal tissues provide all of the omega-6 fatty acids, in proportions similar to our requirements.

Omega-6 essential fatty acid deficiency has never occurred in any population having an adequate intake of animal products. It has only occurred in people fed artificial liquid formulas.

Ancestral diets generally had relatively low but adequate levels of omega-6 linoleic acid compared to modern diets. Before the 20th century, people generally did not consume large amounts of nuts or seeds because these naturally come in shells that are difficult and tedious to remove (a warning from Nature to limit consumption), and we did not have the technology required to extract mass amounts of oils from plant seeds. Populations having a high immunity to diseases of civilization have consumed far less linoleic acid than modern industrial populations.

A basic principle of toxicology is: The dose makes the poison. Most plant-based oils contain high concentrations of linoleic acid. The relatively small absolute amounts of linoleic acid naturally present in unprocessed animal foods or small amounts of paleolithic plant foods (fruits, herbaceous vegetables) may not have any harmful effects, but when extracted from seeds and concentrated in free oils and consumed liberally (instead of natural animal fats) these fats may have multiple harmful effects, such as making skin more fragile and prone to sun damage, promoting inflammation, and perhaps promoting cancer.[128, 129, 130] Diets high in linoleic acid may have a toxic effect of stiffening the heart muscle.[131]

Conversion of linoleic acid to arachidonic acid (AA) is limited. Linoleic acid must be oxidized by the δ-6-desaturase enzyme to produce γ-linolenic acid, but aging, nutritional shortfalls, and other factors can reduce the activity of this enzyme.

Next γ-linolenic acid must be converted to arachidonic acid by the δ-5-desaturase enzyme, but this conversion is limited because δ-5-desaturase prefers ω-3 to ω-6 fats. (This also would promote arachidonic acid deficiency in vegans relying on alpha-linolenic acid from plants for ω-3.) In tracer studies, only about 0.2 percent of LA gets converted to AA.[132] As a consequence, we most easily meet our arachidonic acid requirement by eating animal products rather than depending on plant-based linoleic acid.

Human mothers' milk contains AA, not only LA. Human infants need AA for proper development and function of the retina and central nervous system. We have evidence that infants have a

---

[128] Ravnskov U. Myth 7: Polyunsaturated Oils are Good For You. In: The Cholesterol Myths: Exposing the Fallacy that Saturated Fat and Cholesterol Cause Heart Disease. Washington D.C.: New Trends Publishing Inc., 2000:217-234.

[129] Braden LM, Carroll KK. Dietary polyunsaturated fat in relation to mammary carcinogenesis in rats. *Lipids* 1986; 21:285-88.

[130] Toborek M, Lee YW, Garrido R, Kaiser S, Hennig B. Unsaturated fatty acids selectively induce an inflammatory environment in human endothelial cells. *Am J Clin Nutr* 2002; 75:119-125.

[131] Beam, Julianne et al. "Excess Linoleic Acid Increases Collagen I/III Ratio and 'Stiffens' the Heart Muscle Following High Fat Diets." *The Journal of Biological Chemistry* 290.38 (2015): 23371–23384. *PMC*. Web. 9 Apr. 2017.

[132] Harris WS, Mozaffarian D, Rimm E, et al.. Omega-6 Fatty Acids and Risk for Cardiovascular Disease. Circulation 2009 Feb 16:119:902-907. <http:// circ.ahajournals.org/content/119/6/902>

dietary requirement for AA to develop a healthy immune function.[133] Together with DHA (discussed below) AA forms 20 percent of the dry weight of the brain, and the brain consumes about 17.8 mg daily of AA.

Despite presumably adequate linoleic acid intake, supplementation with AA has improved cognitive functions in autistic children and in elderly individuals,[134] suggesting that conversion of linoleic acid is not sufficient to meet requirements of children or elders.

Arachidonic acid prevents ischemia-induced heart arrhythmia, a major cause of sudden cardiac death, by virtue of its role in regulating ion channels.[135] This suggests that arachidonic acid deficiency plays a role in arrhythmia and sudden cardiac death.

AA makes up 15-17 percent of the total fatty acids in skeletal muscles, AA-derived prostaglandins play an important role in post-exercise recovering and muscle protein synthesis, and AA supplementation may improve body composition, muscle function and power output in strength-training individuals.[136, 137] Blocking

------

[133] Richard C, Lewis ED, Field CJ. Evidence for the essentiality of arachidonic and docosahexaenoic acid in the postnatal maternal and infant diet for the development of the infant's immune system early in life. Appl Physiol Nutr Metab. 2016 May;41(5):461-75. doi: 10.1139/apnm-2015-0660. Epub 2016 Jan 22. Review. PubMed PMID: 27138971.

[134] Tallima H, El Ridi R. Arachidonic acid: Physiological roles and potential health benefits – A review. J Adv Res 2017. **<https://doi.org/10.1016/j.jare.2017.11.004>**

[135] Ibid.

[136] Roberts MD, Iosia M, Kerksick CM, et al.. Effects of arachidonic acid supplementation on training adaptations in resistance-trained males. J Int Soc Sports Nutr 2007 Nove 28;4:21. **< https://www.ncbi.nlm.nih.gov/pmc/articles/PMC2217562/pdf/1550-2783-4-21.pdf>**

[137] Trappe TA et al. Prostaglandins, COX Inhibitors, and Muscular Exercise. J Appl Physiol 2013

production of AA-derived prostaglandins with COX-inhibiting drugs after resistance training has been reported to abolish protein synthesis.[138] AA may also improve neuromuscular signaling.[139]

AA also probably plays a very important role in control of tumors: it inhibits or kills tumor cells, and has been advocated as an anti-cancer drug.[140] This suggests that arachidonic acid deficiency due to insufficient intake of animal products may increase cancer risk.

We produce endocannabinoids from AA. These control neural processes, and endocannabinoid signaling dysregulation is related to neuropsychiatric disorders. In the brain, endocannabinoid-mediated signaling modulates appetite, pain and mood. One of the AA-derived endocannabinoids, anandamide, appears to modulate sperm motility, improve renal functions, and ameliorate chronic inflammatory disorders of the gut by regulating gut homeostasis, motility, visceral sensation, and inflammation.[141]

Some people have claimed that eating arachidonic acid directly from animals creates a pro-inflammatory environment in the body. However, studies of arachidonic acid supplementation with up to about 7 times usual dietary intakes have found either no increase in signs of systemic inflammation, or decreased levels of pro-inflammatory chemicals and increased levels of anti-inflammatory

---

[138] Ibid.

[139] Tallima H, El Ridi R. Arachidonic acid: Physiological roles and potential health benefits – A review. J Adv Res 2017. <**https://doi.org/10.1016/j.jare.2017.11.004**>

[140] Ibid.

[141] Tallima H, El Ridi R. Arachidonic acid: Physiological roles and potential health benefits – A review. J Adv Res 2017. <**https://doi.org/10.1016/j.jare.2017.11.004**>

markers in people having higher blood levels of arachidonic acid.[142, 143]

AA actually plays an important role in the resolution of inflammation as a precursor for mediators having pro-resolution capacity, one of the most important being lipoxin A_4. Lipoxin A_4 has been demonstrated to reduce bronchoconstriction in asthma and decrease eczema severity and duration.[144]

Since the above-mentioned disorders are common in modern populations eating plant-based diets rich in linoleic acid but restricted in arachidonic acid, I believe it is likely that we have a dietary requirement for AA, which we can satisfy only by regularly consuming animal products (in the absence of supplements produced by technology). This in turn means that in Nature we are obligate carnivores.

α-Linolenic Acid

Hypothetically, we require α-linolenic acid (LNA) as a precursor for the biosynthesis of the longer-chain omega-3 fats eicosapentaenoic acid (EPA) and docosahexaenoic acid (DHA). However, research has shown that our ability to convert α-linolenic acid to EPA is

---

[142] Ferrucci L, Cherubini A, Bandinelli S, et al.. Relationship of Plasma Polyunsaturated Fatty Acids to Circulating Inflammatory Markers. J Clin Endo & Metab 2006 Feb;91(2):439-46. <**https://academic.oup.com/jcem/article/91/2/439/2843288**>

[143] Harris WS, Mozaffarian D, Rimm E, et al.. Omega-6 Fatty Acids and Risk for Cardiovascular Disease. Circulation 2009 Feb 16:119:902-907. <**http://circ.ahajournals.org/content/119/6/902**>

[144] Tallima H, El Ridi R. Arachidonic acid: Physiological roles and potential health benefits – A review. J Adv Res 2017. <**https://doi.org/10.1016/j.jare.2017.11.004**>

limited, and the conversion to DHA is even more limited.[145] EPA and DHA are more biologically potent than LNA. We more easily enrich our tissues with EPA and especially DHA if we directly consume these fats (more on this in the section on DHA below, and in great detail in Chapter 9).

Both plant and animal tissues provide the omega-3 fatty acid α-linolenic acid, but only animal products provide EPA and DHA.

DHA

Docosahexaenoic acid (DHA) is a structural constituent of central nervous system cell membranes. Our ancestors consumed land animal fats and seafoods rich in DHA during the period of evolutionary expansion of the brain. It is essential to healthy brain and eye development in children and function in children and adults. Deficiency of DHA very likely plays a role in major psychiatric disorders and cognitive decline with age.[146, 147, 148]

Hypothetically we could produce DHA from α-linolenic acid provided by plant foods; however, when vegetarians increase their α-linolenic acid intake, they do not increase levels of DHA in their

---

[145] Pawlosky RJ, Hibbeln JR, Novotny JA, Salem N. Physiological compartmental analysis of α-Linolenic Acid metabolism in adult humans. J Lipid Res 2001 Aug; 42:1257-65. <http://www.jlr.org/content/42/8/1257.long>

[146] Bradbury J. Docosahexaenoic Acid (DHA): An Ancient Nutrient for the Modern Human Brain . Nutrients. 2011;3(5):529-554. doi:10.3390/nu3050529. <https://www.ncbi.nlm.nih.gov/pmc/articles/PMC3257695/>

[147] Lauritzen L, Brambilla P, Mazzocchi A, Harsløf LBS, Ciappolino V, Agostoni C. DHA Effects in Brain Development and Function. Nutrients. 2016;8(1):6. doi: 10.3390/nu8010006. <https://www.ncbi.nlm.nih.gov/pmc/articles/PMC4728620/>

[148] AGostoni C, Nobile M, Ciappolino V, et al. The Role of Omega-3 Fatty Acids in Developmental Psychopathology: A Systematic Review on Early Psychosis, Autism, and ADHD. Int J Mol Sci 2017 Dec;18(12):2608. <https://www.ncbi.nlm.nih.gov/pmc/articles/PMC5751211/>

blood.[149] Sufficient evidence has accumulated to indicate that we require a dietary source of the omega-3 fatty acid DHA.[150, 151]

Edible plants simply do not provide DHA. In Nature, we must eat animal foods to get adequate intakes; therefore, we are by Nature obligate carnivores.

I discuss how you can meet your need for omega-3 fats eating only conventional grain-finished animal products in Chapter 10.

---

[149] Bradbury J. Docosahexaenoic Acid (DHA): An Ancient Nutrient for the Modern Human Brain . *Nutrients*. 2011;3(5):529-554. doi:10.3390/nu3050529. <https://www.ncbi.nlm.nih.gov/pmc/articles/PMC3257695/>

150 Muskiet FAJ, Fokkema MR, Schaafsma A, et al., "Is Docosahexaenoic Acid (DHA) Essential? Lessons from DHA Status Regulation, Our Ancient Diet, Epidemiology and Randomized Controlled Trials," J Nutr 2004 Jan 1;134(1): 183-186. <http://jn.nutrition.org/content/134/1/183.full>

151 Europeans and Asians almost certainly have a genetically-determined requirement for animal-source AA and DHA: Kothapalli KSD, Ye K, Gadgil MS, et al., "Positive selection on a regulatory insertion-deletion polymorphism in FADS2 influences apparent endogenous synthesis of arachidonic acid," Mol Biol Evol 2016 March 29; 33(7): 1726-1739. doi:10.1093/molbev/msw049 <http://mbe.oxfordjournals.org/content/early/2016/03/09/molbev.msw049.full.pdf+html>

9 THE HYPERCARNIVORE DIET

Do you think you can take over the universe and improve it?
I do not believe it can be done.

The universe is sacred.
You cannot improve it.
If you try to change it, you will ruin it.
If you try to hold it, you will lose it.

TAO TE CHING Chapter 28

In and by Nature, we humans are hypercarnivores, so THE HYPERCARNIVORE DIET (hereafter a.k.a. PRIMAL FEEDING) consists of eating in accord with your True Nature. Your True Nature has two aspects, namely the internal and external. Internal Nature refers to what we call Human Nature as expressed in each individual, consisting of physical, mental, moral and spiritual aspects of a whole. External Nature refers to your Natural habitat, comprising the bioregion you inhabit presently as well as the Natural habitat of your ancestors. To eat and live in harmony with Nature means eating and living in harmony with both your Human Nature *and* your Natural habitat.

Nature, which is our Creator, has a PRIMAL WISDOM and we humans are largely ignorant of How Things Work. Since we are creatures, not the creator, of Nature, our knowledge of How Things Work is always limited. All of the conceptual frameworks we use to try to understand Nature – including modern science – are inherently limited. All conceptual systems consist of concepts which have definitions and rest on assumptions and therefore are limited in scope. Just as a menu can not capture a meal and a map can not fully capture the territory, a conceptual system (science) can not fully capture the Nature of phenomena.

Moreover, we can only sense directly what our perceptual system allows, but we know that other species can sense phenomena that we cannot (e.g. dogs can hear sounds and detect scents that we cannot detect). Because of the intrinsic limits of our perceptual and conceptual systems, we don't know and in principle can never know everything there is to know about Nature, Natural Foods, and how they support our health and fitness.

As Francis Bacon noted: "Nature, to be commanded, must be obeyed." Therefore if we want health and happiness, we must obey or follow Nature.

Nature provides all the foods that we need to thrive (which justifies calling Nature *Providence*). Therefore to maintain health we must understand what Natural conditions (including diet and other environmental conditions) were necessary for the creation of human beings, and what Nature permits and forbids to us.

Nature continuously provides us with guidance to optimal nutrition through 1) our own senses of taste, smell, gastrointestinal comfort or discomfort, and satisfaction, 2) the Nature-given characteristics of our own bodies – particularly our food acquisition and digestive systems, 3) the characteristics of our Natural habitats, and, finally, 4) the various maladies that arise when we deviate from following Nature; e.g. tooth decay warns us not to eat high density carbohydrates, irritable bowel warms us not to consume fiber, etc..

Our problems stem not from a failure of Nature, but from our failure to heed Nature's warnings. Our hubris arises from our unjustified faith in what many call our 'intelligence' which I would rather call cleverness. Literally, the word "clever" means *able to cleave*, that is, able to separate things into parts. A clever creature can break things apart, but not make them whole.

A clever mind thinks itself separate from and superior to Nature. It thinks it can 'improve' on Nature's wisdom or circumvent Her limits by using technology to make edible what Nature has made inedible.

A mind having accessed PRIMAL WISDOM realizes the limits of its abilities. It does not presume to have greater understanding than its Creator.

Nature permits us some foods without restriction: those which we can by Nature acquire, and are by Nature non-toxic, palatable and completely digestible.

Nature puts limits on or forbids us to consume other items by making those items more or less difficult to obtain, bad tasting, indigestible and toxic. If we ignore the warnings of Nature – especially unpalatability and indigestibility in Natural form – and use our cleverness to make edible what Nature made inedible, Nature makes us pay for disobedience by putting us in the portable prison of illness, weakness, ugliness, and unhappiness.

> Life in all its fullness is This Mother Nature obeyed.
>
> Weston A Price

PRIMAL FEEDING involves learning how to follow Nature in order to free yourself, your family and your people from unhappiness, illness, and weakness so you can reclaim health, happiness, strength and beauty, to the greatest extent possible in this lifetime, and even moreso in succeeding generations.

All health and strength comes from good digestion and assimilation of essential nutrients obtained by aligning yourself with Nature. If you have any dis-ease, eat only the permitted animal-source foods and minimize or avoid plant foods until you have regained your health.

HYPERCARNIVORE DIET OVERVIEW

ESSENTIAL & PRIMARY FOODS on average comprise 70-100%
of the diet, variable with season, bioregion and individual needs:

• Any fresh animal meat, organs, eggs, fats and bones
• Water, minerals and salts

OPTIONAL ANIMAL FOODS may comprise a portion of primary
foods for some people:

• Naturally preserved meats
• Some dairy products

OPTIONAL NON-ANIMAL FOODS

Some conditionally non-essential, non-animal foods may comprise
0-30% of the diet, variable with season, bioregion and individual
desire and tolerance:

• Fruits and berries
• Fibrous vegetables and fungi
• Herbs and spices

AVOID/SEVERELY RESTRICT

• Nuts and seeds
• Plant-based oils
• Sugars including honey
• Starchy vegetables (roots and tubers)
• Cereal grains and legumes
• Alcohol
• Man-made foods

ESSENTIAL & PRIMARY FOODS

SUMMARY: Fresh animal meat, organs, eggs, fats and bones along with water and minerals (salts) generally comprise at least 70% of a hypercarnivore diet, with types and amounts variable from day to day and with bioregion, season and individual needs.

MEAT: Nature provides dead animals whether man hunts or not. Humans hunt and trap animals by Nature; virtually all boys and some girls allowed to play outdoors will spontaneously hunt and trap small animals. Nature also equipped us to capture animals. Humans have for millions of years successfully hunted and trapped small and large animals with bare hands and with stones and sturdy sticks (spears) already provided by Nature. Indeed, Nature designed our shoulder girdle (and lopsided brain) for hunting with projectile weapons.

Moreover, raw meat and fat are very tasty, non-toxic, easy to chew and almost 100% digestible. Finally, meat is the only food that can provide complete nutrition by itself.

You can eat all fresh meat, from any animal, whether insect, worm, fish, reptile, bird or mammal, wild or domesticated, including sausages and any type of naturally fatty meat such as brisket or belly.

You may include and benefit from all edible and usable parts of animals, including muscles, organs and bones. The liver is the most nutrient-dense organ. Its name – live-r – reflects its importance to life. If you really want to nourish yourself, regularly consume small amounts of liver, preferably raw, as done by our ancestors. One needs only about one-half to one ounce daily or a total of four to eight ounces each week.

You can eat animal meat and fat raw (e.g. steak tartare, carpaccio, sushi, kibbeh) or cooked conservatively as done in traditional cultures. Conservative cooking uses high heat only briefly, such as for searing or cooking a steak or roast to rare condition, or very low heat for long periods (low slow roasting or simmering).

Conservative cooking methods also preserve nutrients (such as collecting juices in a pan and using them as a topping for the dish). As explained in Chapter 9, Nature has clearly favored people who eat both conservatively cooked and raw animal products.

How much? If you can get your mind out of the way, eventually you can let your hunger and taste guide you, eating as much as tastes good to you, and stopping when it no longer tastes good. However, to get started you will benefit from the following guidelines that will help you avoid eating either too little or too much meat (yes, you can get too much):

Based on protein requirements and protein content of meat, one will need to eat about 6-8 g meat or eggs per kg (3-4 g per lb) lean body weight. For example, a sedentary 68 kg (150 pound) man will need about 400-600 g (15-20 oz) of meat and eggs (which would provide 105-150 g of protein), variable depending on whether he includes protein-rich dairy products (milk, yogurt, cheese) or not.

Nature has set an upper limit to meat and protein consumption. Your digestive tract can only absorb amino acids from whole foods at a limited rate (~5-8 g/h=120-192 g/d). Also, your liver can only deaminate proteins to produce urea for excretion of excess nitrogen at a limited rate. Because of these limits, protein intakes in the range of 200-400 g/d can have adverse effects, including nausea, diarrhea, hyperaminoacidemia, hyperammonemia, hyperinsulinemia, and even death. Historic explorers knew this as "rabbit starvation syndrome" which occurred when men were forced to eat lean meat without added fat. To avoid this acute protein poisoning we may need to limit protein intake to about 2 to 2.5 g per kg per day.[1]

On this basis the *estimated* upper limits of safe chronic protein and meat intake are listed in Table 9.1. Note that the upper numbers are *estimated* maximum tolerable levels, not targets. Your needs and tolerance may vary. Follow Nature which guides you by your senses

---

[1] Bilsborough S and Mann N: A Review of Issues of Dietary Protein Intake in Humans. Int J Sport Nutr and Ex Metab 2006;16:129-152.

of hunger, taste, and satisfaction/dissatisfaction.

Table 9.1 Estimated upper limits for protein and meat intake (g/d)

Bodyweight kg (pounds)	Max protein (g/d)	Max fresh meat (g/d)
45 (100)	90-113	450
50 (110)	100-125	500
55 (121)	110-138	550
60 (132)	120-150	600
65 (143)	130-163	650
70 (154)	140-175	700
75 (165)	150-188	750
80 (176)	160-200	800
85 (187)	170-213	850
90 (198)	180-225	900
95 (209)	190-238	950
100 (220)	200-250	1000
105 (231)	210-263	1050
110 (242)	220-275	1100
115 (253)	230-288	1150

See: Bilsborough S and Mann N: A Review of Issues of Dietary Protein Intake in Humans. Int J Sport Nutr and Ex Metab 2006;16:129-152.

Table 9.2 shows the protein intake from various trimmed cuts of meat with visible fat eaten. Note that 500 g of beef chuck roast provides only 1650 kcal and 500 g ribeye or 80% lean ground beef only about 1250 kcal. One kilogram (2.2 pounds) of either of these would provide 2500-3000 kcal and 230-250 g protein. Chuck roast or steak provides ~70% of energy as fat, ~30% as protein; rib eye roast or steak provides ~55% of energy as fat, ~45% as protein.

Table 9.2 Macronutrients in 500 g various lean meats (visible fat eaten)

Meat	Kcalories	Protein g (% energy)	Fat g (% energy)
Beef chuck or cross rib	1650	116 (30)	128 (70)
Beef T-bone	1455	129 (38)	100 (62)
Beef ground 80% lean	1270	126 (42)	81 (58)
Beef ribeye, sirloin, skirt	1250	134 (46)	76 (54)
Beef ground 85% lean	1200	130 (46)	72 (54)
Beef ground 90% lean	1070	133 (53)	55 (47)
Beef rump, round	1020	153 (60)	45 (40)
Chicken breast with skin	920	137 (64)	37 (36)

Source: USDA, cronometer.com

All of these cuts of meat provide more than 25% of energy from protein. Unless your lean body weight is more than 90 kg (200 lbs), if you eat enough of any of these meats to obtain sufficient calories, you may consume more protein than your body can process efficiently and may experience acute protein toxicity. Most people can't thrive on a hypercarnivore diet consisting of lean meats alone and will need to add separate fat to dilute the protein and meet energy requirements.

I speak from experience. Although I primarily eat ribeye, 80% lean ground beef, and chuck, like Stefansson, I have more than once gotten diarrhea for several days when I consumed too much meat and protein without enough added fat. At a body weight of about 68 kg (150 lb) I found that if I exceeded 200 g/d for several days I would end up with diarrhea for several days thereafter. Consequently I recommend keeping your protein intake around 2 g/kg (1.0 g/lb) of body weight.

One's desire for meat may vary from time to time according to individual needs, bioregion, and season. Generally, desire or taste for meat – especially fatter meats – may increase in colder regions and seasons, and in response to physical injury or increases in demanding physical activity, or decrease in hotter regions and seasons and when you are more sedentary.

ANIMAL FATS: Nature provides some animal fats with all meats, and some of these fats are Naturally separated or easily separable from the lean meats. Some of the animal fats provided by Nature have high density; for example, the kidney fat in oxen and sheep contains about 99 percent fat (mostly saturated fats). Since humans have been consuming these fats since time immemorial, we have evolved taste, appetite and digestive apparatus and ability to cope with high concentrations of fat. We find fats highly palatable and fats are virtually 100% digestible. Therefore Nature clearly permits us to eat animal fats according to hunger and appetite.

You need to eat separated, rendered or concentrated animal fats such as tallow, lard, butter, or heavy cream (fresh or sour) to satisfy your energy requirements and prevent protein overdose. Inuit (Eskimos) dipped their meat and fish in seal oil and ate whale blubber for this purpose.[2]

As a rule of thumb, you need to eat one part added fat for three parts meat. For example, if you eat 300 g meat you should also include ~100 g added fat (butter, tallow, bacon fat, cream, etc). If you are lean and very active, or in a very cold season or climate, you may need an even higher proportion of fat. *Fatigue, failure to thrive,*

---

[2] Price W. Nutrition and Physical Degeneration. Price-Pottenger Nutrition Foundation, 1970. 70-71.

nausea or diarrhea can signify you are eating too much protein and not enough fat.

Nature limits the amount of fat one can eat. The gut can absorb fatty acids at a maximum rate of about 0.175 g per kg per hour.[3] Unabsorbed fat can cause abdominal pain, bloating and diarrhea. Table 9.3 lists estimated daily maximum fat intakes based on the maximum absorption rate.

The upper limit is not a target but an *estimated* boundary. The closer you approach these limits, the more likely you will suffer some adverse digestive effects. Some people may need to stay 10-20% below the maximum tolerable level to function optimally. Others may be able to consume more than the estimated limit without ill effect. Your tolerance may also vary with time.

Due to the limits on protein and fat absorption, some very active people who have high energy requirements may need to include some well-tolerated sources of carbohydrate to get adequate kcalories without exceeding maximum tolerable intakes of protein and fat. For example, suppose a 45 kg woman tolerates up to 100 g protein (Table 9.1) and 170 g fat (Table 9.3) in a day without digestive distress. That would provide 1930 kcal. If she expends 2200 kcal daily, she is going to need 270 kcal from 68 g of digestible carbohydrates. This is one reason THE HYPERCARNIVORE DIET allows consumption of fermented dairy and fresh and dried fruits according to your own need and tolerance.

Observers reported that among Eskimos/Inuit, fat intake varies individually and seasonally. "In warm weather about one-seventh of the meat may be fat, in cold weather, especially when the Eskimos are traveling, one-third to one-half may be taken as fat."[4]

---

[3] Bilsborough S and Mann N: A Review of Issues of Dietary Protein Intake in Humans. Int J Sport Nutr and Ex Metab 2006;16:129-152.

[4] Heinbecker P. Studies on the metabolism of Eskimos. J Bio Chem 1928 Dec 1;80:461-475. <http://www.jbc.org/content/80/2/461>

Table 9.3 Estimated upper limits for total fat intake (g/d)

Bodyweight kg (pounds)	Max fat (g/d)
45 (100)	189
50 (110)	210
55 (121)	231
60 (132)	252
65 (143)	273
70 (154)	294
75 (165)	315
80 (176)	336
85 (187)	357
90 (198)	378
95 (209)	399
100 (220)	420
105 (231)	441
110 (242)	462
115 (253)	483

See: Bilsborough S and Mann N: A Review of Issues of Dietary Protein Intake in Humans. Int J Sport Nutr and Ex Metab 2006;16:129-152.

When you have limited yourself to a carnivore diet for a sufficient period of time, your palate will become a highly sensitive guide to your fat requirements. You will know by taste you when you need more fat added.

BONES: All Natural human and other carnivore diets include bones and bone marrow, either gnawed upon, eaten (small soft bird and fish bones), or in the form of bone broth. You should gnaw on bones, eat soft bones of small animals, or include bone broth made from bones and cartilage in your daily diet.

EGGS: Nature provides bird and fish eggs without any human effort. Humans can easily collect eggs, and eggs are tasty, non-toxic and, for most people, digestible without discomfort. Thus, Nature generally permits us to eat eggs to the limits of our taste and satisfaction. When healthy we may freely eat eggs from any bird or fish.

Like other carnivores, we can also eat egg shells to obtain the calcium and other minerals contained therein. Boil leftover shells for 10 minutes to sterilize. Drain them and leave them to dry overnight. Next day, finish drying them in a 200°F oven for about 10 minutes. Grind the shells to a powder in a coffee grinder. Store in a tightly sealed jar in a cool dry place. One tsp. provides 800-1000 mg calcium. Take in doses of 1/4-1/2 tsp. with meals.

However, if you have any autoimmune or allergic disease, you may need to limit or avoid eggs – especially raw egg whites – until you have healed the condition. Egg whites are a high histamine food and common allergen (cooking reduces their allergic potential). Only you can test and know what works for you. Again, follow Nature, as it guides you through your own desires and responses.

WATER AND MINERALS: Nature permits unlimited consumption of water and the minerals naturally carried by those waters. However, that does not mean that you should consume as much water as possible.

Nature gave you an acute sense of thirst to guide your consumption of water. Your sense of thirst is reliable. It was honed over millions of years to guide you to appropriate intake of fluid. Drink only when thirsty and only enough to slake the thirst. Do not drink arbitrary amounts of water such as 8 glasses a day, just because alleged "authorities" recommend this. Drinking when you are not thirsty is as harmful as eating when you are not hungry. It is acting against

Nature and when you oppose Nature you will receive portable punishment in the form of disease, disorder or degeneration.

If you have ever spent a long time in a pool of fresh water, you will know that doing so causes your skin to shrivel up. Chemists call water the universal solvent because it will dissolve just about any substance, and this is why, if you stay in water long enough, it will actually start to dissolve your skin. Exposing your internal tissues to an excessive flood of fresh water daily by drinking more than thirst demands puts stress on your tissues. Drinking excess water causes your kidneys to work hard to remove the excess water in order to keep the body dry and warm enough to allow normal metabolism to occur. Drinking excess water can also cause water retention, edema and puffiness. Drinking water causes you to urinate more and you lose minerals every time you urinate. This loss of minerals reduces your tissues' ability to retain water (water follows salt). As a result, drinking excess water can actually make you thirsty.

Excess water consumption dilutes the sodium in your blood, which can cause water intoxication hyponatremia, with symptoms of delirium, vomiting, nausea, cerebral edema, noncardiogenic pulmonary edema, seizures, and coma and death in extreme cases.[5, 6] Thirteen percent of runners at the 2002 Boston Marathon developed water intoxication hyponatremia.[7] Dreyfuss reports:

> "The data continue to accumulate showing that hyponatremia is a greater risk to athletes than is dehydration. Every summer in the United States, athletes die and suffer neurological complications from drinking too much...The US Army has seen

---

[5] Farrell DJ, Bower L. Fatal water intoxication. *Journal of Clinical Pathology*. 2003;56(10):803-804.

[6] Rosner MH, Kirven J: Exercise-associated hyponatremia. CJASN 2007 Jan;2(1): 151-161. <http://cjasn.asnjournals.org/content/2/1/151.full>

[7] Almond CSD, Shin AY, Fortescue EB, et al.: Hyponatremia among runners in the Boston Marathon. N Engl J Med 2005;352:1550-56. DOI: 10.1056/ NEJMoa043901.

the same result in a percentage of soldiers. The culprit is hyponatremia and the data suggest that the primary cause is simply drinking too much water."[8]

He goes on to report finding that "There seems to not be a single case of death resulting from sports-related dehydration in the medical literature." These athletes are drinking too much water despite heavy sweating in prolonged endurance events. The average person is not sweating as much, yet many non-athletes are drinking liters of water daily, expressing fear and claims of dehydration.

Not everyone needs as much fluid water – e.g. 8 glasses or 2 liters daily – as claimed by authorities and purveyors of bottled water. Fresh meat, eggs, and dairy products provide large amounts of water. Tea and coffee also provide water – experiments have proven these satisfy fluid requirements as efficiently as pure water.[9, 10]

When you drink very cold water, your body has to use energy to bring the water up to body temperature; then, when you urinate, you lose that heat with the urine, so drinking excess water, especially cold water, drains energy from your metabolism. This is beneficial when you are hot, but not when you are cold. If you live in a cold climate, you may have noticed that when you are exposed to cold, your body starts eliminating water by route of nasal discharge and

[8] Dreyfuss JH. Every year, more athletes are injured by hyponatremia than by dehydration. MDalert.com 2017 Jan 19. <http://www.mdalert.com/article/every-year-more-athletes-are-injured-by-hyponatremia-than-by-dehydration>

[9] Killer SC, Blannin AK, Jeukendrup AE (2014) No Evidence of Dehydration with Moderate Daily Coffee Intake: A Counterbalanced Cross-Over Study in a Free-Living Population. PLoS ONE 9(1): e84154. https://doi.org/10.1371/journal.pone.0084154

[10] Ruxton, C., & Hart, V. (2011). Black tea is not significantly different from water in the maintenance of normal hydration in human subjects: Results from a randomised controlled trial. *British Journal of Nutrition, 106*(4), 588-595. doi: 10.1017/S0007114511000456

urination. This is because water has a natural cooling effect on the body. If you run cool, drinking more water than you need will simply make you colder. When you are damp and cold due to excess fluid in your system, your cells and tissues will not be able to maintain healthy functions.

Bottled water is an environmental nightmare. Unknown to many, at least 50% of water sold in bottles is just tap water repackaged.[11, 12] Bottled water does not have to meet any of the EPA's standards for water quality, and FDA standards (which govern bottled water) are lower than the EPA.[13] Production of water bottles uses 1.5 million barrels of oil annually, and 3 times as much water is used to make the bottle as to fill it up; 25 billion plastic water bottles get landfilled, littered or incinerated every year.[14]

Your ancestors did not run around with a bottle of water at hand at all times. Dehydration is not just around the corner. You don't need to drink water constantly despite lack of thirst, and if you've bought the lie that you have to drink before you feel thirsty to stay hydrated, you've probably been drinking way more water than you need. Follow your thirst and you will likely find you only need a fraction of what you've been drinking.

---

[11] Food & Water Watch: Take Back The Tap: The Big Business Hustle of Bottled Water. <https://www.foodandwaterwatch.org/insight/take-back-tap-big-business-hustle-bottled-water>

[12] Byron K. Pepsi says Aquafina is tap water. CNN Money 2007 July 27. <https://money.cnn.com/2007/07/27/news/companies/pepsi_coke/>

[13] Postman A. The Truth About Tap. Lots of people think drinking bottled water is safer. Is it? NRDC 2016 Jan 5. <https://www.nrdc.org/stories/truth-about-tap>

[14] Gashler K. Thirst for bottled water unleashes flood of environmental concerns. USA Today. <https://usatoday30.usatoday.com/news/nation/environment/2008-06-07-bottled-water_N.htm#>

All Natural water contains minerals – predominantly magnesium and calcium – that the water dissolved into itself by its Natural actions as it flows on Earth. Our ancestors always drank these mineral-rich waters. You also should drink the most mineral-rich water you can obtain, such as spring or well water. If your tap water is not mineral-rich, then you may have to consume additional minerals, particularly magnesium and calcium (eggshell powder).

SALTS: Some people incorrectly believe that no nonhuman wild species requires or uses minerals – rocks – directly for nutrition. In fact, nonhuman species suffering nutritional shortages will go out of their way to consume various non-organic items to supplement salt and other minerals to their regular foods. For example:

- Deer requiring additional calcium or phosphorus to support antler growth will chew on cast-off antlers, eat soil surrounding decayed bones, lick rocks, and drink brackish water to obtain the minerals, if the plants they normally consume do not provide enough.[15]

- When deficient in sodium, African buffaloes will lick salt-encrusted plants, rocks, and other sweaty buffaloes.[16]

- Wherever possible, herbivores seek out bogs, marshes, and rivers for aquatic plants that contain more sodium and other minerals than the land plants on which they primarily feed.[17]

- A biologist witnessed a herd of cattle crowding around a tree and licking its bark; she found that the tree had one copper nail embedded in the bark where the cattle had focused their attention—and that the cattle had a copper deficiency.[18]

---

[15] Engel C. Wild Health: Lessons in Natural Wellness from the Animal Kingdom. Houghton Mifflin Harcourt, 2003. 29.

[16] Ibid., 32.

[17] Ibid.

[18] Ibid., 34.

These examples show that Natural selection has favored the survival of individuals who can detect when their habitual food lacks sufficient minerals and find alternative sources for those nutrients. Several of these examples also show that nonhuman animals will use non-organic sources of minerals (e.g. rocks, soil, metals) whenever necessary; unlike some humans, they do not erroneously believe that only minerals embedded in plant or animal tissues can serve as vital nutrient sources.

Thus, Nature not only permits but sometimes requires animals to obtain salt or other minerals from rocks.[19] Very early human ancestors probably exploited wetland habitats and ate a variety of both aquatic and terrestrial animal foods (including blood) that would have provided an extremely high intake of salt and selected for individuals having a strong taste, tolerance and even requirement for dietary salt.[20, 21]

You must consume adequate salt, especially in the early phase of adopting a hypercarnivore diet, when the dramatic reduction in carbohydrate intake will greatly reduce insulin levels, leading to a marked loss of water and salt. This can lead to muscle cramps, nausea, fatigue, and headaches.

On the other hand, overconsumption of salt can produce excessive thirst, water retention and edema. If you notice water retention or swelling under the eyes or in the limbs, check your salt and water intake.

---

[19] Denton DA, McKinley MJ, Weisinger RS. Hypothalamic integration of body fluid regulation. PNAS 1996 July;93:7397-7404. <http://europepmc.org/backend/ptpmcrender.fcgi?accid=PMC38996&blobtype=pdf>

[20] Russon AE, Compost A, Kuncoro P, Ferisia A. Orangutan fish eating, primate aquatic fauna eating, and their implications for the origins of ancestral hominin fish eating. Journal of Human Evolution 2014;77:50-63.

[21] DiNicolantonio J. The Salt Fix (Harmony Books, New York, 2017): 20-25.

As you adapt to THE HYPERCARNIVORE DIET, you will find that Nature has provided you with a very reliable way to measure how much salt you need: your sense of taste. Simply add salt to taste.

OPTIONAL ANIMAL FOODS

SUMMARY: Some people may tolerate some naturally preserved meats and dairy products and for these people these may comprise some individually determined limited portion of their meat and fat intake. If you have some disease or disorder you wish to heal, you may benefit from avoiding these foods for some time. Each individual must determine his/her tolerance for these foods.

PROCESSED MEATS: Nature occasionally provides meats dried and seasoned by wild fires, smoke and concentrated mineral salts (ashes) (see Chapter 9). Thus, our ancestors probably learned from Nature (wild fires) how to preserve meat using fire, smoke and salts. Prior to invention of refrigeration, all European ancestors (and American Indian tribes as well) depended on dried, salted and smoked meats and fish to sustain health during long winters. Traditionally these did not contain nitrites and nitrates.

Generally, you may consume nitrate- and nitrite- free salted and processed meats such as bacon, ham, preserved sausages, and so on in lesser amounts, for example, perhaps 10% of your total meat intake. However, if you have not seen improvement in your diseases of civilization, you may want to consider eliminating preserved meats from your diet for a period of at least one month to find out if this improves your condition.

DAIRY: As mammals, all humans have the natural ability to digest milk at birth and through childhood. Because Nature through evolution conserves what works, milks from various animals contains the same basic constituents – types of protein, fat and carbohydrate, as well as vitamins and minerals – and only differ in proportions of these constituents.

306

Moreover, milk is derived from blood. Like blood, milk contains animal protein, fat, sugar and cholesterol. Let me emphasize that the sugar in milk and blood is *animal* sugar; lactose is composed of glucose and galactose, both produced by the animal, not derived from plants. Therefore, milk is, like blood, liquid meat.

Some people believe that no other adult animal consumes the milk of another species, and that this proves that consuming dairy products is unnatural and to be avoided. However, the belief that no other adult wild animal consumes milk from other species is false. Wild carnivores (cats and gulls) have been observed to steal milk from lactating elephant seals.[22]

Farm animals such as pigs, lambs and chickens will voraciously consume cow milk as a supplemental feed.[23] They know milk is good food when it is provided; they are just incapable of getting it for themselves.

Moreover, even if no other carnivore has figured out how to get a continuous supply of milk from its prey, this does not prove that it is unnatural, wrong or harmful for us to do it. Nature does not subject us to the same limitations as other species. It is Human Nature to use the mind to create unique solutions to problems. Whether Nature approves of our consumption of dairy products or not is to be judged by whether doing so improves our health and strength or not. If it does, Nature approves; if it doesn't, Nature disapproves.

Symbiosis is quite common in Nature, and Nature has allowed many human groups to establish mutualistic symbiosis with other mammals – cows, goats, lambs, camels, horses, yaks and others – to obtain milk. Not only Europeans but many non-European tribes have traditionally subsisted on or utilized dairy products from wild

---

[22] Gallo-Reynoso JP, Ortiz CL. Feral cats steal milk from northern Elephant Seals. Therya 2010 December;1(3):207-212.

[23] Dougherty S, Dougherty B. The Independent Farmstead. Chelsea Green Publishing, 2016.

and domesticated animals for hundreds or thousands of years, including:

- Among Far East Asians, the Mongols (horse, sheep and goat milk), Tibetans (yak milk), and Chinese minority Kazaks (cow, sheep, and mare milk)
- Among people of the Near East Asians, the Punjabis, and subcontinental Indians (water buffalo and cow milk).
- Among Arabs camel milk is used by the Bedoins and many others
- Among Africans the cattle tribes including Kenyan Maasai, Ariaal, and Turkana; the Nigerian Tuareg and Fulani (the latter also in Senegal); the Tamsheq (Mali), Borana (Ethiopia), Herero (Namibia), and Baggara (Sudan). Also the Wanande (goats) and Baitu (goats and cattle), to name only a few.

Thus, Nature permits us to consume dairy products. However, are milk products beneficial for health?

Individuals vary in their retention of the ability to produce lactase, the enzyme needed to efficiently digest milk sugar and protein, known as lactase-persistence, past childhood. About 75% of adults world-wide are lactase-nonpersistent (LNP). Among North American adults, about 80% of Native Americans, 75% of people of African ancestry, 50% of Hispanics, and 20% of Caucasians are LNP/lactose intolerant.

It is interesting to note that Asians, Arabs and Africans are typically LNP, but as noted above some of them subsist on animal milk products. Since all of these traditional dairying tribes use raw (unpasteurized) milk, some people claim that raw milk contains lactase, making it more digestible for LNP people. However, raw milk does not contain lactase[24] and experiment has proven that raw milk is not more digestible for LNP people than pasteurized milk.[25]

The Maasai and Ariaal (Samburu) of Kenya used large amounts of milk as a staple, obtaining of their 64% and 66%, respectively, of their total energy intakes from milk, despite a high (62%) prevalence of LNP among these people.[26, 27] For children of Kenyan Samburu pastoralists who have been forced into agriculture and plant-based diets, milk provides 50% of micronutrient requirements and low milk consumption results in higher risk of stunting, underweight and wasting. [28]

Most of the traditional dairying tribes already listed, including the Maasai, Mongols, Tibetans, Kazaks, Punjabis, Hindus, and others were/are LNP and yet use (or used) fermented milk as a staple food. Most lactose-intolerant people can consume fermented dairy products (yogurt, cheese, etc.) without experiencing digestive

---

[24] FDA: Raw Milk Misconceptions and the Danger of Raw Milk Consumption. <https://www.fda.gov/food/foodborneillnesscontaminants/ buystoreservesafefood/ucm247991.htm>

[25] Mummah S, Oelrich B, Hope J, et al.: Effect of Raw Milk on Lactose Intolerance: A Randomized Controlled Pilot Study. Ann Fam Med 2014 Mar; 12(2): 134-141. <https://www.ncbi.nlm.nih.gov/pmc/articles/ PMC3948760/>

[26] Jackson RT, Latham MC. Lactose malabsorption among Masai children of East Africa. Am J Clin Nutr 1979 Apr;32(4):779-82.

[27] Little MA, Gray SJ, and Campbell BC: Milk consumption in African Pastoral peoples, in: Drinking: Anthropological Approaches, ed. by Igor de Garine

[28] Iannotti L, Lesorogol C. Animal milk sustains micronutrient nutrition and child anthropometry among pastoralists in Samburu, Kenya. Am J Phy Anthro 2014 Sept;155(1):66-76.

distress, because fermentation reduces the lactose to glucose and galactose, which LNP individuals can absorb without issue.[29, 30, 31]

Moreover, some experiments have shown that most LNP people – including those who claim to be markedly lactose intolerant – can in fact tolerate at least 2 cups of pasteurized, unfermented normal lactose milk daily without digestive distress.

Suarez and associates tested LNP individuals for tolerance of pasteurized milk and found that even those self-described as severely lactose intolerant had negligible symptoms from consuming one cup (240 mL) of milk daily.[32] They also found that about 30% of self-described markedly lactose-intolerant subjects are actually lactose-persistent, have no difficulty digesting lactose and misattribute their gas and bloating to milk. Consequently Suarez and associates hypothesized that LNP individuals could also tolerate two cups of milk daily if taken in two widely divided doses with food, and also that psychologic factors play a role in perceptions of lactose intolerance.

---

[29] Brown-Riggs C. Nutrition and Health Disparities: The Role of Dairy in Improving Minority Health Outcomes. Edberg M, Hayes BE, Rice VM, Tchounwou PB, eds. *International Journal of Environmental Research and Public Health*. 2016;13(1):28. doi:10.3390/ijerph13010028. <https://www.ncbi.nlm.nih.gov/pmc/articles/PMC4730419/>

[30] Jarvis JK, Miller GD. Overcoming the barrier of lactose intolerance to reduce health disparities. *Journal of the National Medical Association*. 2002;94(2):55-66. <https://www.ncbi.nlm.nih.gov/pmc/articles/PMC2594135/>

[31] Gaskin DJ, Ilich JZ. Lactose maldigestion revisited: Diagnosis, Prevalence in Ethnic Minorities, and Dietary Recommendations to Overcome it. Am J Lifestyle Med 2009 May 1;3(3):7.

[32] F L Suarez, D Savaiano, P Arbisi, M D Levitt; Tolerance to the daily ingestion of two cups of milk by individuals claiming lactose intolerance, *The American Journal of Clinical Nutrition*, Volume 65, Issue 5, 1 May 1997, Pages 1502–1506, https://doi.org/10.1093/ajcn/65.5.1502

To test these hypotheses, they administered a lactase-persistence test to volunteers to distinguish true LNP from LP subjects. Then they gave a standardized personality inventory (MMPI-2) to 19 LNP subjects who described themselves as markedly lactose intolerant (S-LNP), 13 LNP subjects who denied lactose intolerance (A-LNP), and 10 lactase persistent individuals who erroneously believed they were lactose intolerant (S-LP). The subjects were then given either 240 mL regular or lactose-reduced milk twice daily for 7 days in a double-blind crossover study, and asked to record their symptoms.

Neither LNP group had a significant increase in symptoms during the regular compared with the lactose-reduced milk periods. In fact, for all LNP subjects, symptom scores for bloating, pain and borborygmi averaged less than 1 on a scale where 1 = trivial, regardless of whether they consumed regular or reduced-lactose milk.

However, the S-LNP reported significantly greater gas and bloating than the A-LNP group during both treatment periods. The psychological inventory showed that both the S-LNP and the S-LP subjects scored high on the "lie" validity scale, which indicates that subjects are exaggerating or defensively concealing information or minimizing their condition. The MMPI-2 presents questions such as "I am never angry" or "I never tell a lie;" positive responses to these yields a high score for dissimulation, and represent a tendency to deny even minor personal flaws or failings and a lack of insight into one's own motivation, inflexibility, and rigidity.

Suarez and colleagues concluded that true LNP subjects tolerate two cups of regular milk daily with negligible symptoms, and that both LNP and LP subjects who describe themselves as markedly lactose intolerant probably have underlying gas and bloating that they misattribute to lactose intolerance. These people's flatulence is probably due to eating sugars, starches and fibers from plants!

Advocates of paleolithic diets argue that "milk is a species-specific endocrine signaling system that activates a central signaling node in cellular metabolism for stimulation of growth and cell proliferation" in newborns.[33] On this basis, they argue that since Nature designed the milk of each species to promote growth and development of the newborns of that species, non-human milk products could be harmful to humans, especially adults.

Whole cow milk products have been reported to promote intestinal injury and bleeding (leaky gut) in infants, contributing to allergies and immune system disorders.[34] However, infants have immature digestive tracts, so it should go without saying that we should make every effort to feed infants only human milk, and milk products may not affect adults similarly.

Opponents of milk consumption point out that milk consumption has been *linked* to hyperinsulinemia, insulin resistance, and elevated serum IGF-1 levels in children and adults.[35,36,37,38] Lactose- and whey protein- rich milk products are unusual among animal products

[33] Melnik BC. Diet in Acne: Further evidence for the Role of Nutrient Signaling in Acne Pathogenesis. Acta Derm Venereol 2012:92:228-231.

[34] Sullivan PB. Cow's milk induced intestinal bleeding in infancy. Archives of Disease in Childhood 1993;68:240-45.

[35] Melnik BC. Linking diet to acne metabolomics, inflammation, and comedogenesis: an update. *Clinical, Cosmetic and Investigational Dermatology*. 2015;8:371-388. doi:10.2147/CCID.S69135.

[36] Norat T, Dossus L, Rinaldi S, et al. Diet, serum insulin-like growth factor-I and IGF-binding protein-3 in European women. Eur J Clin Nutr. 2007 Jan;61(1):91-8. Epub 2006 Aug 9. PubMed PMID: 16900085.

[37] Gunnerud U, Holst JJ, Östman E, Björck I. The glycemic, insulinemic and plasma amino acid responses to equi-carbohydrate milk meals, a pilot- study of bovine and human milk. *Nutrition Journal*. 2012;11:83. doi: 10.1186/1475-2891-11-83.

[38] Melnik BC, Schmitz G, John SM, Carrera-Bastos P, Lindeberg S, Cordain L. Metabolic effects of milk protein intake strongly depend on pre-existing metabolic and exercise status. *Nutrition & Metabolism*. 2013;10:60. doi: 10.1186/1743-7075-10-60.

in having a high insulin index.[39] Some authors allege that consumption of milk products promotes hyperinsulinemia-related maladies such as acne,[40] prostate cancer,[41] skin tags, and others.

However, these associations are statistically and logically tenuous. To illustrate, in the prostate cancer study cited above,[19] the relative risks reported for high vs. low dairy consumers ranged from 1.12 for total dairy products and total prostate cancer incidence, 1.49 for skim/low fat milk and risk of low-grade, early-stage and screen-detected cancers, and 2.17 for whole milk intake and risk of progression to fatal disease after diagnosis. As discussed in the Preface of this book, statistically speaking, any relative risk less than 2.0 is unimportant because it can only represent a truly trivial absolute risk.

Moreover, since this was an epidemiological study, it can only generate some hypotheses to test with randomized trials. This study found only one association possibly worth further investigation, namely that between whole milk intake and progression to fatal disease after diagnosis. Since this was an epidemiological association, it could not establish that whole milk intake was causally responsible for the increased risk. It remains to be determined whether this association is spurious or not.

[39] Elin M Östman, Helena GM Liljeberg Elmståhl, Inger ME Björck; Inconsistency between glycemic and insulinemic responses to regular and fermented milk products, *The American Journal of Clinical Nutrition*, Volume 74, Issue 1, 1 July 2001, Pages 96–100, https://doi.org/10.1093/ajcn/74.1.96

[40] Melnik BC. Evidence for acne-promoting effects of milk and other insulinotropic dairy products. Nestle Nutr Workshop Ser Pediatr Program. 2011;67:131-45. doi: 10.1159/000325580. Epub 2011 Feb 16. Review. PubMed PMID: 21335995.

[41] Song Y, Chavarro JE, Cao Y, et al. Whole Milk Intake Is Associated with Prostate Cancer-Specific Mortality among U.S. Male Physicians. *The Journal of Nutrition*. 2013;143(2):189-196. doi:10.3945/jn.112.168484.

Possibly men who are diagnosed with prostate cancer and drink more whole milk also tend to have some other habit, dietary or not, that increases their risk for progression to fatal disease. For example, perhaps these men got their whole milk intake in the form of milk shakes containing ice cream and therefore sugar; or they consumed milk primarily on top of sweetened breakfast cereals or with cookies. In these ways whole milk could be strongly associated with an adverse outcome actually caused by consumption of plant-based sugars.

A 2015 study that claimed that high intakes of dairy products might increase total prostate cancer risk.[42] However, the "statistically significant" relative risks reported ranged from 1.02 to 1.18 for high dairy consumers compared to low. These *relative* risk increases of 2-18% are insignificant findings. If among the low dairy consumers 5 of 100 subjects got prostate cancer, and among the high dairy consumers 6 of 100 subjects got prostate cancer, the high dairy consumers had a *relative* risk increase of 20% (6 is 20% more than 5), but the absolute risk difference is only 1% (6% vs 5%). In this case, an 18% increased *relative* risk represents an *absolute* risk increase of less than 1%. This is trivial and not indicative of any true adverse effect of high dairy consumption. Most likely these results merely indicate the bias of the authors and reviewers.

In 2016 Thorning and associates assessed the totality of scientific evidence on the effect of milk and dairy products on human health.[43] They found inconsistent evidence for an association between consumption of milk products with prostate cancer, but consistent evidence for an association with reduced risk of colorectal cancer, bladder cancer, gastric cancer, and breast cancer; and no effect on

---

[42] Dagfinn Aune, Deborah A Navarro Rosenblatt, Doris SM Chan, et al.; Dairy products, calcium, and prostate cancer risk: a systematic review and meta-analysis of cohort studies, *The American Journal of Clinical Nutrition*, Volume 101, Issue 1, 1 January 2015, Pages 87–117, https://doi.org/10.3945/ajcn.113.067157

[43] Thorning TK, Raben A, Thostrup T, et al.: Milk and dairy products: good or bad for human health? An assessment of the totality of scientific evidence. Food Nutr Res 2016;60:10.3402/fnr.v60.32527. PMID: 27882862.

risk of pancreatic cancer, ovarian cancer, or lung cancer. All of the relative risk ratios were modest (5-25%) indicating that very likely milk and dairy product intake neither increases nor decreases cancer risk.

A study claiming to link dairy consumption with acne found relative risk increases ranging from 1.12 to 1.44.[44] Another reported relative risk increases ranging from 1.10 to 1.19.[45] Again, these relative risks are well below 2.0 and represent trivial absolute risks so they are most likely statistical noise or a measure of investigator bias, not proof that dairy products promote acne.

A 2013 randomized trial found that a group assigned to consume 4 servings of dairy per day had a 9% reduction in plasma insulin levels and an 11% reduction in insulin resistance (estimated by HOMA-IR) compared with a group consuming no more than 2 servings daily.[46] This casts doubt on the hypothesis that dairy intake causes insulin resistance.

Some evidence suggests that lactose-intolerant non-Europeans who allegedly have no ancestral adaptation to dairy produce may benefit from or at least are not harmed by including dairy in their diets. For example, among elderly Japanese, greater intake of milk and dairy produce (and lower intake of rice) has been linked to lower risk

[44] Adebamowo CA, Spiegleman D, Danby FW, et al. High school dairy intake and teenage acne. J Am Acad Dermatol 2005 Feb;52(2):207-14.

[45] Adebamowo CA, Spiegelman D, Berkey CS, et al. Milk consumption and acne in teenaged boys. *Journal of the American Academy of Dermatology*. 2008;58(5): 787-793. doi:10.1016/j.jaad.2007.08.049.

[46] Rideout TC, Marinangeli CPF, Martin H, et al.: Consumption of low-fat dairy foods for 6 months improves insulin resistance without adversely affecting lipids or bodyweight in healthy adults: a randomized free-living cross-over study. Nutr J 2013;12:56. <https://www.ncbi.nlm.nih.gov/pmc/articles/PMC3651862/ >

of dementia, especially Alzheimer's disease.[47, 48] Among Chinese, dairy consumption (marked by red blood cell levels of trans fatty acids naturally found in dairy products) was found associated with a significantly lower risk of type 2 diabetes.[49, 50] Among Koreans, dairy food consumption was linked to a reduced risk of metabolic syndrome.[51] Heart disease, hypertension, stroke, colon cancer, obesity, and type 2 diabetes disproportionately affect Africans, Hispanics and Asians living in America, and these groups tend to avoid dairy products due to lactose intolerance; but an emerging body of evidence suggests that dairy products may reduce risks of

[47] Ozawa M, Ohara T, Ninomiya T, et al. Milk and dairy consumption and risk of dementia in an elderly Japanese population: the Hisayama Study. J Am Geriatr Soc 2014 Jul;62(7):1224-30. <https://doi.org/10.1111/jgs.12887>

[48] Mio Ozawa, Toshiharu Ninomiya, Tomoyuki Ohara, Yasufumi Doi, Kazuhiro Uchida, Tomoko Shirota, Koji Yonemoto, Takanari Kitazono, Yutaka Kiyohara; Dietary patterns and risk of dementia in an elderly Japanese population: the Hisayama Study, *The American Journal of Clinical Nutrition*, Volume 97, Issue 5, 1 May 2013, Pages 1076–1082, https://doi.org/10.3945/ajcn.112.045575

[49] Zong G, Sun Q, Yu D, et al. Dairy consumption, type 2 diabetes, and changes in cardiometabolic traits: a prospective cohort study of middle-aged and older Chinese in Beijing and Shanghai. Diabetes Care 2014;37(1):56-63. <http://care.diabetesjournals.org/content/37/1/56.long>

[50] Yu DX, Sun Q, Ye XW, et al. Erythrocyte *trans*-fatty acids, type 2 diabetes and cardiovascular risk factors in middle-aged and older Chinese individuals. *Diabetologia*. 2012;55(11):2954-2962. doi:10.1007/s00125-012-2674-2. <https://www.ncbi.nlm.nih.gov/pmc/articles/PMC3681519/>

[51] Kim J. Dairy food consumption is inversely associated with the risk of the metabolic syndrome in Korean adults. J Hum Nutr Diet 2013 Jul;26 Suppl 1:171-9.

these diseases via their provision of calcium, magnesium, potassium and other essential nutrients.[52, 53]

A 2016 systematic review of prospective population studies concluded that consumption of various forms of dairy products has either favorable or neutral associations with cardiovascular-related outcomes including cardiovascular disease, coronary artery disease, stroke, hypertension, metabolic syndrome and type 2 diabetes.[54]

Another 2016 systematic review of the totality of scientific evidence regarding the impact of consumption of milk and dairy products on human health concluded that milk and dairy product intake was consistently associated with a neutral or reduced risk of type 2 diabetes; a reduced risk of cardiovascular disease, particularly stroke; and a beneficial effect on bone mineral density with no association with risk of bone fracture.[55] Moreover this study found no effect of milk and dairy product intake on all-cause mortality.

Most likely, for people of any genetic heritage, increased consumption of easily digested milk products rich in essential animal protein, fat and/or minerals displaces consumption of far more

---

[52] Brown-Riggs C. Nutrition and Health Disparities: The Role of Dairy in Improving Minority Health Outcomes. Edberg M, Hayes BE, Rice VM, Tchounwou PB, eds. *International Journal of Environmental Research and Public Health*. 2016;13(1):28. doi:10.3390/ijerph13010028. <https://www.ncbi.nlm.nih.gov/pmc/articles/PMC4730419/>

[53] Jarvis JK, Miller GD. Overcoming the barrier of lactose intolerance to reduce health disparities. *Journal of the National Medical Association*. 2002;94(2):55-66. <https://www.ncbi.nlm.nih.gov/pmc/articles/PMC2594135/>

[54] Drouin-Chartier JP, Brassard D, Tessier-Grenier M, et al. Systematic Review of the Association between Dairy Product Consumption and Risk of Cardiovascular-Related Clinical Outcomes. Adv Nutr 2016 Nov 15;7(6):1026-1040. doi: 10.3945/an.115.011403.

[55] Thorning TK, Raben A, Thostrup T, et al.: Milk and dairy products: good or bad for human health? An assessment of the totality of scientific evidence. Food Nutr Res 2016;60:10.3402/fnr.v60.32527. PMID: 27882862.

hazardous, high carbohydrate, low nutrient density plant products (like rice), resulting in better overall health, strength and vitality. Thus, dairy products are probably safe and nutritious foods, like other animal products, for anyone who can digest them, and fermenting them makes them digestible for almost all people.

Previous to the invention of the refrigerator, people who consumed dairy products generally consumed them in fermented forms, such as yogurt, koumiss, sour cream, buttermilk, and cheeses. Fermentation digests lactose to simpler sugars (glucose and galactose), rendering soured or aged milk products more digestible and less problematic to the adult human digestive system.

Ghee (clarified butter) contains no lactose and almost no protein. Heavy cream and butter contain little milk sugar or protein; sour cream and cultured butter have been fermented to reduce further their lactose contents.

Table 9.4 lists the carbohydrate, protein and energy content of various dairy products. Ghee, butter, heavy cream, sour cream, mozzarella and fermented cheeses including cream cheese have the lowest amount of total carbohydrate and lactose per total kcalories. Cheeses except for cream cheese have the highest protein contents per kcalorie, but it should be noted that most of the protein in cheeses is casein whereas about 18% of the protein in whole milk and yogurt is whey.

Table 9.4: Carbohydrate and protein in dairy products (g/100 g)

Product	Carbohydrate	Protein	Energy (kcal/100g)	Fermented?
Ghee	0	0.28	876	No
Butter	0.06	0.85	717	Some
Monterey jack cheese	0.68	24.48	373	Yes
Meunster cheese	1.12	23.41	368	Yes

Product	Carbohydrate	Protein	Energy (kcal/100g)	Fermented?
Swiss cheese	1.44	26.96	393	Yes
Mozzarella	2.47	21.6	318	No
Heavy cream	2.74	2.84	340	No
Cheddar cheese	3.09	22.87	404	Yes
Cottage cheese (4% fat)	3.38	11.12	98	No
Sour cream	4.63	2.44	198	Yes
Yogurt (whole milk)	4.66	3.47	61	Yes
Half & half (commercial)	4.73	3.13	123	No
Whole milk	4.8	3.15	61	No
Cream cheese	5.52	6.15	350	Yes

Source: USDA, cronometer.com.

If you have any disease to heal, and especially if your ancestors did not routinely consume milk products, you may want to start your hypercarnivore diet with elimination of all milk products or at least those containing significant lactose, i.e. milk. On the other hand, if your ancestors did routinely consume milk products, you may want to start your hypercarnivore diet with inclusion of any fermented full-fat dairy products you find delicious and readily digestible.

However, I also recommend testing inclusion or exclusion of full-fat fresh milk, fermented milk, and fresh and aged cheeses, to see how either affects your digestion, elimination, health, strength, and vitality. *Individual experimentation is essential. Each individual must evaluate his/her own tolerance for various dairy products.*

OPTIONAL PLANT FOODS

SUMMARY: Some people may choose to include some fruits, berries, above-ground vegetables, fungi (mushrooms), and herbs in a hypercarnivore diet, with types and amounts variable day to day and with bioregion, season and individual needs and tolerance, up to about 30% of the diet volume in any given day.

Permitted plant foods are limited not by rules or ideology, but because we are not anatomically, physiologically, or metabolically designed or adapted to eating large amounts of them. In other words, the limits are set by Nature manifesting through your taste, tolerance, biology and seasonal providence.

FRUITS AND BERRIES: In some regions and seasons, Nature provides some palatable fruits or berries, which are the only plant parts apparently produced specifically for animal consumption. More accurately, plants produce sweet fruits and berries to seduce animals into distributing the plants' seeds.

All great apes, including humans, have taste receptors uniquely adapted to detecting fructose and sucrose, carbohydrates found concentrated in fruits. These sweet receptors emerged in the hominoid primate lineage more than thirty-five million years ago, and probably played a critical role in support of primate brain evolution by improving food search efficiency and dietary selection of energy-rich fruits.[56]

Using common sense, it is very hard to imagine that any of our stone age ancestors would have refused to eat tasty fresh fruits or berries in season. They weren't wedded to any dietary ideology and certainly did not have any idea that they had to avoid seasonal berries in order to remain in the carnivore club or stay in ketosis. Although fruits are

---

[56] Nofre C, Tinti JM, and D. Glaser D. Evolution of the Sweetness Receptor in Primates. II. Gustatory Responses of Non-human Primates to Nine Compounds Known to be Sweet in Man. Chem. Senses 21: 747-762, 1996.

scarce in Arctic regions, Inuit (Eskimos) consumed some berries both in-season and preserved by freezing.[57]

Also, as discussed in the sections on meat and fat, we need either fat or carbohydrate to dilute protein from lean meats, and, due to Nature's limits on protein and fat absorption, some people may need to include some carbohydrate to meet energy needs. Fruits can supply either fat (olives, avocados) or sugar to meet these needs.

Therefore, Nature permits and may even require some people to eat *some* fleshy fruits or berries, in the regions and seasons that provide them, especially whenever or wherever the available meat is too low in fat but fruit is abundant. Therefore, your HYPERCARNIVORE DIET may include fruit at your own discretion, kept within limits set by your own tolerance, taste and satisfaction.

Nature has given us a limited tolerance for fruits and berries, and to avoid adverse effects we need to respect those limits. Further, some people new to a hypercarnivore diet may have disorders or diseases that will not reverse or heal without avoiding or limiting fruits for some indefinite period of time.

Fruits and berries present some hazards. Many contain strong acids that in excess can directly damage the teeth, and sugar that feeds

---

[57] Price W. Nutrition and Physical Degeneration. Price-Pottenger Nutrition Foundation, 1970. 71.

bacteria that produce more acids that damage the teeth.[58, 59, 60, 61] Intolerance to fruit sugars may contribute to irritable bowel syndrome in at least 60 percent of sufferers.[62] Fruits also contain other compounds that can have some toxic effects in humans (as discussed Chapter 5) if consumed in too large amounts.

For example, many fruits, such as plums, contain phytochemicals that mildly irritate (or, depending on quantity, poison) the gut, and indigestible carbohydrates that promote microbial fermentation that produces gases and acids that can also poison the gut. This causes bloating and bowel evacuation, even diarrhea as water moves into the intestines to dilute and remove the toxins. This is one of the most successful reproductive strategies of plants. They entice you to eat the sweet fruit so you will take and distribute the seeds, but they also affect your gut function so that any seeds you ingest are rapidly moved through it, undigested, and deposited in soil with a pile of fertilizer you supplied.

Moreover, many modern fruits have been made larger and much higher in sugar than their wild ancestors through selective breeding;

[58] Ali H, Tahmassebi JF. The effects of smoothies on enamel erosion: an in situ study. Int J Paediatr Dent. 2014 May;24(3):184-91. doi: 10.1111/ipd.12058. Epub 2013 Aug 4. PubMed PMID: 23909804.

[59] Bassiouny MA. Clinical observations of dental erosion associated with citrus diet and intake methods. Gen Dent. 2014 Jan-Feb;62(1):49-55. Review. PubMed PMID: 24401351.

[60] Staufenbiel I, Adam K, Deac A, Geurtsen W, Günay H. Influence of fruit consumption and fluoride application on the prevalence of caries and erosion in vegetarians--a controlled clinical trial. Eur J Clin Nutr. 2015 Oct;69(10):1156-60. doi: 10.1038/ejcn.2015.20. Epub 2015 Mar 18. PubMed PMID:25782429.

[61] Ganss C, Schlechtriemen M, Klimek J. Dental erosions in subjects living on a raw food diet. Caries Res. 1999;33(1):74-80. PubMed PMID: 9831783.

[62] Berni Canani R, Pezzella V, Amoroso A, Cozzolino T, Di Scala C, Passariello A. Diagnosing and Treating Intolerance to Carbohydrates in Children. *Nutrients*. 2016;8(3):157. doi:10.3390/nu8030157.

in other words, they are artificial, not Natural foods (i.e. they would not and could not exist in Nature independent of human artifice). Generally many berries and melons more closely resemble the fruits available to our stone age ancestors. Some fruits contain little carbohydrate, and some – e.g. olives and avocados – are both low in carbohydrate and high in fats (Table 9.5).

If you have any symptoms, condition, disorder or disease related to high insulin (hyperinsulinemic diseases of civilization), you may need to avoid or only occasionally consume the very sweet, high fructose fruits (high or very high carbohydrate in Table 9.5) until you have achieved health.

Table 9.5 Net carbohydrate contents of fruits (g/100 g). portion).

0-5 (very low carbohydrate)

cucumber (1), avocado (2), summer squash or zucchini (2), tomato (3), olives (3), blackberry (5), raspberry (5)

6-10 (low carbohydrate)

eggplant (6), lemon (6), strawberry (6), winter squash (7), cranberry (7), lime (8), watermelon (8), papaya (9), orange (10), peach (10), plum (10)

11-15 (moderate carbohydrate)

tangerine (11), apple (12), blueberry (12), kiwi (12), pear (12), pineapple (12), mango (13), passionfruit (13), sweet cherries (14), persimmon (15)

16-25 (high carbohydrate)

fig (16), grapes (16), banana (21)

50+ (very high carbohydrate)

all dried fruits, including: prunes (54), apricots (55), apple (57), goji berries (63), dates (67), raisins (75), dried cranberries (76)

Source: USDA, cronometer.com

On the other hand, if you are lean or have very high energy requirements you also may find you tolerate or benefit from some high or very high carbohydrate fruits to dilute protein and fat in your diet. Also, fruits and berries are rich in potassium and have cooling properties. Nature makes these available in warmer regions and seasons when we might desire cooler fare and need more potassium in our diets because we are losing more fluids, potassium and sodium in sweat and urine.

In temperate regions, it is probably Natural to consume a little fruit and therefore carbohydrate, but a bit less fat, in the summer and early autumn, when Nature provides ripe, cooling and thirst-quenching fruits but animals are lean. In the winter and early spring, Nature provides little or no fresh fruit but more animal protein and fat.

In tropical regions, fruit is more abundant year round, while fat animals are less common. If you live in or have descended from people adapted to a fruit-rich and hot tropical bioregion, you might feel a need to consume less fatty meat and more cooling fruits. Only you can determine whether doing so is beneficial for you.

In summary, some times, in some places, some people might benefit from including some fruits or berries in their diets. To reiterate, THE HYPERCARNIVORE DIET is ultimately about following Nature, not any dogmatic rules. If you find that you sometimes desire and benefit from including some fruits or berries in your diet, then include them so long as you find them beneficial. However, if you find any adverse effects, avoid them.

If you choose, here are some suggestions for consuming fruits and berries in alignment with Nature:

First, consider limiting yourself to fruits and berries that grow in the type of climate that you inhabit, in the season in which Nature provides them. That means you might consume locally provided fruits in season, if guided to do so by your senses of hunger, taste and satisfaction. Fresh fruit and berries are best consumed in season, when their natural constituents helps us adapt to the season. For example, in the hot summer you may consume locally produced melons. If Nature provides no fresh fruit in your habitat in the winter, you will then consume no fresh fruit, or only limited amounts of those fruits that can sustain long-term cold storage, such as dried berries or apples.

Fruits contain compounds that help them adapt to the local environment. A fruiting plant adapted to the tropics – e.g. the banana tree – can't survive in northern regions, because it is heat-adapted, not cold-adapted. This means its fruits contain compounds that help them dissipate tropical heat. In contrast a fruiting plant adapted to northern climates (e.g. cranberry, blueberry) produces anti-freezing compounds. If a human living in a cold climate eats a fruit adapted to a hot climate, his or her body will be influenced by the heat-dissipating compounds in the tropical fruit. He or she may lose some adaptation to the local environment.

Second, you can remove excess fiber from fruits by peeling (if possible), and reduce the gut irritants in some fruits by cooking them.

FIBROUS VEGETABLES AND FUNGI: Nature provides vegetation, and we can easily collect it and put it in our mouths, but few Natural vegetables are palatable and digestible in their Natural (raw) state.

Since vegetables are largely composed of indigestible fiber and contain bitter toxins, they commonly cause gut discomfort (colic), gas, bloating, diarrhea, and, paradoxically, constipation, especially when consumed raw. Unfortunately, because most people have been programmed to believe that vegetables – especially raw vegetables – are especially nutritious, they fail to connect the consumption of vegetables with their distress and disease.

The vegetables that some people assert are necessary for a 'balanced diet' did not exist for our ancestors. Modern vegetables are products of extensive plant breeding, not spontaneous products of Nature.[63]

---

[63] Chassy BM. The History and Future of GMOs in Food and Agriculture. Cereal Foods World 2007 July-August;52(4):169-172. <http://www.ask-force.org/web/History/Chassy-History-Future-2007.pdf>

As Ray Audette astutely observed in *Neanderthin*, a creature can not require what in Nature it can not acquire. Since in Nature we can't acquire modern vegetables or adequate nutrients from plants, we cannot require fibrous vegetables or their phytonutrients in our diets.

Before being programmed to believe that vegetables are 'good' to eat, most children spontaneously reject consumption of vegetation. Most children must be bribed, tricked, cajoled, or coerced into capitulation by parents who erroneously believe that their kids need to eat unpalatable and indigestible vegetables.

In Chapter 5 I discussed the research which has demonstrated that eating vegetables has little or no antioxidant or general health benefit. Moreover, many vegetables and fungi (mushrooms, yeast) have practically no net energy value to us; that is, it takes more energy to obtain and prepare them than we can extract from them for our own energy needs. However, if they've been sufficiently cooked or fermented and are consumed in small, tolerable amounts, some vegetables can provide some micronutrients (vitamins and minerals). For example, sea vegetables are excellent sources of iodine and other minerals that are scarce in land vegetation.

Cooked or fermented vegetables are more nutritious and less toxic than raw because heat or fermentation destroys their naturally-occurring toxins and releases their nutrients from their indigestible cells. Therefore, I recommend avoiding or severely limiting raw vegetation. Most people will find that they tolerate well cooked or fermented vegetables better than raw vegetables.

In summary, Nature guides us to avoid any vegetable or mushroom we find unpalatable or that produces undesirable digestive effects. Consider starting your hypercarnivore diet with a period of at least 30 days limiting well-cooked or fermented non-starchy vegetable matter to no more than 5% of your diet. Eliminating them altogether will provide the clearest picture. This way you can learn how eating vegetables affects your digestion, elimination and general health and vitality. Once you have established a baseline of comfortable digestion without any gas, bloating, or cramping, experiment to find out how much, if any, well-cooked or fermented vegetables you can consume without adverse effect.

HERBS: As discussed in Chapter 5, Nature not only permits but apparently guides us to use herbs in small amounts as flavorings and medicine. You can consider tea, coffee, and other plant-flavored beverages as well as culinary spices and herbs and medicinal herbs part of this category.

Many people will profit from including digestive bitters or artichoke extract in the diet, especially before fatty meals, to stimulate bile flow and rehabilitate a liver and gall bladder made lazy by long adherence to low fat plant-based diets.

GENERALLY AVOID

No one has a dietary requirement for any of the foods in this category. If you have any undesired physical or mental condition, disorder or disease, you should strictly avoid the following items until you have established satisfactory health. Even if you have established health, you should consider these items more hazardous than the discretionary plant foods, and generally avoid them. You may individually test foods from these categories to see if you tolerate any of them without causing a relapse of your condition.

Nature warns us to avoid the following foods by making them very difficult to obtain, unpalatable, indigestible, or toxic in their Natural (i.e. raw) state. When we ignore Nature's warnings and use 'knowledge' and cleverness to make the inedible edible, we pay the price for our sin (i.e. mistake) against Nature (the Creator) by suffering damage or disease.

NUTS AND SEEDS: Some tribes – including for example the African Ju/'hoansi (a.k.a. !Kung Bushmen), the Australian Aborigines, and South Pacific Islanders – consume large amounts of locally available oil-rich wild nuts or seeds. Mesolithic stone age

Europeans may have used substantial quantities of hazelnuts in season.[64, 65]

The Ju/'hoansi are reported to get 40-50% of their total energy intake from mongongo nuts when they are in season. They also used oil from the nuts as a body rub.

However, nuts and seeds are offspring of their parent plants, so to protect them from predators the parent by Nature packs them in tough shells and fills them with bitter anti-nutrients that can cause oral ulcerations and interfere with digestion and assimilation of proteins and micronutrients. These compounds can cause gut discomfort, respiratory reactions, and skin rashes, by which Nature warns us to limit or avoid eating nuts and seeds.

According to the American College of Allergy, Asthma & Immunology, tree nut allergies are among the eight most common food allergies affecting children and adults, and also nuts are more frequently linked to life-threatening anaphylaxis. Tree nut allergies can manifest via the following symptoms:

• Abdominal pain, cramps, nausea, vomiting
• Diarrhea
• Difficulty swallowing
• Itching of the mouth, throat, eyes, skin or other area
• Nasal congestion or runny nose
• Shortness of breath
• Anaphylaxis

Nature has given some creatures – such as squirrels – special equipment for processing seeds and nuts. We are not among those so gifted.

---

[64] Price TD. Ancient Scandinavia: An Archaeological History from the First Humans to the Vikings. Oxford University Press, 2015: 379.

[65] Holst D. Hazelnut economy of early Holocene hunter-gatherers: a case study from Mesolithic Duvensee, northern Germany. J Archaeologcal Science 2010 Nov;37(11):2871-2880.

Any tongue, mouth or digestive discomfort, including flatulence, after consuming these foods is a warning from Nature to avoid them. For example, when I eat more than a few walnuts, I get mouth sores from the astringent chemicals in the walnuts. Some years ago, during my vegan daze, I ate large amounts of sunflower seeds for a few weeks, and broke out in a rash all over my abdomen which retreated when I stopped eating the seeds. I get gas and cramps if I eat more than a small amount of nuts. Consequently I generally avoid nuts and seeds.

Nuts and seeds require some preparation to reduce their anti-nutrient and toxin content. The Ju/'hoansi prepare mongongo nuts by first steaming the fruits that contain the nuts to soften their skins. Then they cook the fruits in water until the flesh separates from the nuts. Then the nuts are roasted. This preparation method uses water to leach toxins from the nuts, then roasting to destroy remaining anti-nutrients.

Thus, if you want to regularly use substantial amounts of nuts or oil seeds, you should leach and deactivate anti-nutrients by this two-step process: First soak them for 12-24 hours or boil them in a large amount of water for 1 hour. Next, dry them. Finally, roast them.

Even with proper preparation, regular consumption of more than condiment quantities of nuts and seeds may cause digestive discomfort, leaky gut and skin disorders. People seeking to improve health – especially those with skin, respiratory, digestive and bowel disorders – should completely avoid all nuts and seeds for at least the first 90 days on a hypercarnivore diet. Some *healthy* people may be able to tolerate very small amounts of properly prepared nuts or seeds from modern cultivars, which farmers have bred to weaken their shells and remove some of their naturally occurring poisons. You will need to find out how much, if any, you can tolerate *without any digestive, respiratory or skin distress*.

As with fruits, each nut-producing tree is by Nature adapted to a specific climate, and invests its seeds – the nuts – with chemicals that help that seed survive in that type of climate. Nature provides hickory nuts, hazelnuts, pine nuts, and walnuts in northern climates; and it provides coconuts, macadamias, cashews and brazil nuts in the tropics. Unless you are using the item for a specific medicinal property, Nature guides us to eat from local rather than distant sources.

PLANT-BASED OILS: All plant-based oils are refined, processed foods. Since we cannot acquire these oils in Nature, we have no requirement for plant-based oils. Most come from plant parts which Nature clearly marked for limits by giving them hard shells or bitter toxins. Moreover, the fruits and seeds from which we draw these oils were in their Natural state very small and generally lower in oil.

Nature therefore does not permit liberal use of either seed- or fruit-derived derived oils such as hemp oil, sesame oil, canola oil, flax oil, corn oil, olive oil, avocado oil or any other oil derived from seeds including nuts. Almost all contain potentially harmful phytochemicals and most contain potentially hazardous quantities of unsaturated oils.

As discussed in Chapter 7, some vegetable oils have fatty acid profiles similar to animal fats by being low in polyunsaturated fats and high in either monounsaturated or saturated fats. In Table 7.1, the plant fats with less than 10% polyunsaturates are coconut (1.7%), high oleic sunflower (3.8%), olive (9.3%) and palm (9.6%). Of those, high oleic sunflower and olive have the most monounsaturates (84% and 77% respectively), palm has the profile most similar to animal fats, and coconut has the most saturated fats. Avocado oil has only 14% polyunsaturated fat and 71% monounsaturated fat, fairly close enough to animal fats. Some people may tolerate these in larger but still limited amounts compared to oils rich in polyunsaturated fats; however I still recommend caution.

Animal fats are nutritionally preferable to plant fats. If you have any health condition you want to improve, you may need to avoid all plant-derived oils until you are free from disease. Once you have restored your health, as with other forbidden foods, you may find that you tolerate some amount of these foods without apparent ill effect. However you should always regard fluid plant-derived oils as more or less hazardous and best minimized or avoided.

As with other plant foods, consider the native bioregion of the plant when testing your tolerance of these oils. Avocado, coconut and palm trees are native to hot and tropical regions; these contain cooling, moistening properties adapted to hot dry climates and consequently are best for people who inhabit such regions. Nature provides people who inhabit colder northern regions with locally native fruits, nuts or seeds which have properties aiding adaptation to cold moist climates, such as pine, hazelnut, pecan, walnut, and sunflower.

CONCENTRATED SUGARS: Nature does not make concentrated simple sugars freely available. Nature does not offer us maple syrup, but much less concentrated maple sap; we make syrup by boiling down 40 gallons of sap to make 1 gallon of syrup. Nature does not provide concentrated beet or cane sugar or molasses. We obtain these only by processing and refining processes.

Some rock art dated to 25,000 years ago appears to depict honey collection. Our prehistoric ancestors and recent hunter-gatherer tribes seasonally used unfiltered honey containing bee larvae, providing not only sugar but also animal protein and fat.[66] However, Nature originally put limits on honey consumption by making it available only seasonally and protecting it with stinging bees. Taking honey from bees makes them weak and therefore by consuming honey we contribute to the loss of bees that Nature needs to carry out pollination of the flowering plants that feed the animals we are designed to eat.

Eating large amounts of any of these concentrated sugars regularly will promote tooth decay. All are high in hazardous fructose. Nature

---

[66] Crittenden AN. The Importance of Honey Consumption in Human Evolution. Food and Foodways: Explorations in the History and Culture of Human Nourishment, 2011:19(4):257-73.

does not permit us to consume any concentrated sugars without paying a heavy price. To recover health, most people need to avoid all extracted, concentrated, "natural" and refined sugars, including honey. Upon recovery of health you may tolerate small amounts.

STARCHY VEGETABLES: Plants store their future energy supply in starchy fruits, roots and tubers. They don't want you to consume their stored treasure, so they put poisons there to discourage predators. For example, common white potatoes contain about 8 mg solanine per 100 g potato, mostly in the skin. Since the toxic dose of solanine is 20-25 mg, eating 3 medium potatoes or one jumbo baking potato (with skin) can cause acute poisoning (vomiting, diarrhea, abdominal pain).[67] Sweet potatoes are rich in raffinose, an indigestible carbohydrate that causes bloating and flatulence.

We are unable to digest starchy vegetables unless we cook them, which provides evidence that we are not by Nature fundamentally adapted to eating starches. Cooking them is using technology to attempt to make edible what Nature made inedible.

When we digest starches they become sugar and this results in excessive sugar intake that causes hormonal imbalances and metabolic diseases. Thus, to establish and maintain health most people need to habitually avoid all starchy fruits, roots and tubers, including: winter squashes, potatoes (sweet and white), yams, cassava, taro, and so on.

GRAINS AND LEGUMES: Nature does not provide edible cereal grass or legume seeds. These are man-made foods, products of human cleverness taking control of plant breeding and implementing technology to make edible the inedible. No human can digest and assimilate nutrition from uncooked – i.e. unprocessed – grains or legumes. These starchy seeds contain high concentrations of highly toxic chemicals, and in their raw forms can kill humans. They also

_____

[67] US FDA. FDA Poisonous Plant Database. <https://www.accessdata.fda.gov/scripts/plantox/detail.cfm?id=1364>

contain anti-nutrients that interfere with protein digestion and assimilation of essential micronutrients. Therefore, Nature forbids us to eat grains and legumes, and we eat them at our own peril, at the cost of our own health, happiness and fitness. To establish health, you must avoid all cereal grains, cereal-grain like seeds, and legumes (beans, peas, and lentils, including soy).

ALCOHOL: Nature does not provide alcohol in any significant quantity, and alcohol is a poison to the human body and mind. Therefore, Nature forbids regular consumption of alcohol.

MAN-MADE FOODS: Nature forbids any food that exists only because human 'intelligence' deliberately interfered with and modified the nutritional composition of the original, Natural plant or animal material.

SAMPLE DAILY MENU

On the next page I have listed the example amounts of foods that a typical individual will need to eat in a day (or week as specified) to satisfy hunger and nutritional requirements.

Since different animal products concentrate different micronutrients, I recommend including a variety of animal foods to ensure adequate intake of all micronutrients. Traditional sausages include nutrient-rich organ meats that one would not typically consume otherwise.

In 2018, at 68 kg, I typically consumed each day about 300-450 g of meat, 150-300 g of eggs (3-6 whole), 4-6 servings of milk, yogurt or cheese, and 110-120 g of added animal fat sources, mostly cream, sour cream, butter, bacon fat and tallow. Typically I consumed 2800-3200 kcal per day.

At 45 kg, my wife Tracy typically consumed each day about 150-200 g of meat, 100-150 g of eggs (2-3 whole), 4-6 servings of yogurt, milk or cheese, and 60-80 g of added animal fat. She typically consumed 1700-1900 kcal per day.

We also included 1/2 to 1 tsp of egg shell powder daily (or other calcium supplement), a cup of homemade bone broth several times a week, and about 100 g of calf or beef liver weekly. We include kelp or other sea vegetables in our bone broth to ensure iodide intake, and intermittently include small amounts of fruits or vegetables (most of the latter pickled or well-cooked).

THE HYPERCARNIVORE DIET GENERAL GUIDELINES

ESSENTIAL (at least 70% of diet volume):
- Fresh meat or eggs, 5-8 g/kg[68] lean body weight (range ~225-900 g/d, depending on hunger, taste, body weight and activity level)
  - Emphasize fat red meat like beef, lamb, bison, game etc.
  - Include 1-6 or more whole eggs or yolks daily if tolerated
  - Include 225-500 g (8-16 oz) of fatty fish each week
  - Include about ~125-250 g (4-8 oz) liver each week
  - Include sausages or other organs/offal
- Animal fat (tallow, lard, butter, ghee, heavy cream, sour cream, etc.), at least 3 g/kg (range ~80-280 g), guided by energy requirements, taste, digestion and satisfaction
- Include reliable sources of 1500-2500 mg calcium daily:
  - Whole milk (fresh or fermented, ~300 mg/cup)
  - Aged cheese (~200 mg/oz)
  - Eggshell powder (~750-830 mg/tsp)
  - Homemade bone broth (variable)
  - Fish with edible bones (variable)
- Unrefined salt to taste
- Pure water according to thirst
- Magnesium (300-900 mg daily) depending on water source

OPTIONAL & DISCRETIONARY (up to 30% of diet volume):
- Any tolerated local fresh (or dried) fruits or berries
- Any desired and tolerated land or sea vegetables or fungi
- Flavoring or medicinal herbs and spices as desired/needed
- 1-2 cups plant-based tea or coffee as desired

NOTE: Your needs may vary; take this only as a guideline or suggestion, not a prescription. Follow your own senses of hunger, taste and satisfaction.

---

[68] One kg = 2.2 pounds, so about 4.5 g per pound.

10 GRAIN-FED OR GRASS-FED?

Some people wonder if one can safely eat conventional meat and milk from grain-finished animals. Documentary films like *Food Inc*, along with a plethora of anti-meat, pro-vegetarian literature, have given people the impression that conventional meat and milk products contains hazardous amounts of hormones, antibiotics, and pesticide residues. Shall we believe this? Let's take a look, starting with hormones.

Hormones

Do conventional beef, pork or poultry contain hazardous levels of synthetic hormones? Short answer: No. For details, read on.

The USDA prohibits the use of hormones in raising pork and poultry, so pork and poultry raised in the US have no hormone residues. For beef, let's start with an ancestral perspective.

When I was teaching the history of nutrition at the Southwest College of Naturopathic Medicine, I once had a native African explain to me that among her people, they have a taboo against hunting female animals. This taboo makes a lot of sense for a tribe dependent on hunting. If you kill a female, you are eliminating a bunch of potential offspring at the same time; while killing a few bulls will have essentially no effect on the fecundity of the herd. You only need one bull to make many cows pregnant.

In addition, bulls are much larger than cows, providing much more meat per kill. For example, an intact bovine bull weighs about 2,400 lb (1090 kg) whereas a cow weighs about 1,600 lb (725 kg). Thus a hunter would get about 50% more meat from killing a bull than from killing a cow.

So hunters would have preferred eating bulls to cows, and in Europe still today some producers raise bulls. Similarly, in the U.S. we get most of our beef from steer—castrated bulls—while we save the cows for calving and milk production.

Bulls and steer differ hormonally. Bull meat samples tested by Fritsche and Steinhart contained medians of 0.34 mg/kg testosterone and 0.32 mg/kg epitestosterone, while steer meat samples (from unsupplemented steers) contain medians of 0.01 mg/kg testosterone and 0.12 mg/kg epitestosterone.[1] Bull meat had up to 1.05 mg/kg testosterone. Thus, bull meat contains a median of 34 times more testosterone and more than twice as much epitestosterone than steer meat; and bull meat might have up to 105 times as much testosterone as a steer.

This data indicates that at least some of the meat typically eaten by hunter-gatherers would have had between eight and one hundred times more endogenous steroid hormone—in the form of testosterone— than an untreated modern "organic" steer. Thus, we must conclude that through evolution humans adapted to consumption of meat containing considerably greater levels of steroid hormone than what we find in a modern untreated or "organic" steer meat.

Since testosterone promotes muscle tissue growth, a steer has much less growth potential than a bull. However, testosterone also makes bulls aggressive and harder to handle, so we can more easily control steers. Modern husbandry attempts to restore the growth potential without the aggression by substituting for a small amount of the lost testosterone other anabolic but less androgenic steroids, primarily estrogens.

Currently the FDA allows the use of five hormones in cattle for meat production: progesterone, testosterone, estradiol-17β, zeranol, and trenbolone acetate. The first three are natural hormones, the same as produced by an intact animal. Zeranol occurs naturally also,

---

[1] Fritsche S and Steinhart H. Differences in natural steroid hormone patterns of beef from bulls and steers. J. Anim. Sci. 1998. 76:1621–1625. Full text: <jas.fass.org/cgi/reprint/76/6/1621.pdf>

produced by fungi. It acts as a non-steroidal estrogen agonist, meaning it acts like estrogen. Trenbolone acts as an androgenic steroid that promotes muscle growth.

These growth promoters are far less potent than a bull's native testosterone. As already mentioned, an uncastrated bull weighs about 2,400 lb (1,090 kg). As a consequence of lower growth hormone levels, a finishing feedlot steer raised with supplementary growth hormones weighs only about 1,410 lb (640 kg). The bull's testosterone level gives him 1,000 lb (455 kg) more body mass!

Does the use of these in raising cattle result in meat or dairy products with unusually high, potentially harmful levels of dietary estrogens or other steroids?

According to Doyle, four studies have found that muscle meat from an untreated steer provides estradiol in a range of 2.8-14.4 pg/g.[2] Two other studies found estradiol at concentrations of 12 pg/g in liver, and 12.6 pg/g in kidney. Doyle also cites an FAO report finding that meat from implanted steers had 9.7 pg/g estradiol at 15 days after implantation, and 7.3 pg/g at 61 days after implantation. In short, the levels of estradiol in hormone-treated meat falls in the normal range found in meat from untreated cattle. Doyle comments:

> "Estradiol levels in edible tissues of implanted cattle are usually significantly higher than in controls but the increases are small, in the ng/kg range. The greatest increases reported in an FAO report on estradiol residues were 0.002, 0.0065, 0.005, and 0.0084 mg/kg for implanted bulls, steers, heifers, and calves, respectively. These increases are well below the FDA recommended limits listed in the table on p. 2 and well below estradiol concentrations in muscles of pregnant heifers (0.016 to 0.033 mg/kg)."[2]

----

[2] Doyle E. Human Safety of Hormone Implants Used to Promote Growth in Cattle:A Review of the Scientific Literature. Food Research Institute, University of Wisconsin Madison, WI 53706. Full text: <fri.wisc.edu/docs/pdf/hormone.pdf>

Similarly, Hartmann and associates examined the natural occurrence of steroid hormones in food.[3] Using gas chromatography-mass spectrometry, they measured the levels of twelve steroids occurring in market-sourced meats, milk products, plants, yeast, and alcoholic beverages, including both naturally occurring and residues of additional hormones used in production. They tested beef (bull, steer, heifer), veal, pork, poultry, eggs, fish, and plants (potatoes, wheat, rice, soybeans, haricot beans, mushrooms, olive oil, safflower oil, and corn oil).

They found no significant difference in hormone levels between meat from hormone-treated and untreated animals. In the typical diet, meat, poultry, and eggs proved to supply less hormones than dairy products, which were found to be the main sources of dietary estrogens:

> "Meat does not play a dominant role in the daily intake of steroid hormones. Meat, meat products and fish contribute to the hormone supply according to their proportion in human nutrition (average about one quarter). The main source of estrogens and progesterone are milk products (60-80%). Eggs and vegetable food contribute in the same order of magnitude to the hormone supply as meat does."

Thus, if you want to eliminate the greatest dietary source of estrogens, you should eliminate milk products, not meat.
Before you conclude that you must avoid dairy products to avoid estrogenic effects, consider that the amount of estrogens provided by milk products is inconsequential compared to the amount of estrogens your body produces by Nature every day.
For example, a 40 kg prepubertal boy, most vulnerable to adverse effects of excess dietary estrogens, produces about 100 micrograms of estrogen daily (Table 10.1). One kilogram of whole milk or

---

[3] Hartmann S, Lacorn M, and Stienhart H. Natural occurrence of steroid hormones in food. *Food Chemistry* 62(1);7-20. <https://vdocuments.site/documents/ natural-occurrence-of-steroid-hormones-in-food.html>>

yoghurt (about a liter) provides less than 0.15 μg estrogens, and a kilogram of cheese provides less than 0.20 μg.[3] Therefore the amount of estrogens provided by a liter of milk or yoghurt is only 0.15% of what the boy's body produces by Nature.

Beef muscle meat from hormone-treated steers contains less than 0.05 micrograms of estrogens per kilogram. To get from conventional beef an intake of estrogens equal to just one percent of his endogenous estrogen production, i.e. 1 μg, he would have to consume 20 kilograms – 44 pounds – of beef in a day!

Table 10.1: Daily production of steroid hormones in humans compared to total daily intake from conventional animal products

	Progesterone		Testosterone		Estrogens (17ß-estradiol + estrone)	
	Daily production (μgd^{-1})	Daily intake (μgd^{-1})	Daily production (μgd^{-1})	Daily intake (μgd^{-1})	Daily production (μgd^{-1})	Daily intake (μgd^{-1})
Men	420	10.6	6480	0.07	140	0.10
Women	19600	9.0	240	0.05	630	0.08
Boys*	150	8.9	240	0.05	100	0.08
Girls*	250	8.1	32	0.04	54	0.07

* Prepubertal
Source: Hartmann S, Lacorn M, and Stienhart H. Natural occurrence of steroid hormones in food. *Food Chemistry* 62(1);7-20. Table 10.

Further, 90% of dietary estrogens are destroyed in the liver shortly after ingestion. Hartmann et al compared the intake of hormones from diet from all sources to natural human hormone production levels, concluding that the food contents of steroids are insignificant compared to endogenous production:

> "These values [amounts provided by diet] are far exceeded by the human steroid production... Children, who show the lowest production of steroid hormones, produce about 20

times the amount of progesterone and about 1000 times the amount of testosterone and estrogens that are ingested with food on average per day. It has further to be taken into consideration that about 90% of the ingested hormones are inactivated by the first-pass-effect of the liver. This leads to the conclusion that no hormonal effects, and as a consequence no tumor promoting effects, can be expected from naturally occurring steroids in food."[3]

Because 90% of ingested steroids are destroyed by the liver, the lowest observed effect level of exogenous estrogen is 5 μg of estrogens *per kg* of body weight.[2] Thus, a 40 kg prepubertal boy would have to consume 200 μg of estrogens daily to observe an effect; only 10% of this would survive the first pass of the liver, and thus would provide 20 μg estrogens, 20% more than the boy's natural estrogen production. To get this 200 μg of estrogens daily from conventional whole milk, the boy would have to consume more than 1300 liters of milk daily. To get this from conventional hormone-treated beef, he would have to consume more than 100 kg of beef every day. Clearly he isn't going to get excess estrogen by drinking milk or yogurt or eating beef.

Similarly, since a prepubertal girl produces 54 μg of estrogens daily, it is impossible that she would have early puberty as a result of a dietary intake of 0.07 μg of estrogens from meat and milk.

Do Hormones In Animal Foods Cause Early Puberty?

Opponents of the use of hormones in modern animal husbandry often claim that the use of hormones in production of meat and dairy products causes early puberty, obesity, and cancer in modern industrial nations.

If consumption of meat and dietary animal hormones are responsible for early onset of puberty, we should find early onset of puberty among heavy meat- or dairy- eating hunter-gatherer or pastoralist groups. Alas for the hormone hypothesis, among hunter-gatherers eating strictly native foods, including Inuit (Eskimos) eating almost exclusively meat and fat, menarche occurred at an average age of 15 years or slightly more, at least 2 years later than among modernized populations.[4]

Cornell University has fact sheet discussing these consumer concerns about hormones in conventional meat and dairy products:[5]

"Can steroid hormones in meat affect the age of puberty for girls?

"Early puberty in girls has been found to be associated with a higher risk for breast cancer. Height, weight, diet, exercise, and family history have all been found to influence age of puberty (see BCERF Fact Sheet #08, *Childhood Life Events and the Risk of Breast Cancer*). Steroid hormones in food were suspected to cause early puberty in girls in some reports. However, exposure to higher than natural levels of steroid hormones through hormone-treated meat or poultry has never been documented. Large epidemiological studies have not been done to see whether or not early puberty in developing girls is associated with having eaten growth hormone-treated foods.

"A concern about an increase in cases of girls reaching puberty or menarche early (at age eight or younger) in Puerto Rico, led to an investigation in the early 1980s by the Centers for Disease Control (CDC). Samples of meat and chicken from Puerto Rico were tested for steroid hormone residues. One laboratory found a chicken sample from a local market to have higher than normal level of estrogen. Also, residues of zeranol were reported in the blood of some

---

[4] Lindeberg S. Food and Western Diseases: Health and Nutrition from an Evolutionary Perspective. Wiley-Blackwell, 2010. Page 147.

[5] Gandhi R, Snedeker SM. Institute for Comparative and Environmental Toxicology, Cornell Center for the Environment, Program on Breast Cancer and Environmental Risk Factors in New York State. Consumer Concerns About Hormones in Food. Fact Sheet #37. June 2000. <https://ecommons.cornell.edu/bitstream/handle/1813/14514/fs37.hormones.pdf?sequence=1>

of the girls who had reached puberty early. However, these results could not be verified by other laboratories. Following CDC's investigation, USDA tested 150 to 200 beef, poultry and milk samples from Puerto Rico in 1985, and found no residues of DES, zeranol or estrogen in these samples.

"In another study in Italy, steroid hormone residues in beef and poultry in school meals were suspected as the cause of breast enlargement in very young girls and boys. However, the suspect beef and poultry samples were not available to test for the presence of hormones. Without proof that exposure to higher levels of steroid hormones occurred through food, it is not possible to conclude whether or not eating hormone-treated meat or poultry caused the breast enlargement in these cases."

All claims that eating conventional animal products causes early puberty are based on epidemiological studies, which can never establish causal relationships. As discussed in the Preface to this book, most of these studies report false conclusions that merely reflect the biases of the authors, reviewers and scientific community.

To establish a causal link between consumption of meat or milk from hormone-treated animals and any health outcome, it is necessary to perform randomized controlled trials which control all dietary variables, and compare two groups who differ only in the type of meat and milk consumed.

No-one has done any randomized controlled trials comparing the age of menarche in girls who for a lifetime eat meat from hormone-treated animals with the age of menarche in girls who eat for a lifetime meat from untreated animals, with otherwise similar diets. Therefore, we have no evidence to support claims that eating conventional meat or dairy causes girls to have early puberty.

Does Eating Conventional Meat Affect Breast or Prostate Cancer Risk?

If consumption of meat and dietary animal hormones are responsible for apparently hormone-related cancers, we should expect ill effects of hormones in meat to appear in heavy meat-eating hunter-gatherer groups since they ate meat from intact animals, particularly bulls having 10 times as much testosterone as domesticated animals.

Among hunter-gatherers eating strictly native foods, including those eating mesocarnivore and hypercarnivore diets, breast and prostate cancer were exceedingly rare or non-existent.[6, 7, 8] Since these hunter-gatherers ate hormone-rich bull meat on a regular basis, it is unlikely that hormones in meat can account for cancer or any other hormone-related problem in modern people.

All claims that eating animal products increases cancer risk are based on epidemiological studies, which can never establish causal relationships. As discussed in the Preface to this book, most of these studies report false conclusions that merely reflect the biases of the authors, reviewers and scientific community.

To establish a causal link between consumption of meat or milk from hormone-treated animals and any health outcome, it is necessary to perform randomized controlled trials which control all dietary variables, and compare two groups who differ only in the type of meat and milk consumed.

No-one has done any randomized controlled trials comparing the breast cancer incidence in women who for a lifetime eat meat from hormone-treated animals with the incidence of women who eat for a

---

[6] Stefansson, V. Cancer: Disease of Civilization. Hill and Wang, 1960. Available on OpenLibrary.org.

[7] Trowell HC, Burkitt DP. Western Diseases, Their Emergence and Prevention. Harvard University Press, 1981.

[8] Lindeberg S. Food and Western Diseases: Health and Nutrition from an Evolutionary Perspective. Wiley-Blackwell, 2010.

lifetime meat from untreated animals, with otherwise similar diets. Similarly, no-one has done any randomized controlled trials comparing the prostate cancer risk of men who eat civilized diets containing meat from hormone-treated animals to civilized men who eat meat from untreated animals. Therefore, we have no evidence to support claims that eating conventional meat or dairy increases hormone-related cancer risks compared to meat from untreated animals.

Plant Foods and Hormonal Disorders

Cordain, Eades, and Eades point out that current evidence actually implicates high carbohydrate intake as the promoter of these hormone-related disorders.[9] High carbohydrate (i.e. plant food) intake raises insulin levels which increases levels of insulin-like growth factors and increases *endogenous* production of steroids, by far the main source of steroid exposure, while reducing sex hormone-binding globulins that reduce steroid activity. Thus, by changing endogenous hormone production, high carbohydrate diets may alter cellular proliferation and growth in a variety of tissues, promoting diet- and hormone-related conditions including: acne, early menarche, certain epithelial cell carcinomas, increased stature, myopia, cutaneous papillomas (skin tags), acanthosis nigricans, polycystic ovary syndrome (PCOS) and male vertex balding.

Hormones Summary

If for budget reasons you choose to eat conventional meat (hormone treated or not) or milk instead of grass-fed, you don't need to worry that it will have any exogenous hormone content that will harm you in any way. You should worry more that by avoiding the meat, you will consume too many carbohydrates that will much more profoundly alter your endocrine system in harmful directions.

---

[9] Cordain L, Eades M, Eades M. Hyerinsulinemic diseases of civilization: More than just syndrome X. Comparative Biochemistry and Physiology Part A 136 (2003) 95–112.

Some markets sell beef from animals raised on typical feeds (corn, soy, etc.) but without added hormones. Often this is no more expensive than beef from animals raised with hormones.

Antibiotic and Chemical Residues

People critical of conventional animal products often claim or imply that these products carry harmful residues of antibiotics and other chemicals, particularly pesticides.

Based on data supplied by the FDA, some people have gotten quite upset to find that, by crude weight, 80% of all antibiotics used in the U.S. get used in livestock production, the other 20% getting used in human medicine.[10] Opponents of antibiotic use claim that this "overuse" of antibiotics in animals constitutes the main cause of antibiotic resistance in bacteria.

Although I am not a fan of antibiotic use, I find it inappropriate and illogical to evaluate the use of antibiotics on the basis of total tonnage given to either all livestock or all humans in the U.S. Medical personnel give doses of antibiotics according to weight, not according to head. In humans, children get smaller doses than adults based on weight. Pigs, averaging 230 pounds each, would get larger doses than the average 150 pound human, and cattle, averaging 1300 pounds, require even larger doses.

According to USDA data, in 2008 U.S. livestock included:

- 96,035,000 cattle and calves with a live weight of 41 billion pounds.
- 66,708,000 hogs and pigs with a live weight of about 30 billion pounds.
- 5,950,000 lambs and sheep, weighing 440, 286, 000 pounds.

---

[10] Loglisci RF. Animals Consume Lion's Share of Antibiotics. Food Safety News 2010 Dec 27. <http://www.foodsafetynews.com/2010/12/animals-consume-lions-share-of-antibiotics/#.W0pRkIInYd0>

- 9,000,000 dairy cattle, which would have an average live weight of about 4 billion pounds.
- 450 million chickens at an average weight of 5 pounds gives 22.5 billion pounds of chickens.
- 6 billion pounds of turkey

These numbers varied only marginally for 10 years spanning 2000-2009.

Using an average weight for humans of 100 pounds (including children), and a U.S. population of 300 million, we can calculate that the total weight of humans in the U.S. comes to about 30 billion pounds. From the above data, we can see that the weight of livestock in the U.S. is in the range of about 104 billion pounds, about 3.5 times the weight of humans in the U.S.. Adding miscellaneous food animals (bison, ducks, and others) not counted in the USDA data would bring the weight of animals even higher.

Therefore, non-human animals constitute at least 78% of the total mass of animals (non-human plus human) residing in the U.S.. If we used antibiotics in non-human animals at the same rate as we do in humans, we should expect that veterinary use of antibiotics would constitute about 80% of antibiotic use. Since that is in fact what the FDA has reported, it seems there is no grounds for accusing the livestock industry of overusing antibiotics. On a pound for pound basis they use the same amount in livestock as prescribed for humans by medical doctors.

Since antibiotics are dosed by body weight, if we used antibiotics in animals at the same rate as in humans, we would expect that we would annually use three to four times as much antibiotics (by gross weight) in treating animals as in treating humans. The FDA reports that in 2009 we used about 29 million pounds of antibiotics for food animals.[11] A critic of the livestock industry claims that an FDA spokesperson told him that about 7 million pounds of antibiotics were sold for human use in 2009.[10] If so, then the livestock industry uses just about 4 times as much antibiotics in food animals as are used in humans. Since the total weight of livestock is about 4 times the total weight of humans in the U.S., the use of antibiotics in livestock is on a weight basis evidently no different from the use of antibiotics in humans.

According to a 2010 FDA report, 39 percent of the antibiotics sold for use in food production animals were not medically important for humans.[12] Use of these antimicrobials in animals does not contribute to the evolution of bacteria that would be resistant to the antimicrobials used in human medicine.

According to the US Centers for Disease Control, 30-50% of therapeutic antibiotic prescriptions to humans are inappropriate.[13] This contributes to evolution of antibiotic resistant bacteria. These antibiotics and other drugs end up in tap water, either by intentional disposal or by urination and defecation after using the drugs.[14] This direct deposit of drugs into municipal water supplies can in part

---

[11] US FDA. 2009 Summary Report on Antimicrobials Sold or Distributed for Use in Food-Producing Animals. Department of Health and Human Services, September 2014. <https://www.fda.gov/downloads/ForIndustry/UserFees/AnimalDrugUserFeeActADUFA/UCM231851.pdf>

[12] Ibid. Table 5.

[13] Fleming-Dutra KE, Hersh AL, Shapiro DJ, et al. Prevalence of Inappropriate Antibiotic Prescriptions Among US Ambulatory Care Visits, 2010-2011. *JAMA*. 2016;315(17):1864–1873. doi:10.1001/jama.2016.4151

[14] Leonnig CD. Area Tap Water Has Traces of Medicines. Washington Post 2008 March 10. Page B01. <http://www.washingtonpost.com/wp-dyn/content/story/2008/03/09/ST2008030901877.html?noredirect=on>

account for the presence of multiple antibiotic resistant (MAR) bacteria in drinking water.[15]

Why Do Farmers Use Antibiotics?

To treat, control and prevent disease. According to the Animal Health Institute, about 87% of all antibiotics used in animals in 2007 were used for therapeutic purposes.[16] Using antibiotics in livestock prevents human disease as well.

A study compared the rate of infection with Salmonella, Toxoplasma, and Trichnella in pigs raised outdoors without antibotics and pigs raised conventionally with antibiotics.[17] Trichonella was found only in the antibiotic fee pigs, and these also had a 40% higher prevalence of Salmonella and a 7 times higher prevalence of Toxoplasma.

Inspection of retail organic and conventional chickens found that while most of both were contaminated with campylobacters, almost 50% more of the organic chickens were infected with Salmonella.[18]

---

[15] Armstrong JL, Shigeno DS, Calomiris JJ, Seidler RJ. Antibiotic-resistant bacteria in drinking water. *Applied and Environmental Microbiology*. 1981;42(2): 277-283. <**https://www.ncbi.nlm.nih.gov/pmc/articles/PMC244002/**>

[16] Animal Health Institute. Fact or Fiction: Common Antibiotic Myths. <https://www.ahi.org/issues-advocacy/animal-antibiotics/fact-or-fiction-common-antibiotic-myths/#2>

[17] Gebreyes WA, Bahnson PB, Funk JA, et al.: Seroprevalence of Trichinella, Toxoplasma, and Salmonella in antimicrobial-free and conventional swine production systems. Foodborne Pathog Dis 2008 Apr;5(2):199-203. doi: 10.1089/fpd.2007.0071.

[18] Cui S, Ge B, Zheng J, Meng J. Prevalence and Antimicrobial Resistance of *Campylobacter* spp. and *Salmonella* Serovars in Organic Chickens from Maryland Retail Stores. *Applied and Environmental Microbiology*. 2005;71(7):4108-4111. doi:10.1128/AEM.71.7.4108-4111.2005.

From 1997 to 1998, Denmark banned the use of antimicrobial growth promoters in poultry production. During this period, Denmark's poultry production increased by only 7.4% but the number of human cases of campylobacteriosis increased 26.5%.[19]

A cost-benefit analysis of termination of antibiotic use in livestock found that this would prevent not more than 0.03 fatalities and 3.5 excess illness-days due to antibiotic-resistant bacteria annually. However, it would likely cause more than 40,000 excess illness days per year from campylobacteriosis, consisting of 6691 excess cases of infection, 40 of those severe, and 0.54 excess deaths. Thus, the illness cost would greatly exceed the illness benefit: there would be a 40-fold increase in illness, 18 times more fatalities, and a 10,000-fold increase in illness-days.[20]

All uses of antimicrobial drugs, in both humans and animals, contribute to the development of antibiotic resistant strains. Consequently, the FDA has issued guidance calling for voluntary phasing out of the use of medically important antibiotics for non-medical purposes (such as growth promotion) in the livestock industry.[21]

Livestock operations may still use subtherapeutic doses of medically unimportant antibiotics as growth promoters. Currently no one

---

[19] Cox, L. (2005). Potential human health benefits of antibiotics used in food animals: a case study of virginiamycin. Environment International, 31(4), 549-563.

[20] Ibid.

[21] US FDA. Guidance for Industry #213. New Animal Drugs and New Animal Drug Combination Products Administered in or on Medicated Feed or Drinking Water of Food-Producing Animals: Recommendation for Drug Sponsors for Voluntarily Aligning Product Use Conditions with GFI #209. December 2013. <https://www.fda.gov/downloads/AnimalVeterinary/GuidanceComplianceEnforcement/GuidanceforIndustry/UCM299624.pdf>

knows why subtherapeutic doses of antibiotics promote growth.[22] Whatever the mechanism, it results in greater production efficiency. Growth promoters allow us to produce more meat from fewer animals with less food, and this means less manure output and less impact on the environment.[23]

Antibiotic and Chemical Residues in Meats and Dairy?

The Food Safety Inspection Service of the USDA performs random tests of animal products for residues of antibiotics and other chemicals or classes of chemicals, and publishes the findings annually.[24] In 2017, the Service reported testing 7029 domestically produced animals for residues.[25] Of these, 15 – 0.2% – had non-violative residues, and 22 – 0.3% – had lab confirmed violative residues. Put otherwise, 99.5% of items tested had no detectible residues of any of the tested chemicals including antibiotics. According to this same report, of 177,138 total samples taken, 172,976 – 98% – had no detectible residues, and 4162 – 2% – tested positive in a processing plant, but of those, only 681 – 0.4% – were confirmed in laboratory tests.

The USDA FSIS page "Beef: Farm to Table" explains the regulation of antibiotic use in cattle:

---

[22] University of Michigan. Antimicrobial Resistance Learning Site for Veterinary Students. <https://amrls.cvm.msu.edu/pharmacology/antimicrobial-usage-in-animals/non-therapuetic-use-of-antimicrobials-in-animals/use-of-antibiotics-in-animals-for-growth-promotion>

[23] The Poultry Site. How Do Antibiotics Promote Growth in Poultry? 2014 July 02. <http://www.thepoultrysite.com/poultrynews/32623/how-do-antibiotics-promote-growth-in-poultry/>

[24] Chemicals tested include: aminoglycosides, arsenic, avermectins, ßeta-agonists, carbadox, hormones, metals, MRM, nitrofurans, and pesticides.

[25] USDA National Residue Program for Meat, Poultry, and Egg Products. FY 2017 Residue Sample Results. May 2017. <**https://www.fsis.usda.gov/wps/wcm/connect/93ae550c-6fac-42cf-8c11-006748a4d817/2017-Red-Book.pdf?MOD=AJPERES**>

"Antibiotics may be given to prevent or treat disease in cattle. A 'withdrawal' period is required from the time antibiotics are administered until it is legal to slaughter the animal. This is so residues can exit the animal's system. FSIS randomly samples cattle at slaughter and tests for residues. Data from this Monitoring Plan have shown a very low percentage of residue violations. Not all antibiotics are approved for use in all classes of cattle. However, if there is a demonstrated therapeutic need, a veterinarian may prescribe an antibiotic that is approved in other classes for an animal in a non-approved class. In this case, no detectable residues of this drug may be present in the edible tissues of the animal at slaughter."[26]

The same rule applies to all other animal products produced in the US (pork, poultry, etc.). If the USDA finds violative residues in an animal product, the product is impounded and destroyed and the producer is subject to costly penalties, which may include prohibition of any sales of products to either domestic or foreign markets. In short, producers stand to lose their businesses if they produce animals with antibiotic or chemical residues exceeding USDA limits.

U.S. exports beef to Europe, so it must meet not only USDA standards but also European Food Safety Authority (EFSA) standards. Smith and colleagues tested U.S. beef for pesticide and chemical residues for which the EFSA tests.[27] They included conventional, "natural," "organic," "cull cow," and "chronically ill" cattle. The tested chemicals included:

---

[26] USDA FSIS. Beef from Farm to Table. 2015 March 24. <https://bit.ly/2zG7Z0p>

[27] Sofos JN, Aaronson MJ, Schmidt GR, et al.: Incidence of pesticide residues and residues of chemicals specified for testing in U.S. beef by the European Community. J Musc Foods 2007 May;5(3):271-284.

- Anabolic steroids: diethylstilbestrol, zeranol, trenbolone acetate, melengestrol acetate
- Metals: lead and cadmium
- Carasolol (a beta-blocker)
- Clenbuterol (a beta-agonist)
- Tranquilizers: azaperone and propiopromazine
- Sulfa drugs: sulfamethazine, sulfa-dimethoxine, sulfabromomethazine, sulfaethoxypyridazine, sulfachloropyridazine, and sulfamethoxypyridazine
- 25 individual chlorinated hydrocarbon and organophosphate pesticides

All together they performed 1780 chemical tests, and found no residues that would violate EFSA standards.

Schnell and colleagues tested for pesticide residues in beef from cattle fed fruits, vegetables and plant by-products.[28] They performed 2720 tests for potentially cancer-causing pesticides including acephate, benomyl, captafol, cypermethrine, folpet, azinphos-methyl, captan, chlorothalonil, ethyl parathion, and permethrin. The only pesticide found was benomyl, in the fat of cattle that had beef fed apple or pear pomace. Only 8 tests – 0.3% – found residues, but none of these violated USDA standards.

Over a period of two years, Vazquez-Moreno and associates tested for pesticide residues – including nine different chlorinated hydrocarbons (CHC) and nine organophosphates (OP) – in adipose tissue of beef, pork, and poultry from plants located in northwestern Mexico.[29] None of 112 pork samples had CHC residues, but 28 (13%) of the 208 beef samples contained hexacholorobenzene, heptachlor, aldrin or dieldrin, and 7 (33%) of 39 poultry samples

[28] Schnell TD, Sofos JN, Morgan JB, et al.: Pesticide residues in beef tissues from cattle fed fruits, vegetables and their byproducts. J Muscle Foods 1997 June;8(2): 173-183.

[29] Vazquez L, Langure A, Orantes C. Incidence of pesticide residues in adipose tissue of beef, port and poultry from plants located in Northwestern Mexico. J Muscle Foods 1999 Dec;10(4):295-303.

contained CHC residues. However, none of the CHC levels violated either Mexican or U.S. standards, and none of the tests found organophosphate residues above the detection limit.

Therefore, more than 99.5% of U.S. domestic conventional animal products have no detectible residues of antibiotics or any other chemical contaminant of health concern that is known to possibly contaminate animal products. The remainder may have some residues, but at levels that are of no health concern.

Organic Versus Conventional

I am aware of only one study dedicated to comparison of the contaminant levels in organic versus conventional meat and milk. Ghidini and colleagues compared the levels of organochloride pesticides, polychlorinated biphenyls (PCBs), lead, cadmium and mycotoxins in organic and conventional meat and milk. They found that pesticide and PCBs residues were lower than legal limits in both organic and conventional meat and milk, that lead and cadmium residues were very low with no difference between conventional and organic. The only difference found was that some samples of organic milk had significantly higher aflatoxin contamination, but this was not attributable to organic production methods.[30]

Persistent pesticides are ubiquitous hazards these days, and may occur in "organic" and grass-fed animal products as well as conventional. For example, a company producing organic chicken in the UK found residues of nitrofuran, a banned pesticide, in meat from their birds.[31]

---

[30] Ghidini S, Zanardi E, Battaglia A, et al. Comparison of contaminant and residue levels in organic and conventional milk and meat products from northern Italy. Food Addit Contam. 2005 Jan;22(1):9-14. PubMed PMID: 15895606.

[31] BBC News. Probe into chicken contamination. 2004 Oct 21 <http://news.bbc.co.uk/2/hi/uk_news/northern_ireland/3762066.stm>

Plants Versus Animals

As I discussed extensively in Chapter 5, virtually 100% of plant-based foods contain naturally occurring pesticides, at concentrations (ppm) far above the USDA legal limits for synthetic pesticide residues in meat and milk products. As documented by Bruce Ames, 99.99% of the pesticide load consumed by the typical American consists of pesticides that naturally occur in plant foods, which when tested have a toxicity and carcinogenicity similar to synthetic pesticides.[32]

So if you avoid conventional meats in favor of plant foods, you don't avoid pesticides or antibiotics (plants contain natural antibiotics also), and you probably increase your pesticide and antibiotic load. But when you eat meat, as shown by Schnell et al (above), you have put a filter between yourself and the plant sources of toxins.

Relatively speaking, it appears that fresh conventional meat produced in the U.S. or Europe presents a much lower pesticide and antibiotic load than organically grown cabbage. Evidently most domestic U.S. conventional animal products have no antibiotic, pesticide, or chemical residues, and in the small percentage (less than 0.5%) that has residues, they occur in amounts that present no hazard to health.

Antibiotic and Chemical Residues Summary

Simply, there is no evidence that conventional meat and milk have antibiotic residues that might affect your health. Nor is there any evidence that conventional meat and milk have other chemical (heavy metal, pesticide, etc.) residues greater than found in organic or grass-fed products, or that might affect your health. In fact, more than 99% of conventionally produced meat and milk have no

---

[32] Ames BN, Profet M, Gold LS. Dietary pesticides (99.99% all natural). Proc Natl Acad Sci USA 1990 Oct;87:7777-7781.

detectible antibiotic or chemical residues, and the remainder may have some residues but at levels that are no health concern.

Nutrition

The next concern is the nutritional composition of conventional meat and milk from grain-fed animals in comparison to grass-fed or pastured animals. Is there a nutritionally important difference in total fat content, fatty acid composition, omega-6 to omega-3 ratio, and vitamin and mineral content that would warrant avoiding products from grain-fed animals?

Daley and colleagues reviewed the studies comparing the fatty acid profiles and antioxidant contents of beef from either grain- or grass-finished animals.[33]

- *Total fats:* Grass-fed beef is lower in total fat.
- *Saturated fats:* Grass-fed and grain-fed beef have similar total saturated fat content. They differ in ratios of specific saturated fatty acids, but we have little evidence that this would have any effect on health.
- *Monounsaturated fats:* Grain-fed beef consistently has slightly higher concentrations of monounsaturated fats.
- *Omega-6 fats:* No significant difference in absolute omega-6 fat content between the two types of beef.
- *Omega-3 fats:* Grass-finished beef has higher total omega-3 fat content and therefore a lower omega-6/omega-3 ratio than grain-finished (1.53 vs 7.65, respectively). Two studies compared the absolute amount of omega-3 fat in grass- vs. grain- finished cattle in g/100g of fat. One reported that grass-finished beef had 10 g omega-3 per 100 g total fat whereas grain-fed had only 2 g; the other reported that grass-finished had only 1 g omega-3 per 100 g total fat while grain-fed had only 0.19 g. Thus in one study the

[33] Daley CA, Abbott A, Doyle PS, et al.: A review of fatty acid profiles and antioxidant content in grass-fed and grain-fed beef. Nutrition Journal 2010;9:10. https://doi.org/10.1186/1475-2891-9-10

grain-fed beef had twice as much omega-3 as the grass-fed beef in the other study. Thus some grain-fed beef might have more omega-3 than some grass-fed beef.

- *Conjugated linoleic acid:* Grass-finished beef contains about 2 to 3 times more CLA than grain-finished. However, no one has determined the optimal dietary intake of CLA. Estimates for optimal intake of CLA range from 95 mg/day to 3 g/day. Americans consuming typical plant-based diets and conventional animal products get 150 to 200 mg/day, Germans get 300-400 mg/day, and Australians eating more grass-fed animal products get 500-1000 mg/day. There is no known requirement for CLA for specific body functions.[34]
- *Cholesterol:* No material difference between grass- and grain-finished beef nor between beef and any other type of meat.
- *ß-carotene:* Grass-finished beef has about 7 times more ß-carotene than grain-finished. However, the absolute amount of ß-carotene in grass-finished beef ranged from 0.16 to 0.74 μg/g tissue. Taking the median value of 0.45 μg/g, this would mean one kilogram (2.2 pounds) of grass-finished beef supplies 450 μg of ß-carotene, which is 38 μg of retinol activity equivalents (RAE). The US RDAs for vitamin A for men and women are 900 and 700 μg RAE/d. Therefore, a whole kg of grass-finished beef supplies only a very small amount of ß-carotene. There is no evidence to suggest that grass-finished beef would have substantial positive effects on health in comparison to grain-fed beef because of its small content of ß-carotene.
- *Vitamin E:* Grass-finished beef has about 2 times as much vitamin E as grain-fed beef. Over 6 studies, the average content was 4 μg/g tissue, compared to ~ 2 μg/g tissue for grain-fed. The US RDA for vitamin E is 15 mg/d. Therefore one would have to eat 3.8 kg of grass-finished beef daily to obtain the RDA for vitamin E. The RDA is for people consuming large amounts of polyunsaturated fats; a hypercarnivore has a lower but unknown requirement. It is unknown whether the grass-finished meat would confer better

---

[34] National Academies. Dietary Reference Intakes for Energy, Carbohydrate, Fiber, Fat, Fatty Acids, Cholesterol, Protein, and Amino Acids (National Academies Press, 2005). Page 447.

health as a result of its additional vitamin E content. However, there is evidence that grass-finished beef lasts longer in storage than grain-finished due to the antioxidant protection provided by the additional vitamin E.

- *Antioxidant enzymes:* Grass-fed beef contains more glutathione, superoxide dismutase (SOD) and catalase than grain-fed beef. However, these are not known to be essential nutrients. The human body manufactures its own glutathione, SOD and catalase.

Leheska and associates examined the effect of grass-feeding on the nutrient composition of beef.[35] In Table 10.2 (next page) I summarize their report and compare the grass-fed and conventional beef. As shown, the vitamin and mineral content of grain-finished beef is equal or superior to that of grass-finished beef.

Leheska and colleagues concluded their report with these words:

> "Some consumers have been motivated to buy grass-fed beef because sources show that it has a greater ω-3 and CLA content than conventionally raise beef while also having less fat overall...However, the effects on human health of the lipid differences between grass-fed and conventionally raised beef remain to be investigated. Although lean beef has consistently been shown to be beneficial in a cholesterol-lowering diet, it is still questionable whether grass-fed beef would have similar benefits."[26]

---

[35] Leheska JM, Thompson LD, Howe JC, et al.: Effects of conventional and grass-feeding systems on the nutrient composition of beef. J Anim Sci 2008;86:3575-3585. doi:10.2527/jas.2007-0565 <https://naldc.nal.usda.gov/download/26261/PDF>

Table 10.2. Vitamin and mineral content of raw strip steak from grass-finished or grain-finished cattle (per 100 g edible portion)

Nutrient	Grass-finished	Grain-finished
Calcium, mg	8.7	14.0
Copper, mg	0.07	0.10
Iron, mg	1.9	2.94
Magnesium, mg	23.1	20.0
Manganese, mg	0.009	<0.01
Phosphorus, mg	211.9	275.0
Potassium, mg	342.4	376.0
Selenium, μg	21.2	27.0
Sodium, mg	55.0	61.0
Zinc, mg	3.6	7.05
Thiamin, mg	0.052	0.07
Vitamin B12, μg	1.3	2.5
Choline, mg	65.1	74.6

Sources: Grass-fed: Leheska JM, Thompson LD, Howe JC, et al.: Effects of conventional and grass-feeding systems on the nutrient composition of beef. J Anim Sci 2008;86:3575-3585; Grain-fed: cronometer.com, Food #53506, data source CNF2015:6112.

The Omega Issue

Since both omega-6 and omega-3 fats are essential in the diet, it is important to get the correct absolute amount of each type of fat – neither too little nor too much.

The National Academies of Science Institute of Medicine Food and Nutrition Board states that an Adequate Intake (AI) of the omega-6 linoleic acid is in the range of 12-17 g per day, but admits that "intake levels much lower than the AI occur in the United States without the presence of a deficiency."[36]

Linoleic acid is essential as a precursor for other fats generated from it (the main being arachidonic acid, see Chapter 7). Animal fats provide those other, more physiologically potent fats directly, so when you eat a hypercarnivore diet you can meet your omega-6 fat needs with an absolute intake smaller than the AI. The exact absolute requirement for animal-source omega-6 is unknown, but is probably one-half of the AI, i.e. 6-9 g per day.

The Adequate Intake (AI) for omega-3 fats is estimated to be less than 2 g/ day if provided exclusively as linolenic acid found in plants.[37] Linolenic acid is essential only as a precursor for synthesis of EPA and DHA.[38] Animal fats including those from grain-fed animals supply EPA and DHA which are physiologically more potent than linolenic acid.

The absolute requirement for omega-3 provided directly as EPA+DHA has not been determined but is certainly much lower than 2 g per day. The National Academies have recommended that about 10% of the omega-3 AI consist of EPA and/or DHA (i.e. 100-200 mg), and some research suggests that the AI for omega-3 would be

---

[36] National Academies. Dietary Reference Intakes for Energy, Carbohydrate, Fiber, Fat, Fatty Acids, Cholesterol, Protein, and Amino Acids (National Academies Press, 2005). Page 423.

[37] Whitney EN, Rolfes SR. Understanding Nutrition 10th edition. Thomson Wadsworth, 2005. Page 162.

[38] National Academies, op. cit., page 445.

only 500 mg/day provided directly from animal sources as EPA+DHA.[39, 40]

It is important to note that omega-3 fats can be toxic if overdosed. Excess omega-3 fats may suppress the immune system, prolong bleeding time, and increase oxidative damage.[41] Immune suppression has been observed with doses as low as 0.9 g/d for EPA and 0.6 g/d for DHA.[32] Data from treatment studies indicate that increasing EPA+DHA to 7 to 15 times typical US intakes diminishes the immune system's power against pathogens.[32]

According to the European Food Safety Authority, long term intake of up to 5 g daily EPA+DHA may not cause bleeding problems or affect immune function or lipid peroxidation.[42] The US FDA recommends not exceeding 3 g/d EPA+DHA, with up to 2 g/d from dietary supplements.[43]

---

[39] Kris-Etherton PM, Grieger JA, Etherton TD. Dietary reference intakes for DHA and EPA. Prostaglandins Leukot Essent Fatty Acids. 2009 Aug-Sep;81(2-3): 99-104. doi: 10.1016/j.plefa.2009.05.011. Epub 2009 Jun 13. PubMed PMID: 19525100. <https://www.academia.edu/15193858/ Dietary_reference_intakes_for_DHA_and_EPA?auto=download>

[40] Lee JH, O'Keefe JH, Lavie CJ, et al.: Omega-3 Fatty Acids for Cardioprotection. Mayo Clin Proc 2008;83(3):324-332. <http:// www.markobrienmd.com/Omega3.pdf>

[41] National Academies, op. cit., page 487-94..

[42] EFSA: Scientific Opinion on the Tolerable Upper Intake Level of eicosapentaenoic acid (EPA), docosahexaenoic acid (DHA) and docosapentaenoic acid (DPA). EFSA Journal 2012;10(7):2815. <https:// efsa.onlinelibrary.wiley.com/doi/epdf/10.2903/j.efsa.2012.2815>

[43] US NIH, Office of Dietary Supplements: Omega-3 Fatty Acids Fact Sheet for Health Professionals. <https://ods.od.nih.gov/factsheets/ Omega3FattyAcids-HealthProfessional/#h8>

As mentioned above, according to Daley and associates, grain-fed beef provides between 0.2 and 2.0 g omega-3 fats per 100 g of total fat. Therefore as I will show below in detail, a diet containing a sufficient amount of grain-fed beef fat can provide adequate omega-3 without including any fish or fish oil supplements.

As already stated, based on observed health benefits, if provided from animal sources as EPA and DHA, the absolute requirement for omega-3 fats is likely in the range of 500-1000 mg per day. Given these estimated absolute requirements for the omega-6 and omega-3 fats, the rational conclusion is that the ratio should be 6-18:1, or on average, 12:1, ω-6:ω-3. This is much higher than often claimed but it is based on absolute requirements, not fuzzy thinking about ratios.

What do I mean by "fuzzy thinking about ratios"? Let me take for example the claim that the ω-6:ω-3 ratio should be 1:1.

Now imagine you could construct a diet containing just 0.25 g (250 mg) of each type of fat. You would have a supposedly ideal 1:1 ratio of these fats, but probably not enough of either one of them. You would be deficient in both omega-6 and omega-3 fats, with an "ideal" dietary ratio.

On the other hand, if you could construct a diet that had 25 g of each type, you would also have a 1:1 ratio, but this would very likely be too much of both types.

Therefore, talking about ratios without talking about absolute requirements is illogical and unscientific. The proper ratio is determined not by speculations about prehistoric diets, nor by surveys of supposedly healthy modern diets (such as the so-called Mediterranean diet), but by determining exactly how much we actually require of each of the types of fats.

Proponents of the idea that the ω-6:ω-3 *ratio* profoundly affects health (independent of absolute requirements) may refer to animal experiments purporting to demonstrate that a high ratio can have harmful effects. For an example, Massiera and associates performed an experiment in which they fed mice a diet containing 35% of energy as fat, and 28 times as much omega-6 as omega-3 fat, over several successive generations—a situation similar to the typical Western diet.[44] They reported that animals fed this ratio of ω-6:ω-3 developed hyperinsulinemia and got fatter and fatter over four generations.

Now, what caused these adverse effects?

If you have followed me so far, you will have surmised that these adverse effects were not caused by a dysfunctional ω-6:ω-3 *ratio*. If they were caused by the essential fatty acid content of the diet, the problem was either an excess (toxic) dose of omega-6, or a dietary deficiency of omega-3, or both.

In fact, Massiera and colleagues reported: "In our experiments, LA [linoleic acid, ω-6] represented 18% and LNA [linolenic acid, ω-3] 0.6% of the total energy intake compared with 5-7% and 0.8-1%, respectively, recommended for humans by expert committees on nutrition."[45] Therefore the diet they applied provided both an excess of omega-6 and insufficient omega-3.

The body is harmed if it is poisoned by an excess of something, and also if it is deprived of an adequate amount of some nutrient. As I discussed above, specifying a ratio of ω-6:ω-3 will not in itself guarantee that absolute intakes of the fats will be optimal. Therefore, it is illogical to focus on *ratios* of nutrients rather than absolute requirements, toxicity and deficiency.

Further, it is important to note that, unlike a hypercarnivore diet, the diet used in this experiment had a high carbohydrate content. This is

---

[44] Massiera F, Barbry P, Guesnet P, et al.: A Western-like fat diet is sufficient to induce a gradual enhancement in fat mass over generations. J Lipid Res 2010;51:2352-2361. <http://www.jlr.org/content/51/8/2352.full.pdf+html>

[45] Ibid., page 2359.

important because diets such as this – moderate to high in fat and high in carbohydrate – promote high insulin levels, which have deleterious effects on fatty acid metabolism.

In fact, Massiera et al state: "When combined with high carbohydrate content, a linoleic acid-enriched diet was found to be pro-adipogenic in vivo..."[46] Their study does not give us any information about what would happen to animals fed the same ω-6:ω-3 fatty acid ratio, but in a high fat, very low carbohydrate context. Thus, from this study the most we can conclude is that a typical diet with moderate fat content, a high (possibly toxic) amount of omega-6 fats, a deficient amount of omega-3, and a high carbohydrate content may promote obesity and adversely affect gene expression across multiple generations.

Some authors also argue that a high ω-6:ω-3 *ratio* may promote cardiovascular disease, cancer, osteoporosis, liver disease, and several other diseases of civilization. However, again, these diseases are linked to typical Western diets which combine very high absolute ω-6 intakes, deficient omega-3 intakes, and high carbohydrate intakes that one can achieve only by inclusion of grains, nuts, seeds, and processed vegetable oils in the diet.

According to Daley and colleagues, the ω-6:ω-3 ratio in grain-finished beef averages less than 8:1, a far cry from the 28:1 ratio used by Massiera et al.[47] Furthermore, the absolute amount of omega-6 fat in beef is relatively small (Table 10.3):[48]

---

[46] Ibid., page 2352.

[47] Daley CA, Abbott A, Doyle PS, et al.: A review of fatty acid profiles and antioxidant content in grass-fed and grain-fed beef. Nutrition Journal 2010;9:10. https://doi.org/10.1186/1475-2891-9-10

[48] https://ndb.nal.usda.gov/ndb/

Table 10.3 Omega-6 fats in conventional beef

Food	Serving size	Omega-6 (mg)
Grain-finished beef chuck roast, visible fat eaten	100 g	630
Grain-finished beef chuck roast, visible fat eaten	1 pound	2860
Grain-finished ground beef, 80% lean	100 g	440
Grain-finished ground beef, 80% lean	1 pound	2000

Source: USDA , <https://ndb.nal.usda.gov/ndb/>

Thus, eating 1-2 pounds of grain-finished beef chuck (or 80% lean ground beef) will deliver only about 2-6 grams of omega-6 fat. As noted above, the US National Academies of Science Institute of Medicine Food and Nutrition Board recommends a daily intake of 12-17 grams of omega-6 fats to meet requirements.[49] One pound of beef chuck roast provides about 1500 kcal, so if an active man consumed 2 pounds of it in a day to meet his caloric requirements, he would get 8-12 grams of omega-6 fats, some of this in the more potent form of arachidonic acid, so, roughly the recommended intake or less.

Thus, *fatty grain-finished beef does not provide an excessive amount of omega-6, even when consumed in large amounts.*

In ruminants, gut microbes consume or transform most of the omega-6 in feed grains, such that, as noted, the absolute amount of omega-6 in their tissues remains constant regardless of finishing method. Their tissues develop a high ω-6:ω-3 ratio by route of feed grains lacking omega-3s that they would get from grass or other foraged foods. Again, the ω-6:ω-3 *ratio* of grain-fed beef is high

---

[49] Whitney EN, Rolfes SR. Understanding Nutrition 10th edition. Thomson Wadsworth, 2005. Page 162.

because of a low content of omega-3 fats, not because of a high content of omega-6 fat.

Now compare USDA data for lamb and pork (food; weight; omega-6 mg; omega-3 mg):[50]

Table 9.4 Omega-6 fats in conventional lamb and pork

Food	Serving size	Omega-6 (mg)	Omega-3 (mg)
Lamb, composite, trimmed to 1/8" fat, choice, raw	100 g	1000	330
Lamb, composite, trimmed to 1/8" fat, choice, raw	1 pound	5000	1500
Pork, composite of cuts, raw	100 g	1300	90
Pork, composite of cuts, raw	1 pound	6000	400

Source: USDA , <https://ndb.nal.usda.gov/ndb/>

Grain-fed lamb and pork have about 1.5 to 3 times as much omega-6 as grain-fed beef. Lamb has in its favor a relatively high content of omega-3, with a ω-6:ω-3 ratio of 3:1. This makes it a really good choice for a hypercarnivore diet. Pork has a less favorable ratio (15:1), but still has a relatively low total absolute amount of omega-6 fats.

Now take a look at the omega-6 levels in the following (food, serving, omega-6):

- Chicken thigh with skin, one pound, 13.6 g
- Chicken thigh without skin, one pound, 9.5 g
- Chicken breast with skin, one pound, 6.4 g
- Chicken breast without skin, one pound, 2.7 g

---

[50] https://ndb.nal.usda.gov/ndb/

- Walnuts, 1 ounce (14 halves), 10.8 g
- Walnuts, 100 g, 38 g
- Almonds, 1 ounce, 3.7 g
- Almonds, 100 g, 13 g
- Sunflower seeds, 1 ounce, 6.5 g
- Sunflower seeds, 100 g, 23.1 g
- Safflower oil, one teaspoon, 3 g
- Safflower oil, one tablespoon, 10 g.

You can see that chicken, walnuts, almonds, sunflower seeds and vegetable oils provide much greater absolute amounts of omega-6 fat than beef, pork or lamb. Some important comparisons:

- Chicken thigh with skin thus has a little more than twice as much omega-6 as lean grain-finished pork, and nearly 5 times as much as fatty grain-finished beef chuck roast.
- Chicken thigh without skin supplies about 50% more omega-6 than grain-finished pork, and more than 3 times as much as fatty grain-finished beef.
- Chicken breast with skin provides about the same amount of omega-6 as pork and twice as much as the fatty chuck.
- Chicken breast without skin has about the same amount of omega-6 as fatty beef on a weight basis.
- In contrast to grain-finished beef, conventional chicken breast has a ω-6:ω-3 ratio of 18.5.
- Just one ounce of walnuts provides six times more omega-6 than a whole pound of pork, and about 3 times more than a whole pound of fatty grain-fed beef.
- One ounce of sunflower seeds provides as much omega-6 as a whole pound of grain-finished fatty beef chuck roast; ounce for ounce, sunflower seeds are 16 times more concentrated in omega-6 than beef chuck with fat.
- Just one teaspoon of safflower oil provides nearly twice as much omega-6 as a whole pound of pork shoulder, and about the same amount as a whole pound of fatty grain-fed beef. This means on a weight basis safflower oil has an omega-6 concentration about 90 times that of grain-finished beef.

So, if you want to avoid excess omega-6, you should focus on limiting chicken skins; limiting dark meat poultry, pork and chicken breasts; eliminating nuts and seeds; and most importantly eliminating all vegetable oils. If eating grain-finished meats as staples, focus on using beef, pork, and lamb.

Striking The Omega Balance

These data make it very clear that the best way to reduce your intake of excessive omega-6 oils lies in restricting intake of chicken and eliminating most tree nuts and vegetable oils from your diet. If you do this, you can easily attain a healthy total diet ratio of omega-6 to omega-3 even if you eat only grain-finished beef, lamb, pork, and bison, by including some fatty fish like salmon, sardines, or sea bass in your diet.

To reiterate, the estimated adequate intakes for the omega-6 and omega-3 fats on a meat-based diet are as follows:

- Omega-6: 6-9 grams daily
- Omega-3: 0.5-1.0 grams daily

Thus, the ratio should be about 6-18 g of omega-6 for every 1 gram of omega-3, or on average, 12:1, ω-6:ω-3. Again, this ratio is based on estimated adequate intakes, not speculation about dietary omega-3 ratios of ancient hunters. I am unaware of any evidence that reducing omega-6 intake below 9 grams daily or increasing animal source omega-3 above 1 gram daily will substantially improve health. In fact, as discussed above, both excessive restriction of omega-6 and excessive consumption of omega-3 may be harmful, producing deficiency or toxicity, respectively.

As we saw above, a pound of fatty beef supplies only about 2-3 g of omega-6. A pound of pork, lamb, or chicken breast with the skin provides 5-6 g. Thus if the base of your diet is 1-2 pounds of grain-finished beef daily, you will obtain no more than the estimated adequate intake for omega-6. If your daily diet includes 0.5-1 pound of grain-finished beef plus 0.5-1 pound of pork, lamb or chicken breast with the skin, you will get about 5-9 grams daily of omega-6, still no more than the estimated adequate intake. (Remember, the estimated adequate intake of omega-6 if obtained from a plant-based diet is 12-17 g daily.)

If you add up to a quart of milk or yogurt or 4 ounces of cheese, you will add only 1 more gram of omega-6. Your omega-6 intake is still in the safe and adequate range.

Now, what about omega-3?

Table 10.5 shows that you can obtain the estimated adequate intake of omega-3 fats (0.5-1.0 g) from a quart of milk or yogurt, or a pound of either beef chuck or lamb shoulder chops. Evidently, if you eat enough meat and milk from grain-fed animals, you do not need to eat fish or fish oils to obtain adequate omega-3 fat intake.

A menu including one pound of fatty grain-finished beef or lamb and one quart of conventional milk or yogurt will provide 2100 kcal and 2.0 g of omega-3 fats, the latter being 2-4 times the estimated adequate intake. Since we have no evidence that consuming more omega-3 than this will have additional health benefits, we have no reason to believe that the greater omega-3 content of grass-fed beef has clinically important effects on human health.

If you want to increase your omega-3 intake beyond this, you can eat fish or take fish oils. However, beware that it is unknown whether consuming more than 2 grams daily of omega-3 fats will improve your health.

I believe the most cost-effective way to increase omega-3 intake is to take fish oils. I have most consistently used 1-2 teaspoon daily of Carlson's cod liver oil (lemon flavored), which provides ~1 g omega-3 per teaspoon, as well as 4500 IU (1350 retinol activity equivalents) of vitamin A and 450 IU of vitamin D.

Table 10.5: Omega-3 fats in meat, milk and eggs from selected grain-finished animals.

Food	Energy (kcal)	Omega-6 (g)	Omega-3 (g)
Milk or yogurt (1 quart)	595	1.17	0.73
Cheddar cheese (4 oz)	458	1.39	0.16
Beef chuck roast, visible fat eaten (1 pound)	1498	2.86	1.27
Pork shoulder roast, visible fat eaten (1 pound)	1221	7.31	0.14
Lamb shoulder chops, visible fat eaten (1 pound)	1253	5.81	1.27
Chicken breast, skin eaten (1 pound)	835	6.40	0.45

Source: USDA data; **cronometer.com**

Sometimes I have also included a very high omega-3 fish oil, Pharmax Finest Pure Fish Oil, which provides ~2 g omega-3 per teaspoon. Combined with the 1 tsp. cod liver oil, this supplies ~3-4 grams of omega-3 daily, or 21-28 g per week.

On days when I have used both fish oils, my overall ω-6:ω-3 ratio is around 4:1 or less. However, I am uncertain whether taking additional omega-3 has provided me with any health benefit. You can also eat some fatty fish meals. Take a look at the USDA figures for the amounts of omega-3s in these canned fish:

• Salmon, pink, canned, solids with bone and liquid, 100 g, 1.7 g

- Sardine, Pacific, canned in tomato sauce, drained solids with bone, 100 g, 1.7 g

Thus, just 210 g (7.5 ounces) of either salmon or sardines in the week will give you 3.5 g omega-3, the estimated adequate intake for a week. If you consume this in addition to grain-finished beef or lamb and conventional milk or yogurt, you will be getting plenty of omega-3 fats. Keep in mind that whole fish supply a number of nutrients other than omega-3 fats that may promote health, including vitamin D, magnesium, and selenium.

Summary

- Meat from grass-finished cattle, bison, or other ruminants provides higher amounts of CLA and omega-3 fatty acids than meat from grain-finished animals, but we have no known dietary requirement for CLA.
- Feeding ruminants (cattle, bison, lamb, etc.) or hindgut fermenters (e.g. pigs) grain instead of grass results in significantly lower levels of omega-3 fats, but has very little effect on the absolute amount of omega-6 in the meat.
- Meat from grain-finished ruminants has very low levels of omega-6 compared to meat from grain-fed poultry, most tree nuts, or nut or seed oils.
- You can obtain adequate intakes (neither toxic nor deficient) of both omega-6 and omega-3 fats by eating beef or lamb meat and milk or yogurt from grain-fed animals.
- The main sources of omega-6 oils in most diets include grain-finished dark meat poultry with skin, tree nuts, oil seeds, and nut or seed oils.
- If you include grain-finished dark meat poultry in your diet, limit to once or twice weekly.
- Regular intake of fatty fish or fish oils can easily provide enough omega-3 fats to provide an intake double the estimated adequate intake.
- We have no evidence that the greater CLA or omega-3 content of grass-fed meat or milk has clinically important effects on human health in comparison to intakes obtained from a hypercarnivore

diet consisting largely of meat and milk from grain-supplemented animals. Such evidence requires randomized controlled trials that have never been performed. Its up to you to experiment if you wish, but based on the reviewed evidence I think it is unlikely that clinical outcomes will be significantly different for many people.

My own diet has consisted almost exclusively (~90%) of conventional meat and milk from grain-fed animals for more than 12 months. I have on average only eaten a few fatty fish meals monthly. As mentioned, during this time I have experimented with including or excluding 1-2 teaspoons of fish oils daily. However, I have not yet been able to identify any noticeable positive effects on my inflammatory skin condition (psoriasis) from including fish oils or fatty fish, nor have I been able to identify any negative effects from excluding fish oils or fatty fish (this may change with more experimentation). Since cod liver oil has been my staple fish oil, even if I did notice some positive effect, I would be unable to determine whether it was the additional omega-3s, or the vitamin D, which provided the benefit.

Nevertheless, I have had significant relief from my major health concerns – including psoriasis – that in theory could be made worse by consuming an excess of omega-6 fats. In fact, my overall skin condition improved dramatically by eating large amounts (1-2 pounds daily) of meat and eggs from grain-finished animals, and my psoriasis lesions improved the most after increasing my consumption of conventional pasteurized whole milk, mostly consumed as homemade yogurt, to at least one quart daily (as discussed in Chapter 7, calcium evidently plays an important role in regulating skin cell differentiation).

Conclusions

The nutritional differences between meat and milk from grain-fed and exclusively grass-fed animals appear minor. The health benefits of grass-fed animal products are uncertain.

However, the human body needs a highly carnivorous diet to thrive. I would never try to feed a cat or wolf an "organic" plant-based diet just because I could not afford to feed them only grass-fed meats.

Don't major in minors. Its more important to eat a meat-based diet compatible with your physiology than to have that diet composed exclusively of meat, milk and eggs from exclusively pastured animals.

Addendum: Thanks to Matt Schoeneberger for help accessing one of the articles I used as a reference for this chapter.

11 COOKED AND RAW

Is Cooked Food Unnatural?

Every known human tribe cooks at least some of its foods.

Australian aborigines lived largely on antelope kangaroo, marsupial rodents, and fish. All were consumed cooked, mostly roasted directly on coals or baked in an oven made of hot stones.

Evidently the !Kung of the Kalahari never eat raw animal flesh, although they do eat some raw plant foods.[1] Traditionally they simply bury meat in embers or hot sand and leave it to bake for 1.5 hours, or slice it thin and cook it atop the fire.

Stefansson reported that although Inuit (more commonly known as Eskimos) ate some meat raw, they boiled most of their meat, then use the broth created by boiling the meat to make a soup from seal blood.

Nevertheless, some people believe that we should eat only raw foods. They argue that no other animal eats cooked food, and cooking only destroys food, never improves it. Some even believe that cooking food is the primary cause of all diet-related diseases.

There is an important logical error in the argument "No other animal cooks its food, therefore cooking food is unnatural." This argument rests on the assumption that no behavior is Natural unless all animals engage in that behavior. This assumption is false.

Probably every unique species engages in at least one behavior that is unique to that species. For example, cheetahs can run at a top speed of 70 mph. No other species can run that fast. Now consider

---

[1] Tanaka J. The San: Hunter-Gatherers of the Kalahari, A Study in Ecological Anthropology. University of Tokyo Press, 1980.

the argument "No other animal runs at 70 mph, therefore running at 70 mph is unnatural." Clearly this argument is unsound.

Those behaviors that are unique to any species are Natural to that species – part of its unique Nature – even if not Natural for any other species. Running 70 mph is Natural for Cheetahs, even though it is not Natural for any other species.

Likewise, a behavior can be Natural for humans – part of Human Nature – in spite of the fact that no other species engages in the same behavior. We do many things not done by any other species. For example, we use language. No other species uses language. Does that make language use "unnatural"? Of course not. Just as running 70 mph is an expression of Cheetah Nature, using language is an expression of Human Nature.

If we were to jettison every human behavior that is unique to humans, we would be ridding ourselves of Human Nature, exactly what makes us human, a unique species. It would be like trying to make the Cheetah "natural" by depriving it of its unique ability to run 70 mph.

When discussing whether some behavior is Natural for humans or not, we should look not at what other species do, but whether the behavior in question improves Human health and fitness or not. If a behavior improves our health and fitness, and our ability to sustain our species in long-term harmony with Nature, it is Natural, i.e. approved by Nature. If a behavior makes us weak or sick or makes our Natural habitat uninhabitable, it is unnatural (disapproved by Nature).

The fact that no other species is smart enough to control fire does not prove that using fire to prepare food is unnatural and harmful to us. In fact it is irrelevant.

But is cooked food really unnatural? It is true that no other animal has control of fire to produce cooked foods, but is it true that no wild animal eats cooked foods?

376

In *Fire and Civilization*, Goudsblom provides a plausible view of stages leading to human control of fire.[2] First, our ancestors had experience with naturally occurring forest fires. Evidently, forest fires ignited by volcanic eruptions or lightning have occurred for as long as forests have existed, about 350 million years. Forest fires have been so central to life on Earth that they have shaped the evolution of some plants and trees, called *pyrophytes*, which can't propagate and spread successfully without being subjected to fire.

From observations of how animals respond to present-day wildfires, we know that soon after a fire, predators will eagerly enter the burnt area to forage for *cooked food* among the remains. Goudsblom quotes the German explorer and anthropologist Karl von den Steinen who described in 1894 how wild animals reacted to bush fires his servants started by carelessly abandoning campfires:

> "The fires which we lit during our journey often burned for days and spread spontaneously over large distances. Their influence upon the animal world was curious and striking. All sorts of predators took well-considered advantage of the event; they sought and found their victims, not so much by the bright flames, but rather amidst the smoldering ashes in which many a rodent would lie charring. Numerous falcons were hovering over the dark clouds of the *quiemada*, game was running to it from afar to lick at the salted ashes, preferably at night because they could not hide in the barren plain. The ground radiated a comfortable warmth."[3]

Hence, given the opportunity, which is recurrent in Nature, non-human predators do in fact eat cooked meats. However, unlike us, they don't have control of fire to cook foods themselves.

---

[2] Goudsblom J (1992) *Fire and Civilization*. London; New York: Penguin Books

[3] Ibid. 13.

Very early human ancestors were predators and like the non-human predators would have known that a forest fire was also a barbecue. From these Natural barbecues they learned the richer flavor of cooked meat, and probably also that cooked/fire-dried meat lasts longer in storage. In addition, forest fires would have given them access to hot embers and someone would have figured out that they could use these embers to start a controlled fire to produce the flavorful meat at will.

Meanwhile, we know that our ancestors had been making stone tools for hundreds of thousands of years before they domesticated fire apparently about 700 thousand years ago. When you strike stones together to sculpt one to a specific shape, the stones may throw off sparks. Observed at night, such sparks resemble lightening. Probably someone would have accidentally started a fire while shaping stone tools. If not by accident, someone who noticed that lightning could start fires would have deduced also that sparks generated by striking stones could set dry plant matter afire. After some experimentation, someone figured out what stones to use to generate the best sparks to start a fire.

From the above, I conclude first that cooked food is a Natural occurrence; second that non-human animals voluntarily eat cooked meat given the opportunity; third that our ancestors probably first learned of the benefits of cooking meat by exposure to meat cooked by wildfires; and fourth that our ancestors gained control of fire through exercise of their Natural curiosity, which is Human Nature. In other words, controlling Fire and eating cooked meat is Natural for Humans even if not for any other species.

Cooking Starchy Plants Grew Our Brains?

Anthropologist Richard Wrangham has advanced the hypothesis that our ancestors acquired the energy required for expansion of our brain by route of cooking starchy plants. He assumes that some primarily plantivorous hominids – the Australopithecines – were direct ancestors of Homo sapiens, and argues that if they had cooked underground storage organs from plants, they would have obtained more energy than if they had eaten lean raw meat.[4]

Aside from the fact that the idea that Australopithicus is a direct human ancestor and was capable of taming fire is speculative and highly questionable, Wrangham conveniently leaves animal fat, the richest energy source, out of the equation.

Wrangham's hypothesis is logically implausible and has been refuted by empirical evidence.[5]

Logically, it requires that we imagine a creature having the brain size and intelligence of a chimpanzee controlling fire to cook roots and tubers, but not hunting and eating raw meat. Since living wild chimpanzees do hunt and eat raw meat, but don't control fire, and many other carnivores having smaller brains than chimps live entirely on raw meat, Wrangham's suggested scenario is implausible. Clearly, an animal can live entirely on hunting without having the intelligence necessary to be Prometheus. Conversely, only an already highly intelligent, large-brained creature could have controlled fire; in other words, the large brain most likely came before the control of fire, not after. In fact, the fossil record indicates that large increases in primate and hominid brain size occurred

---

[4] Wrangham RW, Jones JH, Laden G, Pilbeam D, Conklin-Brittain N. The Raw and the Stolen: Cooking and the Ecology of Human Origins. Current Anthropology 1999 Dec;40(5):567-94.

[5] Cornelio AM, de Bittencourt-Navarrete RE, de Bittencourt Brum R, et al. Human Brain Expansion during Evolution Is Independent of Fire Control and Cooking. Frontiers in Neuroscience 2016 April; 10(167):1-11.

millions of years before the widespread control of fire that would have made starchy plants digestible.[6]

In addition, from a practical standpoint, cooking meat does not necessarily improve its caloric value as Wrangham has claimed. On the contrary, cooking without pots or pans often leads to loss of drippings containing high-calorie fat. Experiments with mice have demonstrated that they tend to need to eat more cooked meat than raw meat to maintain body mass, indicating that the energy gain from a diet based exclusively on raw meat is similar to or even greater than a diet of cooked meat.[6]

Most importantly, as I mentioned, Wrangham conveniently but erroneously imagines that hunting and scavenging would yield only lean muscle meat, when in fact human ancestors had the wits and tools – simply, stones wielded as hammers – to extract very high calorie fat from bones and organs. Bone marrow has a very high energy density of 8.5 kcal/g, compared to about 2 kcal/g for muscle meat, 1.7 kcal/g for heart, 1.5 kcal/g for brains and only about 1 kcal/g for cooked starches. Human ancestors would have known to break open bones to find fat because they would have witnessed hyenas using their jaws to do this.

How and Why Nature Favors Cooking

If cooking meat does not directly increase the caloric yield from meat, why did Nature obviously favor the reproduction of humans who prefer cooking much of the meat they eat?

Cooking meat offers several benefits. First, cooking reduces exposure to food-borne infections that drain an individual of vitality, or even cause death. Therefore, ancestors who used fire to cook animal carcasses had less risk of illness and death from food poisoning, enabling them to be more productive hunters and have more healthy children.

---

[6] Ibid.

Second, application of fire to large mammals' bones makes them brittle and easier to crack open, making high-fat marrow and brains available to the consumer of cooked meat with less effort compared to the consumer of only raw meat.

Third, proper cooking (low temperature, long duration) makes the tougher cuts of meat easier to chew and digest, so ancestors who cooked meat could get more total (net) energy and nutrients from a single carcass than those who only ate raw meat.

Fourth, in the absence of refrigeration, using fire to dry or cook meat results in less meat lost to spoilage.

In summary, ancestors who used fire on animal carcasses spent less energy in eating and could obtain from any one large mammal's carcass more energy and nutrients with less energy expenditure than those who did not. Therefore, they obtained more energy and nutrient return for each unit of time and energy spent hunting, so had more energy available for hunting and having and raising children.

In short, people who use cooking properly used animal resources more efficiently, with less waste, than those who would eat only raw meat. Nature rewards those who make more efficient use of natural resources.

But Doesn't Cooking Denature Protein?

Sure enough. But people who think that the fact that cooking denatures protein means it renders it useless or harmful may not understand the process of digestion.

The word "denature" probably misleads many people into thinking that cooking somehow takes the Nature out of meat protein. In fact, "denature" is a technical term of chemistry referring to a specific change in the structure of a protein.

Proteins in meat are composed of chains of amino acids. These chains fold upon themselves as a consequence of attraction between amino acids in the chains. These folds make the protein have the specific structure or *nature* it must have in order to function as it does, for example as a muscle fiber, transporter or enzyme.

Now, realize that we eat meat to get essential amino acids, not to get specific proteins with their unique structures. In other words, we don't eat muscles in order to get functional (un-denatured) muscle fibers, transporters or enzymes. In fact, a healthy gut can't/won't absorb whole un-denatured proteins because they are too large to pass the intestinal wall. Unless your gut is so damaged by inflammation that its protective and selective functions are disabled – known as leaky gut – it can only assimilate small peptides and amino acids.

Indeed, if we were to absorb into the blood any whole (un-denatured) protein from any animal tissue, our immune system would immediately recognize it as a foreign protein (antigen) and create antibodies to destroy it. Therefore, Nature designed our digestive process so that it breaks all ingested proteins down into small peptides or individual amino acids.

Exposing a protein to either heat or strong acid breaks the bonds between amino acids that cause the chain to fold upon itself. As a result the protein unfolds and becomes a simple chain of amino acids. Since the unfolded protein can no longer function as a fiber, transporter or enzyme, we say that it lost its nature (i.e. is no longer a functional muscle fiber, mineral transporter or enzyme). Hence the term "denature." It doesn't mean the protein is now unnatural, it just means it is no longer able to function as it did in the living tissue.

As mentioned, both heat and acid will denature proteins. This means that if we eat raw meat, our very strong stomach acid always denatures the protein. In fact, our digestive system *must* denature every ingested protein in order to extract amino acids from it. Our pancreatic enzymes can not efficiently break the essential amino acids off of un-denatured animal protein. The protein must be unfolded – denatured – so that the enzymes can properly latch on to the amino acid chain and break the whole protein down into the constituent amino acids so that we can assimilate them.

You can witness acid denaturing of animal protein by the following experiment. Just take some raw meat, poultry or fish, and soak it in vinegar or lemon juice. You can watch the acid act on the meat; it will gradually change the meat protein so that it looks like you had boiled it.

Your stomach acid is pH 1.5, whereas vinegar is pH 3 and lemon juice has a pH in the range of 2.0-3.0. Since pH is a logarithmic, stomach acid is about 3 times stronger than lemon juice with a pH of 2.0, and 32 times stronger than vinegar with a pH of 3.0. Your stomach acid will denature animal protein much faster and more completely than either lemon juice or vinegar.

Thus, even if you ate only raw animal foods, you would not avoid denaturing the protein in those foods. Your stomach acid will do it even if you don't cook the meat. Proper cooking of meat to denature its protein simply helps your body digest the protein.

In fact, some types of animal protein are much more digestible when denatured via cooking. Some studies show that we can extract only about 50-65% of the protein from raw egg whites, versus 90% from cooked egg whites.[7, 8] Yes, cooking makes some animal products more digestible and nutritious. As already mentioned, this is why Nature favored the reproduction of humans who prefer to cook much of the meat they eat.

---

[7] Evenepoel P, Geypens B, Luypaerts A, Hiele M, Ghoos Y, Rutgeerts P. Digestibility of cooked and raw egg protein in humans as assessed by stable isotope techniques. J Nutr. 1998 Oct;128(10):1716-22. PubMed PMID: 9772141.

[8] Evenepoel P, Claus D, Geypens B, Hiele M, Geboes K, Rutgeerts P, Ghoos Y. Amount and fate of egg protein escaping assimilation in the small intestine of humans. Am J Physiol. 1999 Nov; 277(5 Pt 1):G935-43. PubMed PMID: 10564098.

Destruction Is Necessary To Nutrition

Both acids and fire destroy potential pathogens in food and initiate the digestive process. This is why traditional natural medicine systems such as Chinese medicine described the stomach as a kind of cooking pot, wherein the "digestive fire" purposely destroys whole foods, turning all of them into a 100°F soup so that we can extract from them the nutrients we need.

These functions of protection and controlled destruction of what would otherwise be harmful to us are manifestations of the masculine or yang pole of Nature. We see here how in Nature the yin or feminine and yang or masculine functions are dependent upon one another. The yin or female function of providing nourishment (assimilation) can not take place without the proper assistance of the yang or male functions standing at the border, destroying potential pathogens and converting foreign entities (molecular "immigrants") that will not assimilate in their whole form into bits that we can assimilate. Dropping this yang, masculine guard – for example, eliminating stomach acid – will result in destruction of the whole kingdom by allowing dangerous invaders to pass the gates.

Possible Importance of Raw Animal Foods

That said it is also important to note that overcooking animal foods may make them harmful, and we may need or at least benefit from some raw or lightly cooked animal products to ensure that we obtain certain heat-labile nutrients.

Some epidemiological research has found that people who consume meat cooked well-done, fried or barbecued have higher risks of cancer than those who eat their meat rare or medium-rare, although it should also be noted that other studies have found no association, and animal studies have used doses of the suspected chemicals that were equivalent to thousands of times the doses that a person would consume in a normal diet.[9] Given that we have probably been eating cooked meat scavenged from wild fires since before we gained control of fire, i.e. at least 2 million years, we have probably adapted to exposure to these cooking by-products. Nevertheless, meat provides more of certain heat-labile micronutrients if cooked conservatively or rare to medium rare than if cooked well-done.

Francis Pottenger, M.D., a contemporary of Weston Price, conducted experiments with cats to investigate the effects of heat-processing of animal foods on their nutritive value. His experiments showed that heat-processed meat and milk lose nutritive power and foster degenerative diseases.[10]

Cats fed entirely raw diets maintained excellent health, normal behavior and consistent reproduction over 9 generations. Over their lifespans, cats eating raw diets proved resistant to infections, fleas, and parasites, and had no allergies. They were gregarious, friendly and predictable. When thrown or dropped as much as 6 feet, to test their coordination, they always landed on their feet and enjoyed the play.

In contrast, the first generations of cats fed significant amounts of cooked meat and pasteurized milk developed fatigue, weakness, allergies, asthma, gingivitis, and irritability. They did not have the same physical agility or coordination as the raw food cats. In subsequent generations, these conditions became more pronounced and debilitating.

The second generation of animals fed cooked meat or milk had weak and malformed skeletons, crooked teeth, and malformed and malfunctioning organs and glands. They were afflicted with heart problems; near- and far-sightedness; thyroid disorders; infections of

---

[9] National Cancer Institute. Chemicals in Meat Cooked at High Temperatures and Cancer Risk. <https://www.cancer.gov/about-cancer/causes-prevention/risk/diet/cooked-meats-fact-sheet>

[10] Pottenger FM. Pottenger's Cats: A Study In Nutrition. Price-Pottenger Nutrition Foundation, 1995.

the kidney, liver, testes, ovaries, and bladder; arthritis; skin lesions; worms and intestinal parasites; pneumonia; and nervous system inflammation.

Cats fed cooked, deficient diets lost normal sexual differentiation. Roles reversed: female cats became aggressive, male cats passive, and "abnormal activities between the same sexes" were observed. Cooked meat fed females had ovarian atrophy and uterine congestion, and the males failed to produce sperm. The cats became infertile, prone to miscarriage and spontaneous abortion, or delivered kittens stillborn, or small and frail and incapable of nursing.

Mothers had mammary gland failures and were aggressive toward or had no interest in caring for their kittens. By the third generation the cats fed primarily cooked foods were "so physiologically bankrupt that none survive beyond the sixth month of life, thereby terminating the strain."

Pottenger found that individual cats rendered deficient by cooked food diets could partially regenerate if returned to a raw meat diet. However, he also found that he had to feed the regenerating cats an optimum raw food diet for four generations to completely eliminate the deficiency conditions and restore the lineage to health.

Pottenger observed that the same Natural Laws operate in human health and reproduction. The parallels are quite obvious. Modern civilized people suffer from all the same disorders Pottenger found in the cats fed nutrient deficient diets composed of well cooked meat. In contrast, as Weston Price reported, wild people eating animal-based diets including some raw meat or milk did not have the diseases and disorders of civilization.

Now, we are not cats. Humans evidently have been cooking foods for at least one-half million years, during which time Nature obviously selected humans who thrived while eating some cooked meats. Whereas all wild cats live on exclusively or almost exclusively raw meat diets, no known wild human tribe lived on an exclusively raw food diet.

In *Primal Nutrition*, Ron Schmidt, N.D. notes:

> "A home heated by wood gathers people near a fire for hours in cold months. In caves and later primitive shelters, cooking and sharing meals around the warmth of fire was an everyday routine; it has been so in all native cultures since. And yet in every native culture examined, anthropologists find that customs dictate certain foods be eaten raw. Reasons given by the people invariably relate to preventing disease, ensuring fertility, and promoting optimal growth in children."[11]

Traditional native European and Asian examples of raw animal products include sushi, sashimi, carpaccio, steak tartare, egg nog and raw milk, cream, and cheese. Many people prefer red meat cooked rare or nearly raw. Some cuts of meat taste best eaten raw – e.g. liver – or cooked very rare – seared outside, essentially raw inside – and these can provide animal protein and fats heated only to about body temperature.

Some of the nutrients best supplied by or unique to animal products are sensitive to excessive heat. These include some B-complex vitamins (particularly B6), the amino acid taurine, and the essential fatty acids arachidonic acid, EPA and DHA.

This is why I suggest that Nature favors some *conservative* cooking – cooking that improves digestibility and conserves nutrients – but not *liberal* cooking, which reduces digestibility and destroys nutrients. Conservative cooking uses high heat only briefly, such as for searing a steak or roast to seal in juices before cooking to rare or medium rare, or applies very low heat for long periods (low temperature slow roasting or simmering).

In 2018, we lack evidence to support claims that everyone must eat every scrap of meat raw to achieve health, and have significant evidence that we are by Nature adapted to eating cooked meats.

---

[11] Schmidt R. Primal Nutrition. Healing Arts Press, 2015. 92

Case reports from the Paleomedicina clinic in Hungary (www.paleomedicina.com), as well as testimonies on www.meatheals.com, provide preliminary evidence that people can improve health and sometimes reverse very serious diseases (apparently including cancer) eating hypercarnivore diets composed primarily of cooked meat.

In my view, you should focus on the majors rather than minors, and results rather than doctrine. In 2018, I think the evidence indicates it is more important to eat a diet containing very limited or no plant foods (major issue), than to eat only raw animal food (minor issue). Also, a choice to eat raw animal food should be based on taste and results, not intellectual reasoning. If you get the results you want eating a well cooked hypercarnivore diet, you have no reason to eat raw meat. However, if eating a cooked hypercarnivore diet does not give you all the results you desire, perhaps you are overcooking or sensitive to some of the by-products of cooking. You may want to consider modifying the degree to which you cook animal foods, to include more lightly cooked (medium rare, rare) meat or egg yolks.

12 THE GLUCOGENIC DIET

Very low intake of plant foods and hence carbohydrates can result in a metabolic shortage of glucose, which can change the way the body metabolizes fats, resulting in an increased production of ketones, known as nutritional ketosis. Some people believe that it is necessary to sustain continuous ketosis in order to get all the benefits of restricting dietary carbohydrates. Since the liver can generate glucose from protein, some people following animal-based diets deliberately restrict meat and protein consumption to maintain specific levels of ketosis continuously.

In this chapter I wish to explain why I believe Nature favors a high protein glucogenic diet which probably produces intermittent rather than continuous ketosis.

Gluconeogenesis

Gluconeogenesis – glucogenesis for short – is the generation of glucose from amino acids and glycerol (the back-bone of triglycerides i.e. fats). It is a normal metabolic state in all animals, and even provides about one-third of glucose entering the blood after meals in people on typical carbohydrate-rich diets.[1]

Gluconeogenesis is especially important for meso- and hyper-carnivores. Most ingested amino acids are destined to be transformed into glucose via gluconeogenesis which has been estimated to account for 47-60% of endogenous glucose

---

[1] Jahoor F, Peters EJ, Wolfe RR. The relationship between gluconeogenic substrate supply and glucose production in humans. AJP - Endocrinology and Metabolism 258 (1990)E288.

production.[2, 3] The alternative would be for surplus amino acids to be diverted into de novo lipogenesis, but this path predominates only when the diet includes a high carbohydrate content. It is essential to realize that people eating diets providing limited carbohydrate depend largely or entirely on gluconeogenesis to meet their glucose needs.

As already discussed, when we eat carbohydrate-rich diets, we flood the blood with glucose after every meal. In response, the body releases insulin to store this sugar and stop the utilization of already stored fat. This can result in wide swings of blood sugar levels, alternating between high blood sugar (hyperglycemia) immediately after meals, and low blood sugar (hypoglycemia) after the insulin response to the meal.

Protein providing glucogenic amino acids is the main substrate for gluconeogenesis. Unlike eating carbohydrate directly, endogenous production of glucose from protein is a tightly regulated, demand-driven, slow process that results in gradual restoration of glycogen and release of glucose into the blood without any sudden rise of

[2] Bilsborough S and Mann N: A Review of Issues of Dietary Protein Intake in Humans. Int J Sport Nutr and Ex Metab 2006;16:129-152.

[3] Ackermans MT, Pereira Arias AM, Bisschop PH, et al.: The Quantification of Gluconeogenesis in Healthy Men by 2H2O and [2-13C]Glycerol Yields Different Results: Rates of Gluconeogenesis in Healthy Men Measured with 2H2O Are Higher Than Those Measured with [2-13C]Glycerol. J Clin Endocrin & Metab 2001;86(5):2220-2226.

blood sugar.[4, 5, 6] When glucose produced by gluconeogenesis is released into the blood gradually by the liver there is no rise in insulin levels, because a rise of insulin would suppress glucogenesis and cause hypoglycemia. Thus relying on gluconeogenesis results in stable blood sugar levels, auto-regulated by the liver.

Consumption of just 25 g of potatoes (only 5 g of glucose) causes a dramatic rise in blood sugar levels that will persist for 4-5 hours in normal subjects, and this rise is even greater in diabetics, but 250 g of meat providing about 50 g of protein does not immediately raise blood sugar levels, even in diabetics.[7]

Thus, a high protein intake does not mimic intake of carbohydrates. However, if you restrict dietary carbohydrate, but do not consume adequate meat, your body will be forced consume its own muscle and organ tissue to sustain blood sugar levels and provide glucose for tissues that can't function well without it. This might make it difficult to sustain a very low carbohydrate, animal-based diet.

[4] Conn JW, Newburgh LH. The glycemic response to isoglucogenic quantities of protein and carbohydrate. J Clin Invest 1936;15(6):665-71. <https://www.jci.org/articles/view/100818/scanned-page/671>

[5] P. H. Bisschop, A. M. Pereira Arias, M. T. Ackermans, E. Endert, H. Pijl, F. Kuipers, A. J. Meijer, H. P. Sauerwein, J. A. Romijn; The Effects of Carbohydrate Variation in Isocaloric Diets on Glycogenolysis and Gluconeogenesis in Healthy Men, *The Journal of Clinical Endocrinology & Metabolism*, Volume 85, Issue 5, 1 May 2000, Pages 1963–1967, https://doi.org/10.1210/jcem.85.5.6573

[6] Jahoor F, Peters EJ, Wolfe RR. The relationship between gluconeogenic substrate supply and glucose production in humans. AJP - Endocrinology and Metabolism 258 (1990)E288.

[7] MacLean H. Modern methods in the diagnosis and the treatment of glycosuria and diabetes. Constable, London, 1922. 23-24.

Protein and Ketosis

Some advocates of ketogenic diets suggest that one must limit protein intake to no more than 0.9 grams of protein per pound of lean bodyweight (no more than 2.0 grams per kilogram of lean bodyweight) in order to sustain ketosis.

Experiments refute this idea. In one study that compared the effects of low and high protein intake on ketosis during a carbohydrate-free diet, people produced similar ketone levels (6-10 times baseline) whether they restricted protein to about 100 g protein per day or ate a high protein diet (1.2 g protein per pound body mass daily, ~150 g/d, about 3 times the RDA).[8] However, those who restricted protein to 100 g daily (~0.6 g per pound, about 1.6 times the RDA) ended up in negative nitrogen balance, burning up their own muscle tissue to sustain normal blood sugar levels, whereas those who did not restrict protein maintained a positive nitrogen balance.

Moreover, subjects who consumed the high protein diet lost body fat despite consuming adequate calories. In the authors' words:

> "The fat-sparing action of glucose in normal metabolism is out of proportion to its calorigenic capacity; to date, the practical applications of this knowledge have escaped the clinician….This experiment suggests that a diet adequate in calories, protein and fat but deficient in carbohydrate results in loss of body fat, salt, and water, similar to that of the fasting patient."[9]

This study indicates that a low protein low carbohydrate diet results in loss of lean tissue, whereas a high protein low carbohydrate prevents the loss of muscle, organ, and bone.

---

[8] Azar GJ, Bloom WL. Similarities of Carbohydrate Deficiency and Fasting. II. Ketones, Nonesterified Fatty Acids, and Nitrogen Excretion. Arch Intern Med 1963 Sep;112:338-43.

[9] Ibid.

At least ten other studies have shown that high protein intakes ranging from 120 to 220 g daily do not suppress ketosis and can support ketone levels up to 1.8 mmol/L (0.3 mmol/L is mild ketosis) provided carbohydrate intake is below 40 g daily.[10]

Deliberate restriction of protein to chase deeper ketosis can be harmful because it could restrict supplies of glucose needed for some important processes. In the absence of dietary glucose, we need glucose from gluconeogenesis to replenish compounds essential to energy production in the Krebs cycle. Some of these compounds also participate in additional reactions that synthesize several amino acids (including glutamine), acetyl-CoA, and some lipids.[11] Also, some rapidly replicating tissues, such as hair follicles and white blood cells, appear to depend on glucose supplies to sustain the rapid tissue reproduction or function.[12, 13] When such tissues experience a shortage of glucose, they may malfunction (e.g. hair loss). In addition, some hormones including thyroid hormone, insulin and glucagon are made from amino acids. Restricting protein may lead to shortages of amino acids needed to produce these hormones.

---

[10] Tzur A. How Carbs and Protein Affect Ketosis (Keto Research Review). Sci-Fit 2017 Dec 28. <https://sci-fit.net/carbs-protein-ketosis-research/#Does_a_high_protein_diet_prevent_ketosis>

[11] Bilsborough S and Mann N: A Review of Issues of Dietary Protein Intake in Humans. Int J Sport Nutr and Ex Metab 2006;16:129-152.

[12] "Although fatty acids and ketone bodies were oxidized by the hair follicle, they are poor energetic substitutes for glucose. Nor will fatty acids or ketone bodies sustain hair growth in vitro. " Williams R, Philpott MP, Kealey T. Metabolism of freshly isolated human hair follicles capable of hair elongation: a glutaminolytic, aerobic glycolytic tissue. J Invest Dermatol. 1993 Jun;100(6):834-40. PubMed PMID: 8496624.

[13] Kramer PA, Ravi S, Chacko B, et al. A review of the mitochondrial and glycolytic metabolism in human platelets and leukocytes: Implications for their use as bioenergetic biomarkers. Redox Biology 2014;2:206-210. <https://www.sciencedirect.com/science/article/pii/S2213231714000093>

For example, restricting protein may adversely affect thyroid function through two avenues and head hair growth through those plus a third avenue. First, a shortage of the amino acid tyrosine will impair synthesis of thyroid hormone and lead to thyroid hormone deficiency. Second, when the liver can't produce adequate glucose to meet tissue energy requirements, the body will respond by suppressing thyroid function and glucose-dependent metabolic functions, such as hair growth. Finally, the shortage of glucose will directly impair hair follicle metabolism leading to hair loss.[14]

Wild Hypercarnivores Do Not Sustain Ketosis

As mentioned in Chapter 6, wild non-human carnivores eat very high protein diets. Wild (feral) cats obtain 52 percent of their dietary energy from protein, and 46 percent from fat.[15] Wild wolves obtain 54 percent of their dietary energy from protein, 45 percent from fat, and a mere 1 percent from carbohydrate.[16]

In fact, these animals absolutely require high protein intakes (greater than 30% of energy) to maintain normal blood sugar levels because their livers automatically convert a proportion of ingested protein into glucose.

Dogs (descendants of wolves) fed a carbohydrate-free diet containing only 26% protein become hypoglycemic and ketotic during pregnancy, resulting in stillbirth of more than a third of puppies; but if they have an adequate protein intake (as high as 50%)

---

[14] Ibid.

[15] Plantinga EA, Bosch G, Hendriks WH. Estimation of the dietary nutrient profile of free-roaming feral cats: possible implications for nutrition of domestic cats. Br J Nutr 2011 Oct 12;106(51):535-548. <**https://www.cambridge.org/core/journals/british-journal-of-nutrition/article/estimation-of-the-dietary-nutrient-profile-of-freeroaming-feral-cats-possible-implications-for-nutrition-of-domestic-cats/2E0E827469FFC1AF51387E045C06759A/core-reader**>

[16] Bosch G, Hagen-Plantinga EA, Hendriks WH. Dietary nutrient profiles of wild wolves: insights for optimal dog nutrition? Br J Nutr 2015;113:S40-S54.

they maintain normal blood sugar levels and ability to reproduce.[17] In cats, gluconeogenesis is more or less continuous and peaks in the absorptive phase following meals.[18]

Wild cats and canines evidently are not adapted to sustaining ketosis. This may be because the meat they eat is too lean, very high in protein and not high enough in fat to support continuous ketosis. Instead, they consume very low carbohydrate but very high protein *glucogenic diets* which support continuous hepatic gluconeogenesis.

What about wild human hypercarnivores? Does Nature allow them to continuously maintain diets providing more than 70% of energy from fats, and no more than 25% of energy from protein?

The Inuit/Eskimos eat the fattiest animals on the planet – seal, walrus, narwhal, whale, polar bear, caribou, water birds (cider ducks, auks, and murres), eggs of said birds, musk-ox, caribou, and arctic hare. Among these, "The seal is the animal most constantly and most universally depended upon" and of interest, "Not only is its flesh highly prized but the oil obtained from it furnishes heat and light."[19]

Take note. This means that Inuit used a significant amount of the fat (oil) they obtain from seals to fuel fires and lamps. This gives some indication of the abundance of animal fat available to them. Throughout history people have used animal fats for tanning leather and making candles, soap, salves, balms, lanterns and lamps. This contradicts a commonly heard claim that animal fat was so scarce in Nature that our ancestors had to be eating low-fat diets.

---

[17] Brand Miller JC, Colagiuri S. The carnivore connection: dietary carbohydrate in the evolution of NIDDM. Diabetologia 1994;37:1280-86. <https:// link.springer.com/content/pdf/10.1007/BF00399803.pdf>

[18] [18] Ibid.

[19] Heinbecker P. Studies on the metabolism of Eskimos. J Bio Chem 1928 Dec 1;80:461-475. <http://www.jbc.org/content/80/2/461>

Observers have reported that an average adult Eskimo (Inuit) would consume 4 to 8 pounds of meat in a day, and that their fat intake varied individually and seasonally. "In warm weather about one-seventh of the meat may be fat, in cold weather, especially when the Eskimos are traveling, one-third to one-half may be taken as fat."[20]

The estimated average daily macronutrient intake for Inuit on their native diet was 280 g protein, 135 g fat, and 54 g carbohydrate.[21] Allegedly glycogen in meat provided the carbohydrate, but glycogen in meat degrades to lactate within hours of slaughter so this probably markedly overestimates their carbohydrate intake. Nevertheless, taken at face value, this amounts to 2551 kcal, 43% protein, 48% fat, and 8% carbohydrate. Other investigators have reported protein intakes among Inuit ranging from 43% energy to 56% energy.[22]

These macronutrient ratios are strikingly similar to those reported for wild cats and wolves, suggesting that Nature may not have permitted Eskimos to select a diet providing less than 20% of energy as protein. However, as previously noted, these reports probably overestimated native Inuit protein intake. As previously noted, after living with the Inuit for several years, Stefansson reported that their meals were typically 3 parts lean meat and 1 part fat, much of that seal oil used as a dip for meat, resulting in a protein intake of about 25% of energy.

We now know that the gut and liver can not efficiently process protein intakes of the magnitude (Chapter 8) reported by early observers of Inuit diets. Probably the numbers offered by these early observers (who may not have actually eaten many meals with the Eskimos) reflect some measurement or estimation errors. I would

---

[20] Heinbecker P. Studies on the metabolism of Eskimos. J Bio Chem 1928 Dec 1;80:461-475. <http://www.jbc.org/content/80/2/461>.

[21] Ibid.

[22] Fediuk K. Vitamin C in the Inuit diet: past and present. Master's Thesis. School of Dietetics and Human Nutrition, McGill University, Montreal, Canada, July 2000.

guess that they underestimated the amount of fat consumed by dipping meat into seal oil. Nevertheless, these reports also suggest that Inuit were eating more meat and therefore protein than recommended by some promoters of ketogenic diets. Moreover, a clinical study found that Inuit on their native diets *did not* sustain chronic ketosis, suggesting that Inuit were very efficient at gluconeogenesis.[17]

High Protein Diet and Blood Sugar

Eskimos were also reported to have an average fasting blood sugar of ~120 mg/dL.[17] Although many authorities will identify this fasting blood sugar level as indicating diabetes, Eskimos with this fasting blood sugar level had normal glucose tolerance.[17]

So why would Inuit or anyone else on a very low carbohydrate, high protein diet have a fasting blood sugar of ~120 mg/dL? Here it is important to note that in people eating normal high carbohydrate meals, blood sugar rises to 120-140 mg/dL following meals and is sustained at that levels for some time while tissues absorb the sugar from the blood. In fact, as previously noted high carbohydrate intake results in the liver losing ability to auto-regulate its glucose output.[23]

High blood sugar also occurs in response to intense glycogen-depleting exercises and "It could be argued that a hyperglycemic-hyperinsulinemic response after glycogen-depleting exercise creates the appropriate milieu for at least partial restoration of muscle

---

[23] Clore JN, Helm ST, Blackard WG. Loss of hepatic autoregulation after carbohydrate overfeeding in normal man. *Journal of Clinical Investigation*. 1995;96(4):1967-1972. <https://www.ncbi.nlm.nih.gov/pmc/articles/PMC185834/>

glycogen."[24] It is well known that the release of catecholamines (e.g. epinephrine, nor-epinephrine) during intense exercise will increase blood sugar levels.

Therefore, physically active people eating low carbohydrate diets have to produce glucose from dietary protein to replenish glycogen; they will need a sufficiently high protein intake and gluconeogenesis to meet this need.

The liver's conversion of dietary protein to glucose takes many hours.[25] During an overnight fast the liver converts amino acids from meat into glucose and stores this as glycogen. In the morning, after sleeping and fasting, glucagon, cortisol, epinephrine and norepinephrine levels naturally rise and this results in a release of glucose from the liver to feed glucose to the brain and peripheral tissues. Consequently, people eating a hypercarnivore diet, like the Inuit, may find their morning fasting blood sugar elevated into the acceptable post-meal range – ~120 mg/dL.

Since neither Inuit nor non-human carnivores achieve a "moderate" 15% protein diet or sustain chronic nutritional ketosis, it seems highly unlikely that any hypercarnivorous human ancestors achieved and sustained a such a diet for periods of time sufficient to act as a selection for adaptation to protein restriction. In other words, I think it is unlikely that we are adapted to/designed for carbohydrate-restricted diets that also deliberately restrict protein intake.

---

[24] Marliss EB and Vranic M. Intense Exercise Has Unique Effects on Both Insulin Release and Its Roles in Glucoregulation: Implications for Diabetes. Diabetes 2002 Feb;51(suppl 1):S271-S283. <http://diabetes.diabetesjournals.org/content/51/suppl_1/S271.long>

[25] Bisschop PH, Pereira Arias AM, Ackermans MT, et al. The Effects of Carbohydrate Variation in Isocaloric Diets on Glycogenolysis and Gluconeogenesis in Healthy Men. J Clin Endocrinology & Metabolism 2000 May 1;85(5):1963-67. <https://academic.oup.com/jcem/article/85/5/1963/2660569>

Nature Favors The Glucogenic Diet

Since an insufficient supply of blood glucose will result in unconsciousness progressing to death, Nature has designed our metabolism with multiple redundant mechanisms for establishing a floor to glucose levels. Five hormones including glucagon, growth hormone, thyroxin, cortisol, and epinephrine (also known as adrenaline) work together to keep blood sugar from falling too low by stimulating glucogenesis.

In contrast, so far as we know in 2018, Nature has not given us similar multiple redundant mechanisms for maintaining specific minimum blood ketone levels. As already noted, blood ketone levels are not regulated by hormones, but are by-products of a metabolic shortage of glucose prevents the formation of sufficient oxaloacetate to sustain complete ß-oxidation of fats in the mitochondria. Ketogenesis thus occurs in proportion to the metabolic shortage of glucose. Although restricting protein in addition to restricting glucose might increase ketogenesis compared to just restricting glucose, do we have reason to believe that deliberately maximizing ketone levels is a Holy Grail worth pursuing?

Is Ketosis Key to the Benefits of Ketogenic Diets?

Ketogenic diets have been used to treat epilepsy for nearly 100 years. People have assumed that the anti-seizure effect of a ketogenic diet is produced by ketones. However, some studies have reported a lack of correlation between ketone bodies concentration and reduction of seizures, suggesting that regulation (stabilization) of blood glucose or other mechanisms not yet identified may be at least partly responsible for anti-seizure effects.[26, 27]

A low-glycemic index diet (10% carbohydrate, 30% protein, 60% fat; 40-60 g carbohydrate daily) reduced seizures in children as effectively as a ketogenic diet; the elevated ketone levels produced by a ketogenic diet provided no additional protection against seizures compared to the very low carbohydrate diet.[23] The researchers concluded that "ketosis is not required for excellent seizure control."

A murine study found that a non-ketogenic low carbohydrate diet (approximately 15% carbohydrate and 25% protein) high in branched chain amino acids and using fruits and vegetables for the carbohydrate portion had an anti-seizure effect comparable to a ketogenic diet without elevation of ketones, suggesting that the anti-seizure effect is due to reduction of glucose metabolism (glycolysis), not elevation of ketones.[28]

These studies suggest that some and perhaps all of the positive effects of a ketogenic diet are due to reduction and regulation of glucose or other phytonutrients, not the induction of ketosis. They even support the conclusion that one can obtain the benefits of a ketogenic diet while consuming 10-15% of one's energy needs in the form of carbohydrates from dairy products, fruits or vegetables.

---

[26] Muzykewicz DA, Lyczkowski DA, Memon N, Conant KD, Pfeifer HH, Thiele EA. Efficacy, safety, and tolerability of the low glycemic index treatment in pediatric epilepsy. Epilepsia. 2009 May;50(5):1118-26. doi: 10.1111/j. 1528-1167.2008.01959.x. Epub 2009 Feb 12. PubMed PMID: 19220406.

[27] Neal EG, et al. A randomized trial of classical and medium-chain triglyceride ketogenic diets in the treatment of childhood epilepsy. Epilepsia. 2009;50:1109–17. doi: 10.1111/j.1528-1167.2008.01870.x.

[28] Dallérac G, Moulard J, Benoist J-F, et al. Non-ketogenic combination of nutritional strategies provides robust protection against seizures. *Scientific Reports*. 2017;7:5496. doi:10.1038/s41598-017-05542-3. <https://www.ncbi.nlm.nih.gov/pmc/articles/PMC5511156/#CR28>

Maximized Ketosis ≠ Maximized Fat Loss

A ketogenic diet does not guarantee you will lose fat or avoid gaining fat because the body has a mechanism for storing fat even in the face of very low carbohydrate intake and insulin levels via acylating stimulating protein (ASP).[29] Fat intake stimulates a marked increase in plasma ASP, which is "far more potent than insulin in stimulating triglyceride synthesis in human adipocytes."[30] Moreover, contrary to common belief, dietary fat does stimulate some insulin release, albeit less than protein or carbohydrate.[31] This occurs because one of the roles of insulin is to prevent utilization of stored resources (e.g. body fat) when exogenous resources such as dietary fat are available. If you consume more calories and fat than you burn, you will accumulate more fat in your fat cells, even if you avoid all plant foods and carbohydrates and restrict protein and maintain a deep state of ketosis.

Conversely, some people can achieve good appetite control and sufficiently low insulin levels to lose fat and get very lean while consuming very large amounts of protein along with some whole plant foods and carbohydrates (generally, up to 75 g per day). In fact many, many bodybuilders have for many years used exactly this approach – a diet very high in protein but limited in both fat and carbohydrate – to achieve very low body fat levels. If very high-fat, protein-restricted ketogenic diets were more effective than high-protein, moderately fat- and carbohydrate- restricted diets for

---

[29] Cianflone K, Vu H, Walsh M, Baldo A, Sniderman A. Metabolic response of Acylation Stimulating Protein to an oral fat load. The Journal of Lipid Research 1989 November;30:1727-1733. <http://www.jlr.org/content/30/11/1727.full.pdf+html>

[30] Ibid.

[31] Carr RD, Larsen MO, Winzell MS, et al. Incretin and islet hormonal responses to fat and protein ingestion in healthy men. AJP. Endocrinology and Metaoblism. 2008 Oct;295(4):E779-E-784. <https://www.physiology.org/doi/full/10.1152/ajpendo.90233.2008>

achieving fat loss it is likely they would have become standard practice among competitive bodybuilders, but in fact they have not.

To lose body fat you must ingest less energy than you expend in a day. The best way to do this is to increase your protein (meat and egg) intake to the level necessary to induce satisfaction, while avoiding carbohydrate and limiting fat to just enough to make meals palatable and satisfying. In 1957, George Thorpe, M.D. reported in the Journal of the American Medical Association:

> "The simplest to prepare and most easily obtainable high-protein, high-fat, low-carbohydrate diet, and the one that will produce the most rapid loss of weight without hunger, weakness, lethargy, or constipation, is made up of meat, fat, and water. The total quantity eaten need not be noted, but the ratio of three parts of lean to one part of fat must be maintained. Usually within two or three days, the patient is found to be taking about 170 g of lean meat and 57 g of fat three times a day. Black coffee, clear tea, and water are unrestricted, and the salt intake is not reduced. When the patient complains of monotony, certain fruits and vegetables are added for variety."[32]

If composed of 540 g trimmed beef sirloin steak and 180 g ghee or tallow, this diet would provide 2441 kcal, 162 g protein, 203 g fat, and no carbohydrate to speak of. That is 27% of energy from protein, 73% from fat. This is considerably more protein than recommended by advocates of protein-restricted ketogenic diets.

Assuming the individual has a goal healthy body weight of 160 pounds, this diet provides 1 g protein per pound of body mass, whereas, as already noted at the beginning of this chapter, proponents of protein-restricted ketogenic diets recommend less than 1 g of protein per pound of target body mass. Note also that Thorpe allowed "certain fruits and vegetables" and therefore some

---

[32] Thorpe GL. Treating Overweight Patients. JAMA 1957;165(11):1361-1365.

carbohydrate – hence a hypercarnivore diet – apparently without compromising outcomes.

High Protein Diets Decrease Hunger

Evidently, protein is the most satiating nutrient and fat the least, with carbohydrate intermediate between the two.[33, 34, 35, 36, 37, 38] It appears that people adjust their total food intake to satisfy a need for protein; lower protein intake leads to greater total food and kcalorie intake

---

[33] Holt SH, Miller JC, Petocz P, Farmakalidis E: A satiety index of common foods. Eur J Clin Nutr. 1995, 49: 675-690.

[34] Stubbs RJ, van Wyk MC, Johnstone AM, Harbron CG. Breakfasts high in protein, fat or carbohydrate: effect on within-day appetite and energy balance. Eur J Clin Nutr. 1996 Jul;50(7):409-17. PubMed PMID: 8862476. Abstract.

[35] Westerterp-Plantenga MS, Rolland V, Wilson SAJ, Westerterp KR. Satiety related to 24h diet-induced thermogenesis during high protein/carbohydrate vs high fat diets measured in a respiration chamber. Eur J Clin Nutr 1999;53:495-502. <https://www.nature.com/articles/1600782.pdf?origin=ppub>

[36] Leidy HJ, Ortinau LC, Douglas SM, Hoertel HA. Beneficial effects of a higher-protein breakfast on the appetitive, hormonal, and neural signals controlling energy intake regulation in overweight/obese, "breakfast-skipping," late-adolescent girls. *The American Journal of Clinical Nutrition*. 2013;97(4):677-688. doi:10.3945/ajcn.112.053116. <https://www.ncbi.nlm.nih.gov/pmc/articles/PMC3718776/>

[37] Leidy HJ, Armstrong CLH, Tang M, Mattes RD, Campbell WW. The Influence of Higher Protein Intake and Greater Eating Frequency on Appetite Control in Overweight and Obese Men. *Obesity (Silver Spring, Md)*. 2010;18(9):1725-1732. doi:10.1038/oby.2010.45. <https://www.ncbi.nlm.nih.gov/pmc/articles/PMC4034047/>

[38] Ortinau LC, Hoertel HA, Douglas SM, Leidy HJ. Effects of high-protein vs. high-fat snacks on appetite control, satiety, and eating initiation in healthy women. Nutrition Jouranl 2014;13:97. <http://www.nutritionj.com/content/13/1/97>

which may cause weight gain or inhibit weight loss.[39, 40, 41, 42, 43, 44] Hence, if in a chase after ketosis you deliberately restrict protein and favor dietary fat you may find it difficult to satisfy your hunger. The overemphasis on fat and deliberate restriction of protein may lead you to eat more fat and calories than you need.

Meat Restriction May Cause Potassium Deficiency

Whole meat is the primary source of potassium for a hypercarnivore. Dietary fats such as tallow, lard, butter, cream and the like provide very little or no potassium per kcal.

As shown in the Table 12.1, whole meat, eggs and milk products provide far more potassium per kcalorie than separated fats. In fact, the fats are virtually potassium-free. This means that the greater the

---

[39] Simpson SJ, Raubenheimer D. Obesity: The Protein Leverage Hypothesis. Obesity Reviews 2005;6:133-42.

[40] Gosby AK, Conigrave AD, Raubenheimer D, Simpson SJ. Protein leverage and energy intake. Obesity Reviews 2014;15:183-91.

[41] Gosby AK, Conigrave AD, Lau NS, Iglesias MA, Hall RM, Jebb SA, et al. (2011) Testing Protein Leverage in Lean Humans: A Randomised Controlled Experimental Study. PLoS ONE 6(10): e25929. https://doi.org/10.1371/journal.pone.0025929

[42] Annika M. Felton, Adam Felton, David Raubenheimer, Stephen J. Simpson, William J. Foley, Jeff T. Wood, Ian R. Wallis, David B. Lindenmayer; Protein content of diets dictates the daily energy intake of a free-ranging primate, *Behavioral Ecology*, Volume 20, Issue 4, 1 July 2009, Pages 685–690, https://doi.org/10.1093/beheco/arp021

[43] Martens EZ, Lemmens SG, Westerterp-Plantenga MS. Protein leverage affects energy intake of high-protein diets in humans. Am J Clin Nutr 2012 Dec 5; doi: 10.3945/ajcn.112.046540

[44] Martinez-Cordero C, Kuzawa CW, Sloboda DM, Stewart J, Simpson SJ, Raubenheimer D. Testing the Protein Leverage Hypothesis in a free-living human population. Appetite 2012;59:312-15.

proportion of separated fats in your diet, the lower your intake of potassium. Hence, if you restrict meat to restrict protein, and make a greater portion of your dietary energy intake come from separated fats, you are also restricting potassium intake. If you are relatively sedentary and therefore eat a relatively low energy diet –less than 2000 kcal per day – you may end up getting too little potassium from your food.

Table 12.1 Potassium to energy ratio of meat and fat

Food (100 g)	Protein (g)	Potassium (mg)	Kcalories	Potassium/ Kcal
Chicken breast no skin	31	247	173	1.4
Chicken breast with skin	27	178	184	1.0
Beef chuck steak	23	310	330	1.0
Beef sirloin steak	28	340	250	1.4
Ground beef, 80% lean	25	271	254	1.0
Eggs, chicken (about 2 whole)	13	126	155	0.8
Whole milk	3	132	61	2.0
Cheddar cheese	23	76	404	0.2
Tallow	0	0	902	0
Lard	0	0	902	0
Butter	1	24	717	0.03
Cream	3	95	340	0.28

Source: USDA

Muscles, including the heart, arteries, bladder, stomach and intestines, need potassium to contract. Your nervous system also needs potassium to function. Deliberate protein restriction resulting in potassium deficiency can therefore result in the following symptoms:

- Weakness, fatigue, or cramping in muscles.
- Tingling or numbness
- Nausea or vomiting
- Abdominal cramping or bloating
- Constipation
- Heart palpitations
- Excessive thirst or frequent urination
- Low blood pressure
- Fainting
- Depression, psychosis, delirium, confusion, hallucinations

One can prevent or remedy potassium deficiency by eating enough whole animal-source foods. Since most meats supply about one mg of potassium per kcalorie and we need about 2000 - 3000 mg of potassium and 2000 - 3000 kcalories daily, it follows that one should aim for getting enough whole meats to satisfy potassium requirements. This will result in a high protein intake of 150-200 g per day, depending on whether one eats leaner or fatter meats. That's a protein intake much higher than recommended by some advocates of protein-restricted ketogenic diets.

High Protein Low Carbohydrate Diet Reduces the Insulin to Glucagon Ratio

Some people worry that a high protein low carbohydrate diet will raise insulin levels because one of the functions of insulin is to store dietary amino acids. However, as already emphasized, when dietary carbohydrate is low, the body depends on gluconeogenesis for production of glucose. Since insulin suppresses gluconeogenesis, release of large amounts of insulin in response to dietary protein (amino acids) in the absence of dietary carbohydrate (sugar or starch) would result in hypoglycemia and consequent loss of consciousness.

According to insulin researcher Benjamin Bikman, Ph.D., research shows that dietary protein increases insulin release only if accompanied by a high carbohydrate intake.[45] When carbohydrate intake is low, a high intake of amino acids stimulates the release of glucagon, because in this environment the body needs to stimulate gluconeogenesis.

Bikman reports that the insulin to glucagon ratio of an individual eating a standard mixed diet is about 4, that of a fasting individual 0.8, and that of an individual eating a low carbohydrate diet about 1.3. If a person eating a standard mixed high carbohydrate diet ingests some protein, the ratio will increase to 70, because this person needs insulin to prevent the release of amino acids and glucose from storage depots until blood levels of both amino acids and glucose have declined sufficiently.

In contrast, if the fasting individual eats some protein, the ratio will actually drop, because the body needs glucose and will need to use glucagon and suppress insulin in order to get the glucose from the ingested amino acids. If the individual restricting carbohydrate eats some additional protein, the ratio will remain at 1.3, again because the body needs glucose and fatty acids for fuel and a rise in insulin would suppress the gluconeogenesis and ketosis it needs to function in the absence of exogenous carbohydrate.

---

[45] Bikman B. Why you shouldn't fear protein on keto. Video recorded at the Low Carb Breckenridge conference in February 2018. Published in March 2018 at DietDoctor.com. <https://www.dietdoctor.com/video/presentations/bikman>

A High Protein Diet May Combat Cancer

Insulin is an anabolic hormone that promotes growth and inhibits autophagy, while glucagon favors catabolism and autophagy,[46,47,48,][49] which is the destruction of excess and damaged materials and tissue. Compared to any high carbohydrate diet, a high protein, low carbohydrate diet increases the glucagon to insulin ratio, so it favors autophagy. People on a diet providing protein at 1.87 g/kg daily were found to have a plasma glucagon level 34% higher than people consuming only 0.74 g/kg daily.[50] This might help the body dispose of tumors.

I have already noted previously that some animal research suggests that very high protein, low carbohydrate diets – providing as much as 60-70% of energy as protein and up to 15% carbohydrate – may limit cancer initiation, growth, and metastasis, while not raising

---

[46] Deter RL, de Duve C. INFLUENCE OF GLUCAGON, AN INDUCER OF CELLULAR AUTOPHAGY, ON SOME PHYSICAL PROPERTIES OF RAT LIVER LYSOSOMES. *The Journal of Cell Biology*. 1967;33(2):437-449. <https://www.ncbi.nlm.nih.gov/pmc/articles/PMC2108350/>

[47] Schworer CM, Mortimore GE. Glucagon-induced autophagy and proteolysis in rat liver: Mediation by selective deprivation of intracellular amino acids. PNAS USA 1979 July;76(7):3169-3173. <http://www.pnas.org/content/pnas/76/7/3169.full.pdf>

[48] Shelburne JD, Arstila AU, Trump BF. Studies on Cellular Autophagocytosis. Cyclic AMP- and Dibutyryl Cyclic AMP-Stimulated Autophagy in Rat Liver. Am J Pathol 1973;72:521-540. <https://www.ncbi.nlm.nih.gov/pmc/articles/PMC1904032/pdf/amjpathol00253-0183.pdf>

[49] Ana Maria Cuervo; Calorie Restriction and Aging: The Ultimate "Cleansing Diet", *The Journals of Gerontology: Series A*, Volume 63, Issue 6, 1 June 2008, Pages 547–549, https://doi.org/10.1093/gerona/63.6.547

[50] Bilsborough S and Mann N: A Review of Issues of Dietary Protein Intake in Humans. Int J Sport Nutr and Ex Metab 2006;16:129-152.

ketone levels above those found on typical mixed diets.[51, 52] It seems plausible that high protein low carbohydrate diets may assist in the defeat cancer by route of depriving the tumor cells of glucose, the only fuel they can efficiently use, while lowering insulin and raising glucagon, which favors autophagy.

Intermittent Ketosis

On a hypercarnivore diet, eating little carbohydrate but as much protein as desired by appetite, one will likely naturally cycle in and out of ketosis. During long fasting periods between meals, principally overnight, the body will increase ketone formation to conserve glycogen and prevent the loss of muscle tissue for glucose production. When given adequate dietary protein the liver will generate glucose to restore glycogen and meet glucose demands of the brain, red blood cells and peripheral tissues. Ketone production may drop for a period of time – typically in the morning – when glucose is released from the liver into the blood and delivered to peripheral tissues.

Chasing Ketones May Be Futile

As already mentioned, wherever a particular biochemical condition is absolutely required for sustaining life and health, the body – Nature – has multiple redundant systems that enforce that homeostasis. Since so far as we know at this time no such systems exist for maintaining specific levels of ketones in the blood, I conclude that Nature does not consider continuous ketosis essential.

---

51 Ho VW, Leung K, Hsu A, Luk B, et al., "A Low Carbohydrate, High Protein Diet Slows Tumor Growth and Prevents Cancer Initiation," Cancer Research 2011 July;71(13): DOI: 10.1158/0008-5472.CAN-10-3973 <http://cancerres.aacrjournals.org/content/71/13/4484.full-text.pdf>

52 Ho VW, et al. "A Low Carbohydrate, High Protein Diet Combined with Celecoxib Markedly Reduces Metastasis." Carcinogenesis 35.10 (2014): 2291–2299. PMC. Web. 29 Mar. 2017. <https://www.ncbi.nlm.nih.gov/pmc/articles/PMC4178469/>

In contrast, since we have multiple systems designed to support minimum blood sugar levels through glucogenesis, I conclude that Nature identified glucogenesis as more important than ketogenesis.

Hence, I suggest that efforts to micromanage blood ketone levels are unnecessary as well as futile. So long as you eat the foods you are by Nature designed to eat, and you eat them in harmony with your taste and satisfaction – as much as you desire, no more nor less – you can leave all the metabolic details to Nature.

Summary

No animal needs to calculate ratios of macronutrients on its Natural diet. It just eats what Nature provides and allows it to digest without discomfort, and lets its body's innate PRIMAL WISDOM take care of the details.

Although following a HYPERCARNIVORE DIET may sometimes produce nutritional ketosis, it *does not* involve consciously following macronutrient formulas to chase or sustain ketosis. You follow the guidance of your hunger and taste, which manifest the ancient PRIMAL WISDOM of your True Nature, not clever formulas recently invented by the conscious rational mind which has only a limited understanding of Nature.

On a HYPERCARNIVORE DIET you eat only when you are hungry, which for most people will eventually lead to eating only one or two meals in a day. Consequently, you may alternate between periods of glucogenic metabolism and periods of ketogenic metabolism, without attempting to consciously control your ketone levels.

13 Evolution of Homo Carnivorus

Biologically, man is still a wild animal and there is no reason to suppose that his biology is adapted to anything other than wild foods. There simply has not been time for any selective evolution to have changed mankind as mankind has changed its pattern of eating.

Michael Crawford and David Marsh
NUTRITION AND EVOLUTION

Since we appear closely related to the plantivorous chimps, and we do not belong to the order Carnivora, it is tempting and easy to assume and imagine that the alleged last common ancestor of chimps and humans was more chimp-like than human-like, so must have eaten a plant-based diet like the chimps. Many authors also allege that we are descended from species that appear to have eaten plant-based diets with little or no animal food, such as Australopithecus.

If you assume that chimpanzees resemble our ancestors (or, our ancestors resembled chimpanzees), then you may unconsciously assume that chimpanzees have passed through the last 6 million years with little or no evolutionary change via natural selection, while humans have radically changed during the same time frame.

Yet, we really have no reason or evidence to support the proposition that the chimpanzee we see today represents the last common ancestor of chimps and humans and has not changed in 6 million years. If you think that over the past 6 million years humans have changed from chimp-like creatures into our present form, why would you assume that over the same time period chimps have undergone no evolution by natural selection? As one team of researchers noted in 2016, "it is important to bear in mind that extant living species, such as chimpanzee, gorilla, and macaque, are the endpoints of their own evolutionary lines and not our ancestors."[1]

Moreover, we have no reason or evidence that would justify the assumption that the last common ancestor of chimps and humans was chimpanzee-like and primarily adapted to a plant-based diet. As presented in Chapter 4, the chimpanzees differ from both ourselves and Miocene apes in incisor/molar proportions, molar wear gradient, dentine penetrance into molars, molar enamel thickness, molar occlusal basins, canine crowns, and diastema (spaces between teeth).[2] Chimpanzees have incisor/molar proportions so different from what we find in ourselves and our known ancestors that it is highly unlikely that any alleged common ancestor of humans and chimps had teeth like chimps.[3]

In summary: First, chimps do not re-present the last common ancestor but have been subjected to natural selection and evolved to their present form over the last 6+ million years. Second, we are not very likely descended from any ancient primates – such as Australopithecus – who were chimp-like.

[1] Cornélio AM, de Bittencourt-Navarrete RE, de Bittencourt Brum R, Queiroz CM, Costa MR. Human Brain Expansion during Evolution Is Independent of Fire Control and Cooking. *Frontiers in Neuroscience*. 2016;10:167. doi:10.3389/fnins.2016.00167.

[2] Pickford M. Orrorin and the African ape/hominid dichotomy. In: Reynolds SC, Gallagher A (eds.). African Genesis:Perspectives on Hominin Evolution. Cambridge University Press, 2012. 110.

[3] Ibid., 116.

Connecting Some Dots

The first primates appeared on Earth about 55 million years ago.
They were insectivores, i.e. carnivores, who inhabited Africa, North
America and Asia. By 14 million years ago, in the middle of the
Miocene Epoch (23-5.3 mya), apes made their appearance.

During the Miocene, the Earth went through a progressive cooling
trend. Polar ice caps expanded, drawing water from the oceans and
causing seal levels to drop. Lush tropical forests shrank and sparse
woodlands and dry grasslands expanded.

Expansion of grasslands led to increases in populations of animals
(including insects) capable of exploiting the plants or animals
inhabiting the grasslands. At this time, the group of apes that
included our alleged ancestors was "apparently in the process of
adapting to life on the edges of the expanding savannas in Southern
Europe."[4]

To thrive on a savanna, a creature must either eat grass directly, or
eat creatures that eat grass. To thrive on grass, a creature must have
a gut capable of turning fiber, the main constituent of grass, into fats.
Since no living ape species has such a gut, and those Miocene apes
had insectivorous ancestors, it is highly unlikely that those Miocene
savanna-dwelling apes were successfully adapting to the South
European savannas by eating grass.

However, they very well could have exploited grassland insects (e.g.
grasshoppers, crickets) and other small grass-eating animals (e.g.
snails, gerbils, mice).

According to the currently dominant narrative of human evolution,
while the savannas were expanding and forests shrinking during the

---

[4] O'Neil D. The First Primates. Early Primate Evolution: A survey of Geological
Time and Evolution Leading to Hominins. Behavioral Sciences Department,
Palomar College. 2012. <https://www2.palomar.edu/anthro/earlyprimates/
early_2.htm>

millions of predominantly Ice Age years, natural selection acted on that insectivorous savanna species to favor those individuals that preferred to eat fruits and vegetables that a) didn't exist on the savannas and b) were disappearing due to the cold and dry climate. Ultimately this converted that insectivore into a primarily frugivorous arboreal species that was the last common ancestor of chimps and humans. Then about 2-3 million years ago, natural selection changed course completely, started favoring the savanna-dwelling meat-eaters among those fruit-eaters, and eventually changed the members of this lineage back into a savanna-dwelling naked ape capable of hunting very large game animals, such as mammoths and rhinos.

It should be obvious that this scenario is highly unlikely. Due to the biological reversals required, I would venture that this scenario has a probability near zero.

In *Nutrition and Evolution*, Michael Crawford and David Marsh discuss another problem with the currently accepted story of human evolution: it does not provide any good explanation for our divergence from the great apes in bipedal posture and locomotion, high water requirement, amphibious abilities and strong affinity for coastal habitats.

Regarding our bipedal posture and locomotion, Crawford and Marsh comment:

> "The idea of an upright primate scoring by being able to peer over the tops of the grasses is an appealing one – to anyone who has no experience of hunting. In reality the main difficulty facing any hunter is not spotting his prey but preventing his prey from spotting him. A polar bear, for all its white camouflage, will slip into the icy water and move, virtually submerged, towards the seal lying on the edge of the ice. If you watch a cat stalk a bird, it squeezes its body as close as possible to the ground: it seems to flow forward in controlled, silent motion with its eyes fixed unwaveringly on

the position of its prey. The big cats do the same with frightening ease....

"A hunter stalking antelopes or wild pigs with a modern rifle will do his best to emulate the Tasmanian and the cat. Creeping about the savannah on your stomach is extremely uncomfortable but unless you want your target to spot you first it is what you had better do, even if it means that for much of the time you cannot see the animal you are stalking. Beginners who attempt this method, or still worse try to move crouching on all fours, often betray their presence by their give-away rear end protruding above the grass. Anyone trying it will soon be left in no doubt that the human anatomy, with its upright stance, is not designed for stalking prey."[5]

Now, obviously, modern humans can hunt successfully. In what types of habitat are they most successful? I suggest that an upright posture is advantageous if the hunter primarily inhabits a partially or fully wooded biome. An upright human can hide behind and blend in with upright trunks of trees, or hide up in the canopy of trees. Thus he can succeed as an ambush hunter.[6]

Individuals capable of an upright posture and bipedal locomotion would also have been more successful at wading into water to gather shellfish, and capture slow-moving or densely crowded fish or amphibians by hand, spear, net or hook.

Crawford and Marsh also point out that because savannas are very dry, a savanna habitat naturally selects for species that have low water requirements. In this respect we differ markedly from animals highly adapted to the savanna:

---

5 Crawford M and Marsh D. Nutrition and Evolution. Keats, New Canaan, CT, 1995. 156-157.

6 Bunn HT, Gurtov AN. Prey mortality profiles indicate that Early Pleistocene Homo at Olduvai was an ambush predator. Quaternary International 2014 Feb 16;322-23:44-53.

"In savannah conditions man too is helplessly dependent on a supply of water, though he only needs to drink it....On another expedition in Uganda with Neil Casperd we measured the loss of water from our bodies when we were on a foot safari in Tonia-Kaiso. We discovered that between 10 a.m. and 4 p.m. we were losing it at the rate of 1.6 litres an hour, or over two gallons in six hours. Our African colleagues were losing water at the same rate...

"Animals in an arid environment cannot possibly afford to treat a very scarce resource with extravagance. If man is a savannah species he is the only one that rigidly controls its body temperature and uses a copious loss of water through the skin to do so."[7]

Our use of evaporative cooling provides quite strong evidence that we did not evolve in a dry savanna environment. Our early ancestors most likely inhabited water-rich biomes.

Our brain:body ratio also argues against the idea that our ancestors specialized in a savanna habitat. Our brain constitutes about 2 percent of our body mass. No large grassland animal or landlocked arboreal ape compares.

Large grassland herbivores have very small brains. For example, a horse's brain constitutes only 0.02 percent of its body mass. Although land-locked carnivores have larger brains than the herbivores they eat, they still have limited brains. For example, a lion's brain constitutes only 0.2 percent of its body mass.

Landlocked apes also have small brains. A gorilla's brain constitutes only 0.2 percent of its body mass, and a chimp's brain constitutes only 0.6 percent of its body mass.

---

[7] Crawford M and Marsh D. Nutrition and Evolution. Keats, New Canaan, CT, 1995. 167.

Among large animals, the dolphin comes closest to us in brain:body ratio. It has a brain constituting about 1 percent of its body mass.

So our brain is proportionately twice the size of the dolphin's, 3.3 times the size of the chimp's, 10 times the size of a lion's or gorilla's and 100 times the size of a horse's.

However, smaller mammals have brain:body ratios similar to us. For example, a mouse's brain constitutes about 2.5 percent of its body mass, and a squirrel's about 2.2 percent. The brain:body ratio in other small mammals is much the same as the mouse, squirrel and human.

As Crawford and Marsh remark: "There is simply no evidence of any of the savanna or forest species doing anything other than losing out in terms of brain capacity and the allometric calculations simply confirm this conclusion."[8] Thus, it seems possible that as Nature's selection increased the body mass of landlocked animals, it could not keep brain mass in the same proportion as found in small mammals, for lack of something.

So we have these facts:

- Small-bodied land mammals maintain large brains relative to body mass, indicating that they are able to access resources necessary to sustain those large brain:body ratios.
- Large-bodied land mammals, including carnivores, dramatically sacrificed brain mass relative to body mass en route to large bodies, most likely indicating that their habitats do not provide resources necessary for sustaining large brains.
- The large-bodied dolphin is able to maintain a larger brain:body ratio in the marine environment, compared to terrestrial carnivores, suggesting that the limiting factor on land is less limited in the seas.

These facts together suggest three conclusions:

---

[8] Ibid, 161.

1. Both marine and landlocked habitats taken alone lack some resource necessary for to sustain a large-bodied animal with a brain constituting 2 percent of body mass.
2. The most limiting resource on land must be abundant in the dolphins' marine food chain, but the dolphins' marine food chain must lack some resource which put a cap on the evolution of the dolphins' brain size at 1 percent of body mass.
3. If an ancient small-bodied mammal inhabited a biome that provided nutrient resources from both land and marine food chains, natural selection could favor an evolutionary path that conserved the brain:body ratio of ~2 percent while also increasing total body mass.

Crawford and Marsh suggest that we need to update our view of human evolution:

> "The classical interpretation of evolution is of 'improvements' step by step through selective advantage. What possible advantage can it have been for a chimpanzee or a lion to lose relative brain capacity to such a massive extent?

> "The classical view sees *Homo sapiens* as evolving a big brain from a little one. The typical image was portrayed in the 'just Genius' advertisement for the black beer Guinness. The picture depicted a row of apes, starting with a stooped, virtually four-legged version of the pin headed chimp. The next figure was slightly more upright, but still with huge brow ridges and sloping cranium clearly indicating not much inside. The further figures were progressively more upright in stance with the bigger and bigger brains, and finally bowlder-hatted *Homo sapiens* holding a glass of Genius.

> "Now supposing that story was false. Supposing it was the other way round. As the lions and gorillas became bigger, their brains became smaller in relation to the size of the

body and the basic physiological demands it imposed. Then the line that became Homo sapiens did not need to evolve a bigger brain at all. All he did was to keep what he had as a small mammal.

"He simply kept his brain when all around were losing theirs. When one recognises that the savannah species 'lost' relative brain capacity and man retained it, then one can view the origin of man's brain afresh."[9]

The classical view maintains that our lineage started out as a mouse-sized insectivore with relatively large brain, which gradually evolved into an ape similar to a chimp having a smaller brain:body ratio, then finally grew back a bigger brain to become human.

But evidently savannas simply do not readily provide the resources needed for building big brains. No forest or savanna species has the combination of large brain and large body that we have. The only other large animal with a large brain capacity is the dolphin.

Whereas the land food chain is relatively poor in omega-3 fats but rich in omega-6 fats, including arachidonic acid so necessary for full human brain development, the marine food chain is relatively poor in omega-6 fats and rich in omega-3 fats, including the DHA so necessary for full human brain development. Perhaps we have a far greater brain capacity than either the animals confined to land or those confined to sea because we come from a lineage that specialized in eating both terrestrial and aquatic animals.

The Amphibious Ape

Sir Alister Hardy first proposed the so-called aquatic ape hypothesis of human evolution. He pointed to a number of unique human characteristics which we share with aquatic mammals but are absent from and of no adaptive value to a strictly land mammal.

---

[9] Ibid, 160.

First is our exceptional swimming ability. People can swim 22 miles across the English channel and back again. No strictly land mammal can swim (or needs to) this well.

Moreover, people can swim well below the surface and navigate exceptionally well underwater with no artificial gear. Pearl and sponge divers can reach depths of 175 feet simply by holding their breath and using stones to carry them downward. Again, no land-locked species needs such an ability.

Marine mammals have a diving reflex. When seals, dolphins, and whales dive, their heartbeat slows down to 10-12 beats per minute. We have the same reflex. Animals adapted to forest or savanna but not water life have no such reflex.

Our ability to swim appears to be innate. If infants are put in water before they reach six months of age, they will swim spontaneously with eyes wide open and breathing controlled.

Like amphibious and marine mammals (e.g. rhinos and seals, respectively), we have much reduced body hair. Loss of hair provides a hydrodynamic advantage of less drag in swimming. Also, our skin has a large number of eccrine glands, a characteristic we share with water-going animals, whereas land animals have few of these glands.

African forest and savanna species have little subcutaneous fat, whereas we, like marine mammals, have lots of subcutaneous fat, especially when infants. This fat provides buoyancy and insulation in water, but has little utility, or may even be detrimental, in a hot, dry savanna habitat.

Unlike many other land animals, we have a love of water. As Crawford and Marsh write: "Water both excites and soothes us like no other element. We wash in it, dive into it, use it as a playground wherever it is warm enough to do so (and often in places where it is not). Children, like hippos, put their heads under it and blow bubbles and, despite our Victorian inhibitions, the greatest pleasure is to swim naked in it."[10]

Crawford and Marsh add these observations:

- We have plenty of evidence that the oldest human settlements were at the interface of land and water. We have built all of our greatest cities close to the sea, rivers or lakes. We have built small and large water vessels, and with them we have crossed the oceans, and circumnavigated the world. We could not have done any of these things without having a high level of comfort with large bodies of water.

- All human cultures have used marine foods as much as possible. There exists a general agreement that people benefit from eating seafood at least a few times weekly.[11] People across cultures enjoy fishing as a simple pastime. They will sit for hours by the water and compete to see how many fish they can catch; the experience is so fulfilling that they will even consent to put the fish back in the water.

Crawford and Marsh sum this up:

> "We have, then, four facts to deal with: (i) we humans have a close connections with water which includes a continuing reliance on water-borne foods; (ii) anatomically and physiologically, we have features in common with the aquatic mammals that other, purely land-going species do not possess; (iii) we alone among land mammals have retained our relative brain size as our bodies evolved to their present size; (iv) the only other species to have done

---

[10] Ibid: 168.

[11] American Heart Association. Fish and Omega-3 Fatty Acids. 2016 Oct 6. <http://www.heart.org/HEARTORG/HealthyLiving/HealthyEating/HealthyDietGoals/Fish-and-Omega-3-Fatty-Acids_UCM_303248_Article.jsp#.WniTX4Jrwd0>

the same is aquatic [the dolphin]. Can we put these facts together?"[12]

An Alternative Hypothesis

Now, consider an alternative human evolution hypothesis and narrative:

While the savannas are expanding and forests shrinking (starting towards the end of the Miocene, up to ~ 6 mya), some insectivorous primates capitalize on the lush habitats where land and water meet along streams, rivers, lakes and seas. Ancestral hominins probably gravitated towards wetlands and feeding on aquatic animals and plants in response to the late Miocene's drying climate, increasing wet-dry seasonality, and climate changes.[13]

These insectivores would have been able to collect and consume small amphibians, fish and invertebrates – such as freshwater worms, tadpoles, clams, minnows and crayfish – either opportunistically or inadvertently entangled in any vegetation they chose to eat. On land they could have exploited the increasing abundance of grass-eating terrestrial insects and invertebrates such as grasshoppers, crickets, ants, locusts, snails, worms, grubs, and so on. The aquatic plants they consumed would have had a sodium content 500 times that of land plants.[14, 15] This would have exerted a Natural selection for

---

[12] Crawford M, Marsh D. Nutrition and Evolution. Keats, New Canaan, CT, 1995. 175.

[13] Russon AE, Compost A, Kuncoro P, Ferisia A. Orangutan fish eating, primate aquatic fauna eating, and their implications for the origins of ancestral hominin fish eating. Journal of Human Evolution 2014;77:50-63.

[14] DiNicolantonio J. The Salt Fix (Harmony Books, New York, 2017): 20.

[15] Denton DA, McKinley MJ, Weisinger RS. Hypothalamic integration of body fluid regulation. PNAS 1996 July;93:7397-7404. <http://europepmc.org/backend/ptpmcrender.fcgi?accid=PMC38996&blobtype=pdf>

hominins with a taste, tolerance and even requirement for substantial intake of dietary salt.

Table 13.1: "Daily amount of major food groups (in kilograms), arranged from low to high, minimally required for five brain-selective minerals: Iodine, iron, copper, zinc, and selenium (I, Fe, Cu, Zn, and Se) after Cunnane (2005)." Abridged.

	I	Fe	Cu	Zn	Se
shellfish	0.7	0.8	*0.9*	0.5	0.3
eggs	0.2	0.6	*2.5*	0.9	0.9
fish	0.2	*3.5*	3.1	2.7	0.7
meat	1.5	0.8	1.7	0.9	*5*
nuts	1.5	0.8	0.9	0.5	*5.5*
vegetables	4.2	2.1	2.7	*8.7*	6.7
fruit	6	3.7	4.8	*9.3*	6
milk	6.7	24	12.5	*47*	5.5

The figure in **bold italic** identifies the most limiting nutrient in each food group.

From: Verhaegen M, Munro S, Vaeechoutte M, et al.. The Original Econiche of the Genus Homo: Open Plain or Waterside? In: Ecology Research Progress, ed by Sebastian I Munoz. Chapter 6. Nova Science Publishers, Inc, 2007.

Plants and especially animals from wetlands, lakes, rivers and seas would also have provided an abundance of iodine, iron, copper, zinc and selenium, all important for brain development and function (Table 13.1). Verhaegen and associates remark:

> "Of all the major food groups, shellfish requires the least amount (900 grams) to meet the minimum requirement for all five minerals, and is also the food group for which these requirements are most evenly distributed. Eggs (2500 grams) and fish (3500 grams), both more abundant at the waterside than in terrestrial environments, are next, while 5000 grams

of meat, five times more than shellfish, would be needed to meet the minimum requirement for all five minerals [Table 13.1]"[16]

Thus by hanging out by the shore our early ancestors could have met their requirements for brain-selective minerals much more easily than by relying only on land animals. The environment would have naturally favored those with genetics favoring larger brains.

As the members of this lineage gained body size they graduated to hunting small grass-eating mammals (various rodents such as rabbits and gerbils) along with small fish. They would have graduated successively from occasionally opportunistically catching fish by hand, to deliberately and regularly searching and catching fish by hand, to finally using tools to catch fish. Their wetland habitats probably provided large populations of catfish and other slow-moving fish that they could easily obtain when washed ashore, trapped in drying ponds, injured or otherwise disabled.[13]

Then, as they become larger and smarter over generations, they go on to larger and larger, more and more energy-dense, fat-rich game both on land and in water. Eventually they are able to hunt any land or marine animal they desire, including the largest on land (mammoths, elephants, rhinos) or in the sea (whales).

Over generations they gradually gain body size to become one of the megafauna, but, unlike land- or sea- locked species, they had access to large supplies of both land-based omega-6 arachidonic acid, and marine-based omega-3 EPA and DHA, as well as the brain-specific minerals mentioned above. This would have enabled them to retain the same brain:body ratio as their smaller, insectivorous ancestor even while gaining total body mass.

---

[16] Verhaegen M, Munro S, Vaeechoutte M, et al.. **The Original Econiche of the Genus Homo: Open Plain or Waterside?** In: Ecology Research Progress, ed by Sebastian I Munoz. Chapter 6. Nova Science Publishers, Inc, 2007.

In this way, over thousands of years, Nature could have transformed the originally tiny predatory primate (the insectivore) into *Homo sapiens*, the always carnivorous *and* amphibious ape.

Meanwhile the chimpanzee lineage went up into the trees, and adapted to a fruit-based diet less rich in omega-6 and omega-3 fats and brain-specific minerals. Over generations they developed larger and larger bodies, but they didn't have access to enough essential fatty acids and minerals to maintain the relative brain:body ratio of the last common (insectivorous) ancestor. So their plant-based strategy made their brains shrink (relative to their body mass).

The fact that the majority of remains of early man have been found inland does not prove that man evolved inland. Archaeological remains suffer from preservational bias. Organic materials, such as remains of plants or feces, generally do not survive for millennia simply because organic processes quickly recycle such materials. Bones can survive for millions of years, although frequently in a more or less disintegrated condition. Stone tools survive the passage of time in many environmental conditions, but tools made of organic materials (e.g. wooden spears) only survive under unusual conditions.

Moreover, animal bones may survive millions of years in a dry environment, but not in a humid environment. This preservational bias inevitably preserves more fossils in dry savannas than in humid forests or shorelines. Consequently, archaeologists are more likely to find something in dry rather than humid places; so they are more motivated to dig in dry versus wet lands.

Moreover, shores change with time; repeated natural cycles of expansion and contraction of wetlands, streams, rivers, lakes, and seas destroys evidence of shoreline habitation.

Crawford and Marsh explain:

> "We have few, if any, fossils of intermediate dolphins as they evolved from land to marine forms, and the reason is

obvious. The seashore is in constant flux, being eroded, changing shape and shifting place. It is very unlikely that a fossil will endure for millions of years in such conditions, whereas in a dry place inland it is far more probable."[17]

Thus, Nature's preservational bias tends to bias archaeology and anthropology toward a story of human ancestors dwelling inland rather than along bodies of water.

Furthermore, we have incredibly small amounts of fragmentary fossil evidence available to us. In the words of the paleontologist Stephen Jay Gould, "Most hominid fossils, even though they serve as a basis for endless speculations and elaborate storytelling, are fragments of jaws and scraps of skulls."[18] Although we have a few more complete specimens, and they do provide some evidence for an apparent evolution of hominins over time, they do not provide us with a complete recording of prehistory, let alone a journal of daily food intake for representatives of each species over the previous 6 million or more years since the alleged last common ancestor of humans and modern ape.

Wood and Harrison have pointed out that fossil evidence is plagued by the problem of homoplasy: skeletons having significant structural similarities may not have shared evolutionary history because, from a Darwinian perspective, similar environments may select for similar traits in only distantly related lineages.[19] Since the fossil record presently only yields skeletal remains, Wood and Harrison admit that providing convincing evidence for hypothesized evolutionary relationships may actually be impossible:

> "So why do researchers persist in trying to solve a phylogenetic problem that may well be at the limits of, or

[17] Ibid: 176.

[18] Gould SJ. The Panda's Thumb. WW Norton and Company, 2010. 126.

[19] Wood B, Harrison T. The evolutionary context of the first hominins. Nature 2011 Feb 16;470(7334): 347-352. 350.

even beyond, the analytical capabilities of the data and the available methods? The reason is that our own ancestry matters to us. Most vertebrate palaeontologists would be content to accept that the ancestry of *Homo* resides in *Australopithecus*, without needing or expecting to unravel the topological complexity of the different species within the latter genus. We are not advocating that researchers abandon trying to draw inferences about the phylogenetic relationships of hominins at the finest scale possible. However, we do suggest that those who present and accept these hypotheses need to be aware that such inferences, especially ones about stem taxa, are likely to be inherently prone to refutation and subsequent revision."[20]

In contrast, the study of modern human nutritional requirements using living humans is not "at the limits of, or even beyond, the analytical capabilities of the data and the available methods."

Given the severe limits on archaeological research, our well-established knowledge of the anatomy, physiology, metabolism, and nutritional requirements, preferences and practices of contemporary humans – particularly those who lived without civilization – should take precedence when forming any hypotheses about the subsistence strategies and alleged biological evolution of human ancestors.

In short, we ourselves are the living 'fossils' produced by the process of reproduction over thousands of generations. The physical and mental characteristics that enabled our ancestors to survive and thrive in the past are actually present – re-present-ed – in our own bodies and behavior.

---

[20] Ibid.

14 Carnivore Ecology

Food Supply and Population

Of all environmental problems, rapid human population growth has been identified as the most detrimental. Continuous expansion of the human population increases human demands on ecosystems, exacerbating all environmental problems. As human numbers increase, more pollutants are dumped into land, water and air, and more land and water resources are consumed. Thus, environmental degradation is a by-product of increase in human population size.

In 2016 the UN estimated that 815 million people of the 7.6 billion people in the world, or 10.7%, were suffering from chronic undernourishment.[1] Many people believe that we must continuously increase our food supply to support the growing population. However, the production of food entails consumption and pollution of land, water and air resources. Therefore, producing more food means more environmental stress.

Advocates of vegan, vegetarian and other of plant-based diets point out that livestock use large amounts of resources and produce wastes. In the US in the mid-1990s, livestock consumed 130 million tons of grain annually; advocates of plant-based diets allege this to be enough to feed about 400 million people. On this basis they assert that we should reduce or stop production of animal foods, and adopt plant-based diets with animal products extremely limited or excluded, in order to provide more food for more people.

This may sound logical, but it ignores a couple of very important facts:

First, most of the feed grain we produce goes to feed monogastric animals including chickens and pigs, not dairy and beef cattle, which

---

[1] <https://www.worldhunger.org/world-hunger-and-poverty-facts-and-statistics/#hunger-number>

consume grass and other forage that humans can't eat. In other words, stopping the use of grain in livestock feeding would primarily affect our production of pigs and poultry, not ruminants like cattle, yaks, bison, goats and sheep. Since cattle consume foods humans can't digest (grass, hay, etc.), but produce foods humans can digest (milk and meat), they produce 10-30% more human-edible protein than they consume.[2]

Second, if we were to increase the supply of plant food in this way we would likely fuel further undesired population growth.

Prior to the adoption of agriculture about 10,000 years ago, our ancestors' population was, like that of other carnivores, limited by the availability of prey animals for food. Carnivores always maintain a small population in comparison to their food resource base; for example, big cat or wolf populations are always much smaller than the populations of their routine prey species. On average, for a human hunter-gatherer society, food supply restricts population density to less than 1 person per square kilometer (less than 3 people per square mile).[3]

The adoption of agriculture and plant-based diets by some humans supported dramatic increases in population size because agriculture produces much more food per unit area. Traditional farming methods can support 100-1,000 people/km[2] (260-2,600 people/mi[2]), two to three orders of magnitude greater than hunter-gatherers.[4]

Noncontracepting lean !Kung hunter-gatherer women who eat a diet rich in animal protein but low in starch have an average of 4-5 live births per reproductive lifetime. In contrast, noncontracepting

---

[2] Capper JL. Should we reject animal source foods to save the planet? A review of the sustainability of global livestock production. South African Journal of Animal Science 2013; 43(3):233-246.

[3] Hill E. Agriculture. Chapter 16 in: Environmental Science (McGraw-Hill, Dubuque, IA, 2016)

[4] Ibid.

agricultural women eating starch-based diets have much more body fat and may have as many as 11 children per reproductive lifetime.[5] Evidently women on low carbohydrate diets accumulate the body fat stores required to support resumption of menses, a pregnancy and lactation much more slowly than agricultural women eating large amounts of carbohydrate, resulting in a birth interval of 4-5 years for hunters versus 1-2 years for agriculturalists.

Moreover, biologists have empirically proven that, for any species, every increase in food supply promotes population growth. Conversely, reductions in food supply result in decline of populations.[6] Simply, the birth rate of any animal population is determined by how much food is available to each individual. As food supply increases, fatness increases, and as fatness increases, so does fertility.

The body directs food energy to four different compartments: maintenance, growth, energy storage (body fat), and reproduction. Needs for maintenance must be met before growth can occur, essential growth must be completed before body fat will be stored, and body fat must reach minimum levels to support reproduction. Hence, restriction of the food energy available to a population results in less energy available for body fat accumulation and reproduction, so the birth rate drops to maintain equilibrium with the food base.

Food supply experts Russell Hopfenberg, Ph.D., of Duke University (Durham, North Carolina), and David Pimentel, Ph.D., of Cornell University (Ithaca, New York) explain this is why natural populations fluctuate without starvation:

> "Under natural conditions, as the feeder population increases, the food population decreases. This leads to a

---

[5] Huss–Ashmore, R. (1980). Fat and fertility: Demographic implications of differential fat storage. American Journal of Physical Anthropology, 23(S1), 65-91.

[6] Hopfenberg R. Pimentel D. Human population numbers as a function of food supply. *Environment, Development, and Sustainability* 2001;3:1-15. <http://www.bioinfo.rpi.edu/bystrc/courses/biol4961/foodpop.pdf>

decrease in the feeder population which is then followed by an increase in the food population. This increase in food availability again produces an increase in the feeder population. In quarternary consumer species, the so-called 'top of the food chain' [apex predators like us], this occurs primarily through fluctuations in birth rates."[7]

In view of this fact, Hopfenberg and Pimentel explain why the vegetarian idea is misguided:

"Certainly there would be even more human food available if dependence on livestock was decreased. However, because human population is a function of food availability, the resulting increase in available human food would induce a commensurate rise in population. This population increase would ultimately exacerbate the starvation and malnutrition predicament."[8]

Birth rate statistics confirm that low animal protein intake is associated with high birth rates. In 1952 Josué de Castro reported the data in Table 14.1 in his book *The Geography of Hunger*.[9]

[7] Ibid.: 4.

[8] Ibid.: 6.

[9] William RJ. Nutrition Against Disease. Pitman, 1971: 141. Citing DeCastro J. The Geography of Hunger. Little, Brown, 1952.

Table 14.1: Dietary animal protein and birth rate (From de Castro, 1952)

Nation	Dietary animal protein (g/day)	Birth Rate (per 100,000)
Formosa	4.7	45.6
Malay States	7.5	39.7
India	8.7	33
Japan	9.7	27
Yugoslavia	11.2	25.9
Greece	15.2	23.5
Italy	15.2	23.4
Bulgaria	16.8	22.2
Germany	37.3	20
Ireland	46.7	19.1
Denmark	59.1	18.3
Australia	59.9	18
United States	61.4	17.9
Sweden	62.6	15

Source: Williams RJ. Nutrition Against Disease. Pitman, 1971: 141. Citing DeCastro J. The Geography of Hunger. Little, Brown, 1952.

This 1952 data predates the release of the birth control pill (first marketed in 1960) so we can't attribute these differences to use of the contraceptive pill in industrialized nations. It also predates the widespread use of hormones in livestock production. This data seems to show that human birth rates increase in a dose-response fashion as animal protein intake decreases and carbohydrate (plant food) intake increases. Probably high carbohydrate diets favor fat storage and influence sex hormone levels which alter birth rates.

Although one might think high birth rate always signifies health, each species is adapted to a specific birth rate that maintains the species in equilibrium with its natural habitat and food sources. If a species that once maintained a population in equilibrium with its habitat and food source is found to be reproducing at a rate unsustainable by its environment, this suggests that its reproductive biology has been adversely altered by some factor. If so, we should find that the higher birth rate also adversely affects the females and their offspring.

We have evidence that women and children are harmed by the higher birth rates found in agricultural populations. A woman who has 5 or more children in her lifetime – more than the average among noncontracepting hunter-gatherers – is called *grand multiparous*. Evidently, grand multiparous women have a markedly increased risk of any obstetric complication, neonatal morbidity, and perinatal death starting with the 5th pregnancy onward. In comparison to women who have had no more than 4 children, grand multiparas have:[10, 11]

- a doubled risk of malpresentation
- a threefold higher prevalence of meconium-stained liquor and placenta previa
- a 3.6 fold greater risk of premature rupture of membrane
- a 3.8 fold greater risk of intrauterine growth retardation
- a greater risk of breech presentation, preterm labor, placental abnormality, and post partum haemorrhage

------

[10] Mgaya A, Massawe SN, Kidanto H, Mgaya HN. Grand multiparity: is it still a risk in pregnancy? BMC Pregnancy Childbirth 2013;13:241. <https://www.ncbi.nlm.nih.gov/pmc/articles/PMC3878019/>

[11] Alhainiah MH, Abdulijabbar HSO, Bukhari YA: The prevalence, the fetal and maternal outcomes in grand multiparas women. Mater Sociomed 2018 Jun;30(2): 118-120. <https://www.ncbi.nlm.nih.gov/pmc/articles/PMC6029909/>

Infants delivered by grand multiparous women have a three-time greater risk of low APGAR (Appearance, Pulse, Grimace, Activity, Respiration) score signifying increased risk for neonatal mortality.[12]

Lahti and associates examined the risk of severe mental disorders in adult offspring of grand multiparous women.[13] Adult children of grand multiparous women were found to have significantly increased risks of mood disorders, non-psychotic mood disorders (doubled risk) and suicide attempts (nearly 4-fold risk). Women born to grand multiparous mothers had significantly increased risks of any severe mental disorder; non-psychotic substance use disorders (nearly tripled risk); schizophrenia, schizotypal and delusional disorders (more than doubled risk); non-psychotic mood disorders (nearly tripled risk); and suicide attempts (5-fold increased risk). These risks were found to be independent of maternal age and body mass index at childbirth, year of birth, sex, childhood socioeconomic position, and infant birthweight.

Thus, the birth rates found in non-contracepting agricultural populations may exceed the level that a woman's body can support to produce physically and mentally healthy children. In other words, the birth rates found in noncontracepting agricultural populations may be unnatural for our species. This may also imply that an agricultural diet produces hypersexuality in humans, i.e. sexual activity beyond what the human organism is by Nature adapted to. Hence I hypothesize that high-carbohydrate, plant-based diets alter human hormonal function and reproductive behavior to favor increased sexual activity and consequent birth rates that both harm women and children, and increase the population growth rate beyond the level of natural adaptation, with the result that the species as a

---

[12] Alhainiah MH, Abdulijabbar HSO, Bukhari YA: The prevalence, the fetal and maternal outcomes in grand multiparas women. Mater Sociomed 2018 Jun;30(2): 118-120. <https://www.ncbi.nlm.nih.gov/pmc/articles/PMC6029909/>

[13] Lahti M, Erikssson JG, Heinonen K, et al.: Maternal Grand Multiparity and the Risk of Severe Mental Disorders in Adult Offspring. PLoS One 2014;9(12):e114679. <https://www.ncbi.nlm.nih.gov/pmc/articles/PMC4262418/>

whole becomes disharmonious with its natural resource base, i.e. overpopulated.

Although we may not yet know the exact mechanism, converging evidence indicates that non-contracepting humans tend to have more babies when on low protein, high carbohydrate, plant-based diets than when eating high-protein, low carbohydrate animal-based diets. Hence, plant-based agricultural diets seem to be the root source of excessive population growth and the consequent strain on natural resources.

These data indicate that the vegetarian prescription to shift to a more plant-based diet is likely to increase human population, greatly exacerbating all environmental problems. On the other hand, shifting toward a more animal-based diet will likely limit human birth rates and population growth, resulting in a gradual amelioration of all environmental problems. This can occur without people starving or suffering the nutrient deficiencies typically induced by highly plant-based diets.

If we stabilize our food production and focus on increasing reliance on ruminant products (milk and meat), the population can stabilize without any increase in hunger. Studies of monkeys show that when food supply is kept relatively constant, starvation does not occur.[14] Daniel Quinn, author of *Beyond Civilization*, has explained why: If the food supply is held constant at an adequate level, even if the population increases at a rate of 1 to 2 percent per year, the reduction

---

[14] Hopfenberg R, Pimentel D. Human population numbers as a function of food supply. *Environment, Development, and Sustainability* 2001;3:1-15. <http://www.bioinfo.rpi.edu/bystrc/courses/biol4961/foodpop.pdf>

in caloric intake for each individual is so small it is practically unnoticeable for up to 9 years.[15, 16]

Hopfenberg and Pimentel explain:

> "For example, if a populations consists of 1,000 humans and food availability for this population is held constant forever, and allows for 3,000 calories per person per day (holding other vital nutrients constant relative to calorie count), this is a total calories count of three million calories per day. If the number of people increases to 1,014, the number of calories per person per day is reduced to 2,959. If the same amount of population growth occurs the next year, the population will grow to 1,028. The calories per person per day will then drop to 2918. Repeated twice more, the calories available per person per day will drop to 2,879 and then to 2,838. After 4 years of 1.4% population growth, calories per person per day is reduced by only 162. After a total of nine years, the reduction in calories is only 353, to a level of 2,648 calories per person per day. The impingement of the food and nutrient limitation, although subtle, will eventually serve to curb human reproduction. This may occur through social mechanisms, choice behavior or reproductive-biological mechanisms. In other words, halting increases in food production [or energy availability] will halt the increases in population by means of a reduced birth rate."[17]

Regardless of the nutritional quality of foods eaten, such gradual caloric reduction can reduce body fat levels, fertility, and reproductive activity. The birth rate and population can gradually

---

[15] Ibid.

[16] Quinn D. Reaching for the Future with All Three Hands. Accessed on the World Wide Web on 8/7/2003 at: <**www.ishmael.org/Education/Writings/ kentstate.shtml**>. See also Quinn's books *Ishmael, My Ishmael, The Story of B*, and *Beyond Civilization*.

[17] Hopfenberg R, Pimentel D, op. cit.

decline in equilibrium with the decreasing food supply, without any increase in malnutrition. If we wisely focus on reducing production and consumption of unnecessary and empty calories—such as white sugar—people could be both leaner and healthier.

The alternative is to continue vainly increasing food production, focusing on caloric quantity instead of quality (nutrient density). That will generate an even larger population with a higher proportion malnourished and malformed. Many of those people will die of diseases resulting from poverty and pollution.

Moreover, as human population increases, humans consume an increasing proportion of the world's biomass. In the mid-1990s, humans utilized about 50% of the world's biomass. As more land is devoted to production of human food and the number of humans increases, the land and biomass available for other species and therefore biodiversity must decrease. Do we really want an Earth populated only by humans, rice and bean plants?

Hopfenberg and Pimentel conclude:

> "Thus, there appears to be two available systemic methods of population control. One is to continue to fuel population growth through increased food production and allow biological mechanisms such as malnutrition and disease to limit the population by means of an increased death rate. The other is to cap the increases in food production and thereby halt the increases in population by means of a reduced birth rate."[18]

By eating a greater proportion of your diet as animal products, you increase the nutrient density of your own diet, thereby improving your own health, while simultaneously reducing the total amount of food energy available to the world population. Thus, you are doing

---

[18] Hopfenberg R. Pimentel D. Human population numbers as a function of food supply. *Environment, Development, and Sustainability* 2001;3:1-15. <http://www.bioinfo.rpi.edu/bystrc/courses/biol4961/foodpop.pdf>

your part to put a cap on food energy availability. As more and more people do this, we will eventually reduce food energy availability enough to produce a reduction in the human birth rate. A hypercarnivore diet therefore is the most ecological diet, because it attacks the fundamental cause of environmental degradation, the excessive human birth rate evidently produced by high-starch, low-protein plant-based diets.

Ruminants Rejuvenate the Land

Some authors claim that raising livestock, especially cattle, is a misuse of land, causes global warming, ground water loss and pollution, loss of species diversity, and depletion of fossil fuels.[19] They say it is more ecological for humans to eat a grain-based, largely or totally vegetarian diet.

It is important to note that most beef cattle in the US and Canada spent their first 8 to 16 months of life on pasture. They are in feedlots for only 120 to 150 days. Thus, most cattle (as well as other ruminants) spend about 70% of their lives on pasture (grass) and 30% getting grains. In contrast, conventionally raised chickens and pigs are fed virtually 100% grains.

Only about one-third of the Earth's land mass can be used for food production. Of that, only about one-third (or about one-ninth of the total land mass) is suitable for growing crops. Suburban sprawl and erosion from row cropping will continue to take away from this area. The remaining two-thirds of the usable land only supports growth of plants that are not edible for humans, but are edible for ruminant animals such as bison, cattle, deer, elk, zebras, elands, sheep, goats, and the like.[20] If we stopped raising ruminants we would lose all the food value they provide from grasslands.

---

[19] For example: Rifkin J. Beyond Beef: The Rise and Fall of the Cattle Culture (Plume, 1993).

[20] Department of Animal Science, Oklahoma State University, <www.ansi.okstate.edu/breeds>

Grazing ruminants release methane, a greenhouse gas, but their pastures are much more effective than cultivated fields at removing carbon-rich greenhouse gases from the atmosphere.[21] "Grazing land soils in the Great Plains contain over 40 tons of carbon per acre, whereas cultivated soils contain only about 26, on average... Cultivated lands replanted to grasslands plants as a part of the USDA Conservation Reserve Program (CRP) were found to have added an average of 1,000 pounds of carbon per acre per year during the first 5 years after planting, which means that the CRP alone is removing 18 million tons of carbon from the atmosphere each year."[22]

The highest rates of below ground carbon accumulation occur when cropland is converted to grassland with management-intensive grazing. When cultivated soils are returned to pasture with management-intensive grazing, they gain an almost incredible average of 8.0 Megagrams (8 tonnes) of carbon per acre per year for the first 5 years after restoration, and also gain soil water holding capacity by 34%.[23] Within a decade of management-intensive grazing practice, soil carbon levels return to those of native forest soils.

Thus, returning row-cropped land to grassland helps combat atmospheric carbon accumulation. To do this, we need to eat more food produced by grasslands – namely, ruminant meat and milk – and less cropland products, such as grains and legumes.

----

[21] North Carolina State University. "Scientists Find That Grasslands Can Act As "Carbon Sinks"." ScienceDaily. ScienceDaily, 15 January 2001. <www.sciencedaily.com/releases/2001/01/010111073831.htm>

[22] USDA Natural Resources Conservation Service. <https://www.nrcs.usda.gov/wps/portal/nrcs/detail/national/technical/nra/dma/?cid=nrcs143_014209>

[23] Machmuller MB, Kramer MG, Cyle TK, et al.: Emerging land use practices rapidly increase soil organic matter. Nature Communications 2015 April 30;6:6995. <https://www.nature.com/articles/ncomms7995>

Most cultivated plants, including grains and legumes, have sparse root structures and are planted relatively far apart; non-cultivated plants (weeds) naturally fill the gap, but farmers fight back with herbicides. Wind and rainfall can't be stopped and carry exposed soil and chemicals off the farm and into our waterways.

Native grassland plant species do not require chemical input. They have dense root structures that prevent weed growth and erosion, enable the soil to retain water, refill subterranean aquifers, and protect surface waterways. Compared to cultivated lands, properly managed pastures make almost no contribution to soil erosion, ground water loss, or water pollution. In fact, they are essential for proper ground water management.

Properly managed grazing also results in natural distribution and incorporation of animal urine and feces into the soil. Factory farms and feedlot produce high concentrations of wastes that often end up in waterways. Fortunately, wastes from these operations can be successfully incorporated into pasture lands, helping reduce the water pollution problem.

Do grazing cattle damage range lands? Only if improperly managed. Ruminants are a natural, essential part of healthy grassland ecology. If they are managed in a way that mimics natural patterns of native animals (deer, elk, bison, etc.), grazing cattle can improve rangelands. Well-managed grazing increases the number and vigor of native perennial grasses, reduces weed species, improves the vegetative cover of stream banks, hastens manure decomposition, and extends the pasture's growing season.

Grazing lands also constitute the most extensive wildlife habitats in the United States. Wildlife are dependent on grazing lands for habitat. It is estimated that about two-thirds of wildlife is produced on private grazing lands.

In addition, grazing lands serve as recreational areas providing open spaces, scenery and beauty.

Grasslands need grazing ruminants to stay healthy. According to the USDA's Agricultural Research Service, ungrazed grass lands are degraded through loss of native plant species diversity, increased weed growth, and reduced carbon storage. Pasture plants, ruminant animals, and apex predators are symbiotic by Nature's design. By raising and eating ruminants we contribute to the health of rangelands.

Energy Efficiency

Raising animals entirely on pasture is probably the most energy efficient of all food production methods. In raising row crops, farmers commonly invest 5 to 10 calories of fossil fuel (for large machinery used for tilling, planting, and harvesting) for each calorie of food or fiber harvested. Pasture-based animal husbandry is 10 to 20 times more energy efficient, producing 2 calories of energy profit (food, fertilizer, and fiber) for every calorie of fossil fuel invested.[24]

Why? Diverse grasslands complete with ruminant animals are ecosystems evolved by Nature. It requires little human effort to maintain these systems. Vast single crop farms are artificial and can be maintained against Nature's design for diversity only by investing enormous amounts of human labor and energy.

Meat, eggs, and milk are all edible with little or no processing or cooking. In contrast, grains and legumes all require extensive, energy-intensive processing such as grinding or cooking. This is true even of so-called quick-cooking rice and cereals, which are "quick" because they are processed and precooked by the food industry. Farming uses less than one-fifth of the energy consumed

---

[24] USDA Natural Resources Conservation Service. <https://www.nrcs.usda.gov/wps/portal/nrcs/detail/national/technical/nra/dma/?cid=nrcs143_014209>

by our food system. The other 80 percent is spent in processing, packaging, distributing, and preparing the food.[25]

In 1994 the food processing industry was the fifth-largest U.S. industrial energy user, behind petroleum and coal products, chemicals and allied products, paper and allied products, and primary metal industries. The largest single consumer of energy in the food processing industry was wet milling of corn, the process used to extract starches, sweeteners, alcohols, gluten meal, proteins, and oil from corn. Corn milling consumed 15% of the total energy used in the food industry. Next came beet sugar processing, soybean oil mills, malt beverages, and meat packing plants, in that order. Meat packing plants consumed only 5% of the total energy consumed in the food industry. Corn milling alone consumed 3 times as much energy as meat packing plants; corn milling, beet sugar processing, soybean oil mills, and malt beverages altogether consumed 33% of all the energy used in food processing, 6 times as much as consumed by meat packing plants (Figure 14.1, Table 14.2, next page).[26]

---

[25] Center for Sustainable Systems, University of Michigan. 2017. " U.S. Food System Factsheet." Pub. No. CSS01-06. <http://css.umich.edu/sites/default/files/U.S._Food_System_Factsheet_CSS01-06_e2017.pdf>

[26] Drescher S, Rao N, Kozak J, Okos M: A Review of Energy Use in the Food Industry. Agricultural and Biological Engineering Department, Purdue University. 1997. American Council fo an Energy-Efficient Economy. Research Report IE981. <https://aceee.org/files/proceedings/1997/data/papers/SS97_Panel1_Paper02.pdf>

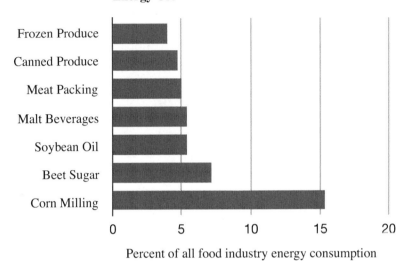

Figure 14.1: Top Eight Energy Consuming Food Industries by Percentage of Total Food Industry Energy Use

Percent of all food industry energy consumption

Table 14.2 Total energy consumption by fuel type of selected food industries

Industry Groups	Total Energy Consumption
Food and Kindred Products	922
Wet corn milling	141
Beet sugar	67
Soybean oil mills	50
Malt beverages	50
Meat packing plants	48
Canned fruits and vegetables	44
Frozen fruits and vegetables	40

Source: Energy Information Administration via Drescher et al.: A Review of Energy Use in The Food Industry. Purdue University. Reference 26.

In a report prepared for the American Council for an Energy-Efficient Economy, Purdue University scientists identified wet corn milling, soybean oil milling, and the dairy industry as the top industries having "many opportunities for energy conservation and waste minimization."[27] However, they noted that in the dairy industry production of spray dried milk, roller dried milk, and casein consumed the most energy. Production of fluid milk used less energy than any other dairy product by far, less than 4000 BTU per gallon compared to 116,462 BTU per gallon of roller dried milk , 69,891 BTU per gallon of spray dried milk, and 97,052 BTU per gallon of casein. Production of spray dried milk, roller dried milk, casein, and anhydrous milk fat consumed 7.5 times as much energy as production of pasteurized milk, butter, and cheese (296,026 BTU vs. 39609 BTU).

Evidently some fluid milk plants implement inefficient boilers operation for pasteurization which results in wastage of 52% of fuel energy. Drescher and colleagues state that boiler fuel requirements could be reduced from 57 billion BTU per year to only 1 billion BTU per year using various heat recovery options.[28] If so then production of pasteurized fluid milk would be even less energy costly than stated here. The bottom line is that the majority of energy used in dairy production goes to highly processed dried milk products, not fresh milk, butter, or cheese.

All told, the industrial production of highly processed plant foods consumes far more energy than the production of fresh meat or milk products. We highly process these plant products because we aren't very capable of digesting them ourselves. Instead of spending fossil fuels to convert corn, beets and soybeans into nutrient-poor

---

[27] Drescher S, Rao N, Kozak J, Okos M: A Review of Energy Use in the Food Industry. Agricultural and Biological Engineering Department, Purdue University. 1997. American Council for an Energy-Efficient Economy. Research Report IE981. <https://aceee.org/files/proceedings/1997/data/papers/SS97_Panel1_Paper02.pdf>

[28] Ibid.

processed foods, we could feed these crops to cattle and other animals capable of biologically converting them into highly digestible and nutrient-dense meat, milk and eggs. Thus we would avoid expending the fossil fuels on processing plants, and at the same time produce more high quality foods for ourselves, which would in turn improve human health.

When you buy fresh or frozen raw animal products, the total energy spent in getting it to your plate is a tiny fraction of what's spent in the industrial food loop, especially if you have the opportunity to buy directly from the farmer. By avoiding corn products (starch, sweeteners, oil, etc), sugar products, soybean oil, and malt beverages a hypercarnivore goes a long way to reduce his or her energy-consumption footprint compared to people eating typical plant-based diets.

What About Grain-Finished Livestock? Isn't That Inefficient and Unsustainable?

No. Animal scientist Judith Capper conducted several studies on the sustainability of beef production. In one, she compared the environmental impact of conventional (grain-finished with growth-enhancing technology), natural (grain-finished with no growth enhancing technology) and grass-fed (forage fed with no growth-enhancing technology) beef production systems.[29] She found that increased productivity in the conventional system reduces the cattle population required to produce a given volume of beef. The conventional system required 56.3% of the animals, 24.8% of the water, 55.3% of the land and 71.4% of the fossil fuel energy required to produce an equal volume of beef in the grass-finished system. The carbon footprint of beef was lowest in the conventional system, intermediate in the natural system and highest in the grass-finished system. Although the grass-finished system had the potential advantage of greater carbon sequestration per acre of land used, this

---

[29] Capper JL.: Is the Grass Always Greener? Comparing the Environmental Impact of Conventional, Natural and Grass-Fed Beef Production Systems. Animals 2012;2:127-143; doi:10.3390/ani2020127.

was offset by the greater amount of land needed to produce each unit weight of grass-finished beef.

Conclusions

1. A hypercarnivore diet is more ecological than a plant-based diet because it reduces the total food energy supply for humans, thereby attacking the root cause of environmental degradation by placing a cap on human population growth.
2. A hypercarnivore diet based on ruminant meat and milk makes use of agricultural grasslands that otherwise would not be able to produce edible human food.
3. Proper grazing of ruminants is necessary to health of grasslands, and grasslands are one of the most effective ways – if not the most effective way – of sequestering atmospheric carbon.
4. Grasslands do not require the herbicide or pesticide applications required by croplands, so the more we rely on ruminant meat and milk, the less chemicals we use in agriculture and the less we pollute ground water and surface waterways.
5. Grasslands stocked with grazing ruminants perform multiple essential ecological services better than croplands, including: prevention of soil erosion, retention and filtering of water, promotion of native grass growth, and provision of wildlife habitat and recreation areas.
6. Raising ruminants on grasslands is far more energy efficient than row cropping.
7. In our current food system processing of plant foods such as corn, beets and soybeans to produce nutrient poor products consumes far more energy than processing of nutrient-dense fresh meat and milk. Feeding corn, beets and soybeans directly to cattle processes these crops into edible meat and milk, thereby avoiding the large fossil fuel energy expenditure needed for food industry processing of these plants.
8. You can eat either conventional, natural, or grass-fed beef and milk products with a clean ecological conscience, but conventional products evidently have the smallest ecological cost.

15 QUESTIONS AND ANSWERS

Why should I trust you?

I don't want you to trust me. I've provided hundreds of references you can consult yourself to evaluate the information in this book. But ultimately I don't want you to trust those sources either.

I want you to start trusting your own direct experience and Nature. I want you to trust that if you get any negative effects from eating plants, Nature is guiding you to stop eating those plants. I want you to entertain the idea that Nature gave you senses of hunger, thirst, taste, and satisfaction to guide you to select the Natural foods that are most compatible with your digestion and nutritional requirements. I want you to trust that distaste, gas, bloating, and other gut discomfort and pain are Nature's way to warn you when you have eaten something that is harmful to your health and fitness.

So, I'm not setting myself up as the authority. I am trying to direct you to assume sovereignty over your own health. I want you to do a 30 day hypercarnivore experiment and find out for yourself.

I have started the hypercarnivore diet, eating meat, milk and eggs, with very little plants. I no longer have the gas, bloating and flatulence that I had when eating larger portions of plants, but have been on it for X time period, and I am having difficulty moving my stools when I get the urge. What can I do about this?

Constipation refers to difficulty evacuating the bowels, regardless of frequency. Diets high in plants or fiber promote growth of fermentative bacteria in the colon. These bacteria produce gases and acids that can damage the colon, and the large stools produced by indigestible carbohydrates can overstretch the colon. These factors can cause irritable bowel syndrome, and make the colon so weak and distorted that it is incapable of properly moving a smaller stool out.

Also, long adherence to low fat diets can result in poor bile production and flow. A healthy liver produces adequate bile and a healthy gall bladder releases it in adequate amounts to facilitate fat digestion when you eat high fat meals. Bile naturally stimulates bowel movement.

Hence eating a typical plant based diet for years can render your bowels incapable of natural functions. I had this happen to me. Whatever you do, don't take fiber as this will only increase the size of the stool, making it more difficult to move, and continue to poison and distort the intestines.

Magnesium deficiency contributes to this problem. Many municipal water supplies are low in magnesium compared to the waters our ancient carnivore ancestors would have used.

To correct this problem and help your body restore the colon to healthy function, I recommend first using 300-600 mg of elemental magnesium daily, in one or two 300 mg doses. Magnesium stimulates bile production and flow, and enhances water retention in the colon, both facilitating easier evacuation.

Start with 300 mg of magnesium daily for a week, taken in the morning. If this does not improve the situation increase to 600 mg daily in two doses, morning and evening. If after a week you still need help, increase to 900 mg. This alone will solve the problem for most people.

If 900 mg of magnesium daily does not solve the issue or you also occasionally feel some queasiness or nausea after eating high fat hypercarnivore meals, you may need to use an herbal cholegogue (bile stimulant). I recommend digestive bitters before meals, or artichoke extract.

Be patient with this. It can take 6 months or more for the colon to regain healthy function after years of plant-based diets and irritable bowel syndrome.

Is it really safe to eat conventional organ meats, milk, and eggs?

Yes. As discussed in Chapter 10 we lack evidence to support claims that these products are unsafe, contaminated or unhealthful in comparison to natural, organic, or grass-fed products. The USDA prohibits farmers from milking or butchering for food use any animal that has been treated with antibiotics or hormones until sufficient time has passed to allow the animal to metabolize and eliminate these items.[1]

What kind of fitness training do you recommend?

Since all physical activity consumes energy and time and imposes a stress on the body, one should do the minimum amount of physical training required to obtain the desired results.

Since muscular strength is the foundation for all physical activity, progressive resistance training (calisthenics, weight training) should be the foundation of every fitness program, If you only have time for one method of physical training, you should devote it to strength training, because strength training produces better overall fitness than either endurance or flexibility training. Properly performed resistance training can significantly improve strength,

---

[1] USDA FSIS. Beef from Farm to Table. 2015 March 24. <https://bit.ly/2zG7Z0p>

cardiorespiratory fitness[2, 3] and flexibility[4, 5, 6, 7] whereas endurance training does not improve strength or flexibility (actually tends to reduce them), and flexibility training does not improve endurance or strength. Progressive strength training "produces greater strength, gait and balance improvements in elderly people than a flexibility exercise program."[8] Resistance exercise also improves self-esteem, mood, body image, and fatigue.[9]

[2] Artero EG, Lee D, Lavie CJ, et al. Effects of Muscular Strength on Cardiovascular Risk Factors and Prognosis. Journal of cardiopulmonary rehabilitation and prevention. 2012;32(6):351-358. doi:10.1097/HCR. 0b013e3182642688.
<http://www.ncbi.nlm.nih.gov/pmc/articles/PMC3496010/>

[3] Steele J, Fisher J, McGuff D, et al. Resistance training to momentary muscular failure improves cardiovascular fitness in humans: A review of acute physiological responses and chronic physiological adaptations. J Ex Phys (online) 2012 June; 15(3):53-80.

[4] Fatouros IG, Kambas A, Katrabasas I, et al. Resistance training and detraining effects on flexibility performance in the elderly are intensity-dependent. J Strength Cond Res 2006 Aug;20(3):634-42.

[5] Morton SK, Whitehead JR, Brinkert RH, et al. Resistance training vs. static stretching: effects on flexibility and strength. J Strength Cond Res 2011 Dec; 25(12):3391-8.

[6] Santos E, Rhea MR, et al. Influence of moderately intense strength training on flexibility in sedentary young women. J Strength Cond Res. 2010 Nov;24(11): 3144-9. PubMed PMID: 20940647.

[7] Monteiro WD, Simão R, Polito MD, et al.. Influence of strength training on adult women's flexibility. J Strength Cond Res.
2008 May;22(3):672-7. PubMed PMID: 18438255.

[8] Barrett C, Smerdely P. A comparison of community-based resistance exercise and flexibility exercise for seniors. Aus J Physiother 2002;48(3):215-19.

[9] Taspinar B, Asian UB, Agbuga B, et al. A comparison of the effects of hatha yoga and resistance exercise on mental health and well-being in sedentary adults: a pilot study. Complement Ther Med 2014 Jun;22(3):433-40.

In addition, strength training does more for health and longevity than endurance or flexibility. Muscular strength "has an independent role in the prevention of chronic diseases whereas muscular weakness is strongly related to functional limitations and physical disability."[10] Muscular strength reduces the risk of premature death from cancer and all causes in men,[11] and women.[12] Strength training is the only physical training method proven to retard and even reverse aging of muscles.[13]

As already mentioned, properly performed strength training itself improves cardiorespiratory endurance. Sprint interval training is the most time-efficient way to produce cardiorespiratory fitness.[14] Sprint interval training involves not only less time but also less total body strain than conventional medium intensity endurance training. For example, a sprint interval training program would involve as little as 400 yards of sprinting once weekly. In contrast, a medium intensity endurance running program would involve jogging or running 1-5 miles weekly, which amounts to 4 to 20 times more

---

[10] Volaklis KA, Halle M, Meisinger C. Muscular strength as a strong predictor of mortality: A narrative review. Eur J Intern Med 2015 June;26(5):303-10.

[11] Ruiz JR, Sui X, Lobelo F, et al. Association between muscular strength and mortality in men: prospective cohort study. BMJ: British Medical Journal. 2008;337(7661):92-95. doi:10.1136/bmj.a439. <**http://www.ncbi.nlm.nih.gov/pmc/articles/PMC2453303/**>

[12] Rantanen T, Vopato S, Ferrucci L, et al. Handgrip strength and cause-specific and total mortality in older disabled women: Exploring the mechanism. J Am Geriatrics Soc 2003 April 29;51(5):636-41.

[13] Melov S, Tarnopolsky MA, Beckman K, et al.. Resistance Exercise Reverses Aging in Human Skeletal Muscle. PLOS 23 May 2007. <**http://journals.plos.org/plosone/article?id=10.1371/journal.pone.0000465**>

[14] Gillen JB, Martin BJ, MacInnis MJ, et al. Twelve Weeks of Sprint Interval Training Improves Indices of Cardiometabolic Health Similar to Traditional Endurance Training despite a Five-Fold Lower Exercise Volume and Time Commitment. PLoS ONE (2016);11(4): e0154075. doi:10.1371/journal.pone.0154075

stress and strain on for example the knee joints. Over a lifetime this means the medium intensity program involves far more wear and tear on body structures. Since a sprint interval training program puts less total stress on the body, yet produces equal or better results, it is more desirable.

An in-depth introduction to proper resistance training is beyond the scope of this book. I have laid out the basics of proper, brief, infrequent high intensity resistance training on my website www.fullrangestrength.com or **www.donmatesz.com** and on my Full Range Strength YouTube channel. Eventually I will produce a book on this topic. Subscribe to my website to stay updated.

I don't like red meat. Can I eat poultry and fish instead of ruminants?

Ultimately only you can answer this question by your own experiment. Perhaps this would work for some people. However, I believe most people will need to base their hypercarnivore diet on red meat from large mammals, such as beef and lamb, in order to sustain themselves over the long term.

To sustain a hypercarnivore diet, you must get adequate fat, especially saturated fat, from your food. Fat is your main fuel. Generally speaking, poultry and fish – except very fatty fish like salmon and mackerel – do not provide enough total fat and calories to serve as the staple foods for a hypercarnivore diet.

Some people give the impression that the Inuit (Eskimos) lived on a fish-based diet. In fact, sea and land mammals providing fatty red meat – such as seal, whale, moose and caribou –were their principal foods.

Moreover, poultry and fish are not be best ecological choices either. According to the UN Food and Agriculture Organization (FAO), ocean fish stocks are being depleted. Of 600 marine stocks monitored by the FAO, 52% are fully exploited, 17% are over exploited, 7% are depleted and 1% are recovering from depletion.[15]

In addition, you have to kill a very large number of fish to get the same amount of meat you would get from one large mammal. A very large salmon will weigh about 125 pounds, of which about 75% or 94 pounds is edible. A 1000 pound steer will yield about 425 pounds of edible beef. Therefore you have to kill a minimum of 4 unusually large salmon to get the same amount of meat as you would get from a single steer. Most salmon are much smaller.

Birds do not convert grass and other abundant plant matter into edible human foods as efficiently as ruminants. In addition, you have to kill a very large number of birds to get the amount of meat you would get from one large steer. A typical dressed chicken provides only about 4 pounds of meat, so you have to kill 100 chickens to get the amount of meat provided by one steer. In addition, because bird muscle has less fat and calories than large mammal muscle, you need to eat more poultry than beef to meet your needs.

Most people will find that once they remove starches and sugars from their diets, meals based on poultry or fish alone are simply not as satisfying as meals based on beef or other mammal's meat.

So, in summary, you can try eating only poultry and fish if you want, and maybe it will work for some people, but I think it is unlikely it will work for very many people over a long term.

If someone has historically had issues with dairy how do you recommend introducing it?

If you came to the conclusion that you have some intolerance of dairy products while eating a plant-based or plant-rich diet, you may have misattributed the effects of eating plants, particularly fiber, to

---

[15] UN FAO. General situation of world fish stocks. <http://www.fao.org/ newsroom/common/ecg/1000505/en/stocks.pdf>

dairy products. After reduce your plant food intake to a level that frees you of bloating, gas, flatulence and other irritable bowel symptoms, you may find that you can tolerate some fermented dairy products.

For most people, the main problem with dairy products is digestion of lactose. As discussed in Chapter 8, studies have shown that most people can digest fermented dairy products like yogurt and cheese, because fermentation predigests, reduces or removes lactose.

Therefore if you want to experiment with dairy products, start by using small amounts of aged cheese or yogurt, such as 15 g (half an ounce) of aged cheese, or half a cup (125 ml) of yogurt. Pay attention to your response. Test at least three times, to rule out coincidental symptoms.

This is not a balanced diet. How can it be good?

The idea that we need some balanced diet composed of a variety of foods that were unavailable to our pre-agricultural ancestors lacks credibility. As Ray Audette astutely observed in *Neanderthin*, a creature can not require what in Nature it can not acquire.

The vast majority of foods that 'experts' assert are necessary for a 'balanced diet' – such as grains, legumes, modern vegetables, large fruits, sugars – did not exist for our ancestors. These supposedly essential components of a 'balanced diet' are products of extensive plant breeding, not spontaneous products of Nature.

As Bruce Chassy, the assistant dean for Science Communications in the College of Agricultural, Consumer and Environmental Sciences and former head of the Department of Food Science and Human Nutrition at the University of Illinois notes: "Plants such as strawberries, wheat, cabbage, corn, and almost all the rest of our crops descended from ancestors that are not recognizably similar to the plants we grow today."[16]

No non-human species on Earth eats what is typically suggested to be a balanced diet. Each species relies on a very limited number of foods or types of foods. Most rely on one staple food and only include very small amounts of other foods on an irregular basis. This is especially true of carnivores.

My definition of "balanced diet" is: The food or selection of foods that produces healthy function and fitness in the organism in question by providing the measures of nutrients required by that organism. According to this definition, the hypercarnivore diet consisting largely or entirely muscles, organs, fat, bones and eggs (with shells) or dairy products is a balanced diet for humans, just as it is for any carnivore, because it provides the balance of nutrients the human organism requires.

Can I eat X fruit, vegetable or nut as a hypercarnivore?

To reiterate, a hypercarnivore diet can include any fruit or vegetable you tolerate, up to 30% of your diet. Regarding any particular item, you can probably can put it in your mouth, chew, swallow and to some extent digest it. However, I don't know if you will benefit from or be harmed by doing so. Nor can anyone else, other than you yourself, answer your question.

Individuals vary within a range in their level of tolerance for fruits and vegetables. Each individual must honestly evaluate his/her own response to consumption of any food (plant or animal). If the food is incompatible with your health, your body will notify you with more or less immediate responses such as:

• discomfort of the mouth, bad taste or aftertaste

---

[16] Chassy BM. The History and Future of GMOs in Food and Agriculture. Cereal Foods World 2007 July-August;52(4):169-172. <http://www.ask-force.org/web/History/Chassy-History-Future-2007.pdf>

- discomfort, sensitivity or softness of the teeth, unpleasant residual film on the teeth
- stomach discomfort, belching or regurgitation (body trying to eject the unwanted matter)
- post meal abdominal fullness, gas, bloating, flatulence, cramping, loose stools
- recurrent loss of energy, mental clarity, or emotional stability after eating
- dissatisfaction with the meals, cravings for more of something
- nasal itching, drainage or congestion

Longer term use of foods incompatible with your health results in skin issues, joint stiffness and pain, poor sleep quality, and more.

The hypercarnivore takes responsibility for his/her own health. Its your job, not mine, to determine what foods you can and can't include in your diet. As an apex predator, you eat what is useful and avoid the rest.

What about blood tests? When will you get a blood test? Etc.

Blood tests can't tell me (or you) whether I (or you) have tooth decay, acid stomach, belching, gas, bloating, flatulence, loose stools, blocked stools, skin issues, joint pain, fatigue, weakness, poor healing, propensity to injury, nail fragility, lack luster hair, disturbed sleep, chronic unexplained depression, inability to concentrate, dissatisfaction with food or food cravings, or any other of a large number of symptoms indicating poor nutrition.

If you experience none of the listed signs of digestive distress, your skin, hair and nails are getting healthier and stronger, your aches and pains are diminishing, you have growing or stable high energy and strength, you heal easily, you have good physical strength, and you have good sensory and mental function (within bounds set by genetics and previous injury), then you are healthy or getting healthier. What more will a blood test tell you?

I know most people have been convinced that blood tests reveal whether you are healthy or not, but I do not accept this idea and suggest that you should not either. When I was vegan I achieved a total blood cholesterol of 154 mg/dL, which some experts claim to be ideal, but I had almost constant gut distress, excess waist fat, poor exercise recovery, propensity to injury during exercise, slow injury healing, loss of strength and muscle mass, ongoing skin disease, nail fragility, tooth decay and sensitivity, gum recession, accelerated loss of visual acuity, and other symptoms of poor health.

After I changed to a hypercarnivore diet, my total blood cholesterol increased to 419 mg/dL, which some people believe indicates poor health and high risk of cardiovascular mortality. Meanwhile my gut was quiet and painless, my skin was getting healthier, my previous injuries were healing, my exercise tolerance was improving, my waist fat was melting away, my strength and muscle mass were increasing, my nails were growing strong and rapidly, I no longer had tooth sensitivity and my teeth stopped decaying.

Blood tests measure the composition of your blood. I am more interested in how I look, feel and function than in the chemical composition of my blood.

My doctor/dietitian/other health care expert says this is an unhealthy diet. What do you say to that?

Most doctors, dietitians and other health care experts have good intentions, but bad information provided to them by entities that profit from the promotion of foods that do not promote health and fitness.

Very few if any physicians, dietitians or other health care providers get proper education in comparative digestive anatomy and physiology, or archaeology and anthropology, that would prepare them to understand the evolution and nature of the human digestive tract.

Physicians get very little training in nutrition. A 2010 survey of 109 U.S. medical schools found that although 103 required some form of nutrition education, only 26 (25%) required a dedicated nutrition course (down from 32/30% in 2004). Overall, medical students received only 19.6 contact hours of nutrition education during their medical school careers, and only 28 (27%) met the minimum of 25 required hours set by the National Academy of Sciences.[17]

Dietitians receive much more nutrition education, but this education lacks grounding in comparative digestive anatomy and physiology, archaeology and anthropology. They are taught that humans need a so-called balanced diet as prescribed by the USDA and other government bodies. The Academy of Nutrition and Dietetics accepts funding from processed food industries, and promotes processed foods.[18]

Regardless of training, no health care professional knows what works best for you. The hypercarnivore plan is based on directly experimenting yourself, not following experts.

The bottom line is, if you aren't confident and willing to take control of your own health destiny, then you can remain a follower of experts who have inadequate education and understanding of human biology.

On the other hand, if you are confident and willing to take control of your own health destiny for just a few weeks, just ignore your doctor, dietitian or other health care provider long enough to perform the hypercarnivore diet experiment yourself for at least 30 days. If you feel and function better, you will have discovered that your

---

[17] Adams KM, Kohlmeier M, Zeisel SH. Nutrition Education in US Medical Schools: Latest Update of a National Survey. Academic Medicine 2010 Sept; 85(9):1537-1542. <https://www.aamc.org/download/451374/data/nutriritoneducationinusmedschools.pdf>

[18] Nestle M. Dietitians in turmoil over conflicts of interest: it's about time. Food Politics (Blog) 2015 Mar 18. <https://www.foodpolitics.com/2015/03/dietitians-in-turmoil-over-conflicts-of-interest-its-about-time/>

health care expert is misinformed. If you don't thrive, you can always go back to following the advice of the experts.

16 FOLLOW NATURE

In the foregoing chapters I have provided an evidence-based argument for THE HYPERCARNIVORE DIET consisting primarily of meat and fat with optional, discretionary, limited inclusion of plant matter in harmony with Nature's guidance.

However, I do not want you to adopt a new ideology or follow a formula called "hypercarnivore diet" or "primal feeding." I don't want you to adhere dogmatically to any formula or guidelines you might believe that you found in this book. I want you to go beyond ideology to direct experience. I want you to follow Nature as it guides you through your own body and mind.

If you grew up and were educated in any civilization on Earth, you probably have been trained to ignore your Nature and follow rules and formulas provided by 'authorities' who neither have your best interest at heart nor inhabit your body. How can they know what *you* need to eat?

Without doubt, diets of civilized man depart from mankind's Natural diet. Most medical and nutritional authorities study only civilized and therefore sick people, then try to determine which civilized – that is, plant-based – diet causes the least damage. This is like studying a population in which everyone smokes tobacco and has lung disease, then trying to determine which brand of tobacco and method of smoking causes the least lung damage.

Moreover, we now know that plant-based diets fail to support brain regeneration due to shortages of brain-specific nutrients. We know that we have lost and are continuing to lose brain mass and neurons due to civilized diets. Degenerative brain diseases causing dementia affect a majority people in modern nations, and these diseases appear to be caused by dietary deficiencies of animal-source nutrients (vitamin B12, arachidonic acid, and omega-3 DHA at a minimum). Therefore, probably many of these authorities promoting this or that plant-based diet are themselves suffering from some degree of brain deficiency or damage due to consuming civilized diets.

Probably people suffering from brain degeneration due to these nutritional deficiencies have more trouble understanding Nature (Reality) and its laws than someone without those deficiencies, so they make lots of mistakes. Moreover to become an approved 'authority' one must obtain certification from the current authorities, which requires accepting their mistakes and opinions as truths. In addition the need to earn status and money from the Powers That Be (PTB) encourages 'authorities' to fall in line with approved opinions (biases) even if they are without factual foundation. Given this context it is not surprising that, as I noted in the beginning of this book, "Most Published Research Findings Are False."[1]

If you want to understand how to avoid suffering the diseases of civilization, you need to study and emulate uncivilized people: the "barbarians" living the ancient hunter-gatherer way of life, who were never programmed by the PTB, and, like every other wild animal, never measured their health by numbers from a blood, urine or saliva test.

Like all other creatures, you have an innate guidance system, provided by Nature, to enable you to choose the right kind, amount and proportions of food for your needs. If you go against Nature, your body – which *is* Nature – warns you by giving you immediate signals: distaste of the food, mouth or tongue reactions, bad taste in the mouth after swallowing, digestive discomfort, skin reactions, energy crashes, mood disorders, head and body aches, thermal discomfort (excess heat or cold), and so on. Its your job to heed the warnings of Nature, connect the dots, and stop doing what Nature warns you not to do.

PRIMAL FEEDING begins with and leads to greater and greater freedom. Not the imaginary freedom the immature ego desires – to do whatever one wants without consequences – but freedom from limitations and suffering created by acting against Nature. When

---

[1] Ioannidis JPA (2005) Why Most Published Research Findings Are False. PLoS Med 2(8): e124. https://doi.org/10.1371/journal.pmed.0020124

you oppose Nature, Nature will crush you, but when you align with Nature, Nature empowers you. Large ocean waves can beat or kill you if you try to oppose them, but when a surfer aligns with the ocean, the ocean powers the surfer. Meeting strong winds head-on will deplete your energy, but when a sailor aligns his sail with the wind, the wind powers the sailor.

You begin by freeing yourself from false beliefs installed at mass indoctrination centers called public schools and via the mass media's regularly scheduled *programs*. You realize that the PTB want you confused so that you will continue to eat junk that keeps you weak, sick, dumb and easy to manipulate and milk for money. You stop following the 'authorities,' and start following Nature.

You learn to distinguish between mankind's Natural foods and man-made pseudo-foods. By paying attention you will learn directly that only animal products will satisfy your taste and hunger, and provide vigor and strength, without leaving you damaged or depleted. Then you eat as much of them as you need to satisfy taste and hunger at any point in time. You may or may not use some fruits or other tolerable plants for a portion of your energy requirements, flavor, seasonal adaptation or medicine.

As you recover your health through alignment with your True Nature, you will tap into your own PRIMAL WISDOM. You don't need to worry about the details. You don't dogmatically follow inflexible formulas. When you stay true to your Nature you remain fluid and adaptable to Nature's inevitable changes. You make adjustments as needed and dictated by Nature.

Now that you know that Nature made you an apex predator, its time to leave the flock of sheep and rejoin the wolves.

Stay strong, awake, aligned, wise and FREE!

ESSENTIAL RESOURCES

Books

Allen CB and Lutz W. *Life Without Bread*. Keats, 2000.

Audette R. *NeanderThin*. St. Martin's Press, 1999.

Crawford M and Marsh D. *Nutrition and Evolution*. Keats, 1999.

Matesz T. *The Trust Your True Nature Low Carb Lifestyle*. Create Space, 2018. (To be republished as *The Hypercarnivore Diet Companion Guide*)

Price W. *Nutrition and Physical Degeneration*. Price Pottenger Nutrition Foundation, 1970.

Taubes G. *Good Calories, Bad Calories*. Anchor Books, 2008

Voegtlin WL. *The Stone Age Diet*. Vantage Press, 1975.

Websites

www.donmatesz.com
www.meatheals.com
www.shawn-baker.com
http://www.burnfatnotsugar.com/
http://www.empiri.ca/
www.justmeat.co
https://www.paleomedicina.com/en
www.dietdoctor.com

Made in the USA
San Bernardino, CA
11 January 2020